THE RULES OF THE GAME

TAVISTOCK

The International Behavioural and Social Sciences Library

SOCIOLOGY & SOCIAL POLICY
In 10 Volumes

THE RULES OF THE GAME

Interdisciplinarity, Transdisciplinarity and
Analytical Models in Scholarly Thought

EDITED BY TEODOR SHANIN

First published in 1972 by
Tavistock Publications Limited

Reprinted in 2001 by
Routledge
2 Park Square, Milton Park, Abingdon, Oxon, OX14 4RN
Simultaneously published in the USA and Canada by Routledge

711 Third Avenue, New York, NY 10017

Transferred to Digital Printing 2007

First issued in paperback 2013

Routledge is an imprint of the Taylor & Francis Group, an informa business

© 1972 Teodor Shanin and individual contributors

The publishers have made every effort to contact authors/copyright holders
of the works reprinted in the *International Behavioural and Social Sciences
Library*. This has not been possible in every case, however, and we would
welcome correspondence from those individuals/companies we have been
unable to trace.

These reprints are taken from original copies of each book. In many cases
the condition of these originals is not perfect. The publisher has gone to
great lengths to ensure the quality of these reprints, but wishes to point
out that certain characteristics of the original copies will, of necessity, be
apparent in reprints thereof.

British Library Cataloguing in Publication Data
A CIP catalogue record for this book
is available from the British Library

The Rules of the Game

ISBN 978-0-415-26502-7 (hbk)
ISBN 978-0-415-86908-9 (pbk)

Contents

v

PART TWO

*Order, Consciousness, and Meaning:
the broader theme*

Contents

We have endeavoured . . . to observe a kind of perspective, that one part may cast light upon another.

Francis Bacon

In so far as one can speak about scientific image of nature, one has to treat it not so much as an image of nature but rather as the image of our relation with nature.

Werner Heisenberg

When the understanding of scientific models and archetypes comes to be regarded as a reputable part of scientific culture, the gap between the sciences and the humanities will have been partly filled. For exercise of the imagination, with all its promises and its dangers, provides a common ground.

Max Black

The 1972 Foreword (amended)

This volume concerns itself with some major conceptual troubles-pots of contemporary scholarship. It's particular focus is that of disciplinarity and interdisciplinarity in scholarly thought, but it opens out to range over the whole field of knowledge-about-knowledge and it's crucial subject-object relations axis. It is not the work of professional philosophers of science, but reflections of scholars of various disciplines about the more general aspects of their trade. While it is written to stand scrutiny by the scholarly community, it keeps to language comprehensible to well-educated laymen, for each of us is a layman in fields other than his own. To explain why and how such a publication took shape we shall begin with an intellectual experiment by a group of researchers and present the way of reasoning and self-questioning, which brought this group into being.

Why do people pursue knowledge? Material needs and the quest for power to control fellow beings, which knowledge can serve, form basic determinants that are easy to detect. However, these are not sufficient to account for all the persistence of human search. They interrelate with more general and subtle needs and tendencies of human mind: the need to orient oneself in an infinitely complex reality, the tendency to order the endless particularity of human experience and to look for some essences behind the facts, the wish to attach meaning to being-in-the-world and also sheer intellectual curiosity -

the thirst for knowledge for it's own sake. The entrenched, if ambiguous, division between applied knowledge, embodied in technology, and the realm of "pure theory", provides both an indication of and the primary distinction between the different types of knowledge and different aims of it pursued.

An ideal of the "Renaissance man" expressed the happy symbiosis of specific technological skills with the abstract knowledge to which the artistic expressions and creative ability were often added as a matter of course. In our times we seem to be moving away from such an ideal towards division and specialization of knowledge with it's marvelous scientific achievements, but also with some unease at knowing more and more about less and less. One should not dismiss just as an utopian dreams the lingering wish of many scholars to search for more general knowledge transcending pragmatic needs, the tendency to cross-cut through accepted disciplinary boundaries and to look for deeper essence beyond appearances and common sense. The development of contemporary scholarship has been particularly fruitful at the interdisciplinary boundaries, while abstract theorizing have repeatedly turned out to be of more practical value than the technicians of science could have ever dreamt of. Moreover, practical considerations apart, the very fact of persistent existence of such tendencies raises doubts about any attempt to disregard them. To be sure, one can live an effective scholarly existence without ever reaching into those depths. It has been said, the "every person is either Platonist or an Aristotelian". The scholars' camp must have both, and more, while to those bitten by the bug of theoretical concerns, the contemporary feeling of decomposition of the rapidly growing field of scholarship has been particularly disturbing.

Half a century ago, five people met at the campus of Sheffield University: Shulamit Ramon, Michael Barratt-Brown, Paul Clark, Mark Pargeter and Teodor Shanin. Both their similarities and differences between them were significant: they belonged to three different universities and represented four distinct disciplines: psychology, physics, economics and sociology, yet, in spite of the differences of disciplinary languages, aims and prejudices, a common denominator clearly emerged in (1) the feeling of corresponding conceptual confusion in a number of disciplines (2) the consequent wish to explore cross-disciplinary problems and characteristics of scholarly analysis and (3) the belief that a better understanding of subject-object relations in inquiry is necessary for the future advancement of knowledge. None of those present felt himself/herself competent to consider such issues single-handed. Could an interdisciplinary team take on the role of a collective "Renaissance man" at the contemporary levels of complexity? In a good academic fashion, the five decided on an experiment. Invitations to meet and talk it over were sent out to an additional dozens of scholars in a variety of disciplines. A decision was taken that, if at least ten come, an attempt would be made to establish a regular interdisciplinary seminar. More than double of that number turned up.

The character of the seminar those created was very much the result of spontaneous development. The founding members were propelled into position of an informal managing committee with the initiator Teodor Shanin chairing and Mark Pargeter taking on the burdens of the seminar's secretary. We agreed to call ourselves the "Subject-Object Relations Group". A wide variety of disciplines and fields of study were by now represented: physics, biology, mathematics, psychology, sociology, economics, philosophy, theology, statistics, creative arts, linguistics, mass communication. Meetings multiplied, with some of the group members travelling hundreds of miles to make it. Each meeting consisted of an opening paper by one of the participants and several more hours for a round-the-table discussion by scholars from different disciplines. The only limitation accepted was metaphorically to speak in a way which could be followed by a well-educated laymen, for each of us has been a laymen in some of the fields far from our own. The discussion increasingly moved towards consideration of analytical models in diverse disciplines, their possible links and issues of knowledge about knowledge. The debate was always lively and instructive, at times "hot", at some moments sparkling. A wish eventually was voiced to try to present all that to the broader audiences - a de-facto argument for increasing inter-disciplinary contacts.

The 2018 Foreword
Looking Back at Interdisciplinarity

At the beginnings of 1970's the term "interdisciplinarity" and its' semantic "kinsmen", such as transdisciplinarity, cross-disciplinarity etc.., burst into European scholarly debate. It challenged the well-solidified vision of academic scholarship as a system of autonomous disciplines matched by university departments of the day. Each of these disciplines/departments undertook the study of an aspect of reality, the exclusivity of which was assumed. Each of them carried a basic definition, some fundamental texts and a set of prescribed methods of inquiry and verification. Each embraced teams of professional and technical personnel, audiences of students and some supporting budgetary arrangements.

This general image of academic scholarship was challenged at an international and interdisciplinary seminar, which met in 1970 in Nice under the auspices of the Organization of Economic co-Operation and Development (OECD). The counter-arguments came there from the eminent Swiss psychologist Jean Piaget, the Austrian-American astrophysicist Erich Jansch and the French mathematician Andre Lichnerowich. In their view the links ("bridges") rather than the divisions between academic disciplines were of major significance for the future of academic research. Different terminologies were used but the term "interdisciplinarity" was seemingly the most generic in describing that issue.

The critical approach to disciplinarity at the Nice seminar was not solitary. The topic of interdisciplinarity was clearly "in the air". A PhD thesis submitted in that period at the International University in San Diego has made separately some of the points considered by Erich Jansch. Broader in scope was the 1970-71 years-long seminar by Subject-Object Relation Group in Sheffield, UK, which was concerned with many of the issues raised in Nice. By 1972 two books in parallel followed the seminars in Nice and in Sheffield: Interdisciplinarity: Problems of Teaching and Research in Universities (OECD Publications, Paris, 1972) and The Rules of The Game (Tavistock press, London, 1972). Yet, the seminars of Nice and of Sheffield were clearly oblivious of each other: a manifest case of serendipity.

Looking at it from the distance of half-a-century, those were harbingers of a new turn in the way the very structure of academia was being approached. Following the Nice seminar, one can trace a rapidly growing wave, concerning interdisciplinarity, expressed in numerous publications, conferences and the setting up of new research institutions. The character and the path of the Sheffield seminar differed.

***

The Subject-Object Relation Group's seminar in Sheffield of early 1970's was already mentioned in the initial foreword to the book. This seminar focused on considering similarities, differences and links between the academic disciplines. Its' participants were mostly members of the academic staff of the university of Sheffield but a number of them came over to each session from other universities. It was set up and developed with no grants and no employed staff – a fully "voluntaristic" setting. This informality went side-by-side with high levels of participation and lively debate in which even the controversial issues were fully explored while disagreements were ever taken in good spirit. The seminar was planned to take place about once a month, but it's meetings did become actually more frequent, following the wishes of its' members. The seminars' sessions usually begun by presenting paper of analytical model concerning one of the academic disciplines and proceeded for about three hours.

The discussion of analytical models of academic disciplines resulted in the growing significance given to the debate concerning interdisciplinarity and its' different forms. Also it often "overspilled" into considering more general issues of academic scholarship and the general problematic of knowledge about knowledge.

The end of the seminar of Subject-Object Relation Group came as the result of both its' informality and the patterns of mobility within the British universities of the day, linked to patterns of academic promotions. For many the move to a different university, or even to a different country, was usual and "good for advancement". The abler and the better known a scholar, the higher was the possibility of his\her disappearance at the end of the academic session. The end of Subject-Object Relation Group came not through its' decay, the seminar kept well the interest of its' members, but as the result of "promotional" disappearance of the hard core of its' members. Those left behind tried to keep the seminar going but failed.

It has been initially assumed that the seminar will last for 3 years. When it became clear that many of its' members plan to leave Sheffield at the end of that academic session, it was agreed to try to publish some of the contributions to it. It was also decided to add to the text a Part II devoted to works, which influenced our debate or else were specifically ordered to express a view presented by a member of the seminar. A contract was signed with the Tavistock Publishers. We selected the books' title which amused us. Looking back, it did not make sufficiently clear the book's content, which contributed to its' reaching a fairly narrow academic circle.

Models and Thought

TEODOR SHANIN

> *. . . the lens of mankind through
> which men see, the medium by which
> they interpret and report what they see.*
>
> C. Wright Mills

I. THE CREDIBILITY GAP IN SCHOLARSHIP – AN ASPECT OF THE SCIENTIFIC REVOLUTION

The major axis of cultural history seems to lie in the mutual causation of constant new experience and, just as constant, an attempt to generalize and formalize whatever passes for knowledge in society. Scholarly disciplines embody the formalization aspect. The very word 'discipline' conveys the images of order, control, and rigid training. It reflects, on the one hand, the need of the human mind for rationalizing and for orientation in an immensely complex reality, to be achieved by building up systematic and coherent general images and symbolic schemes.[1] It represents, on the other hand, a closed, self-supporting, and to a great extent self-validating group of specialists who reproduce themselves by initiating into their circle those youngsters who respond well to training. Qualities, of mind and of social organization, find expression in the stability of the paradigms of science, i.e. the 'universally recognized scientific achievements that for a time provide model problems and solutions to a community of practitioners'.[2] More than that, such paradigms delineate the very fields of the specific disciplines and determine the extent of their crystallization in scholarship. Outside the natural sciences the

1

heterogeneity is greater, yet the disciplinary order, control, and training operate on very similar lines. Suitably formalized and reified language provides powerful reinforcement of the existing disciplinary system.

Kuhn has lucidly described how the order of accepted knowledge in science is constantly disturbed by new 'anomalies' of experience, i.e. the type of evidence that does not fit into an accepted system of explanation. 'New' minds (often outsiders to the disciplinary establishment) which somehow manage to escape the security checks of selection and pressures for conformity in the scholarly community act likewise. As a rule the first challenge of new evidence or new understanding does not make much headway either with the practitioners of the discipline or with the laymen. The systems of intellectual and administrative control act here as powerful defences of the *status quo*. Yet, if the pressure grows, the credibility gap between, on the one hand, new insights and more or less formalized evidence and, on the other hand, the accepted knowledge may make the ruling paradigm crumble. Then comes the period of revolutions. In actual fact the ensuing crisis leads first to a variety of compromises and readjustments within the existing conceptual scheme, which may succeed. If, however, the credibility gap is too huge to be bridged and the subversion by nonconforming anomalies and the pressure of 'new forces' too substantial to be contained, paradigms of science collapse in a 'scientific revolution'. The essence of such a revolution is in a 'qualitative leap', an 'epistemological break' – a rapid closing of gaps between evidence and accepted knowledge through basic reconceptualization of reality. The old paradigm may be kept at times as a theoretically degraded but pragmaticly useful approximation of certain situations, while a new and different view of reality becomes generally accepted as 'knowledge'. The extent and 'broadness' of this reconceptualization vary, from overhaul of a sub-branch of scholarship in which 'unanticipated anomalies and strategic data became the occasion for development of new theory',[3] as far as what was referred to as axial stages of human history, when crucial upheaval in social structure meets with and is comprehended through shattering changes in the general *Weltanschauung* of society.[4] Yet whatever the magnitude of change in the paradigms of thought, the post-revolutionary period seems to display some basic similarities. The new ideas are rapidly welded into a consistent pattern, which acquires once more self-stabilizing defensive characteristics. Many of the rebels of yesterday become 'establishment figures' of today. The disciplines (in many cases newly created by 'the revolution') crystallize, the bulk of their practitioners close ranks and minds, new credibility gaps start to grow, a new qualitative leap is in the making.

The period in which we live has seen a more or less constant crisis of knowledge, a 'permanent revolution', to keep to the somewhat metaphorical language. On the one hand, the immense spread and professionalization of research, the heavy investment in the research business, the developments in communication, the mass production of literature, and the spread of universities, related to constant and rapid social and technological change, have created a ceaseless flood of information and potentially anomalous data. On the other hand, although the existing organization of the scholarly community has in many cases been highly effective in solving the puzzles defined by the existing paradigms, it has also displayed a number of serious limitations. Bureaucratization and outside controls have created rigid disciplinary structures limiting the very creativity they profess to advance. Super-specialization into an increasing number of disciplines and subdisciplines, which come to handle increasingly complex pictures of narrower and narrower aspects of reality, has proved time and again to be counter-productive in terms of better understanding of the broad context of the subject-matter. An unparalleled 'insulation' of 'mature scientific communities' from 'laity'[5] came into being while the comprehension and affirmation of the scientific wonderland through categories of pragmatic knowledge became increasingly doubtful, or impossible. The enormous prestige acquired by science and the scientist aggravated this tension. The problems of conceptualization, now permanent, became related to, and further increased by, the political and moral crisis of the generation of nuclear weapons, Vietnam, the moon race, and race riots. They bring into question the very quality and purpose of rationalism on which Western scholarship was based. Both images and self-images of scholarship moved from the devilish Dr Faustus of the Middle Ages through the benefactor of mankind of nineteenth-century evolutionism and optimism and back again to that of a fiend, or at least the tortured soul of a contemporary Oppenheimer.

One of the results of the atmosphere of permanent intellectual crisis has been the increasing interest of scholars in knowledge about knowledge, i.e. the full range of methodologies of discipline, psychology of perception and creativity, sociology of knowledge, and epistemology. The history of science and the major modes (or archetypes, or super-paradigms) of scientific explanation have provided here a possible comparative conceptualization in terms of sequences and 'directions of development'. Aristotle's quest for an explanation of nature in terms of purpose has been compared, for example, to explanations in terms of sufficient conditions adopted in later ages. Probably the best known is Bronowski's division of post-sixteenth-century history of science into three major periods in which order, causality, and chance played in turn the role of the central idea of science.[6] However, the contemporary conceptual crisis seems to be much broader in scope than the natural sciences alone on which scientific historiography seems to rest. It seems also 'deeper', for 'unconfident' scholarship has on the whole led to a more general philosophical concern with its own epistemics, to which simple historical relativism seems somewhat insufficient as an explanation. A number of crucial epistemological problems cut across the whole field of contemporary scholarly thought. Among these the relation between theory and experience or data, analytical methods versus the holistic approach (closely related to the issue of reduction) and the problems of levels of knowledge as distinct from those acknowledged by the 'official' methodology, all reflect the more general issue of subject–object relations, i.e. the relation between the observer or student and the object of his observation or study. It is this syndrome of knowledge about knowledge and its particular expression in models of thought that form the focus of our discussion.

II. THE INTERDISCIPLINARY PROBLEMS OF SUBJECT–OBJECT RELATIONS

The first problem is the relationship between theory and fact. The optimistic belief of the nineteenth century in the ability of scientific induction to close the gap between reality and theory (and to dispose of 'the need of metaphysics') seems in our times naïve if not superficial. Theorizing and empirical research still form separate worlds, at least as far as formalized procedures are concerned. It is the awareness of the depth of this gulf and of an ultimate if partial separateness, that poses again the paradoxes of Cartesian dualism, Hume's scepticism, and Kant's 'gnesology' concerning the basic differences between the 'logical' and the 'real'. In so far as one can judge, this is reflected today in the conclusions of the theoreticians right across the disciplinary boundaries from Heisenberg's 'uncertainty principle' in physics as far as to the discussion of 'theories of middle range' in sociology, with Gödel's theorem in mathematics as a further extension of it.[7] The unending efforts 'to close the gap' by positivist reductions and the post-factum impositions of 'hypothetico-deductive' language on scholarly work are but another recognition of the problem.[8] Several other epistemological issues are related here. First, is reality structured in a way that can be learned by the human mind or, on the contrary, 'since the word unity contradicts both reality and its cognition',[9] is it only the human mind that establishes systematic order? Secondly, can causality be established at all, or is the 'black box' of input–output analysis the only possible object of study? And so on.

The relation between the whole and the parts provides the second major interdisciplinary problem of contemporary scholarship. In scholarly jargon the word analysis has by now become synonymous with thought, study, knowledge itself. The synonymity reflects here the fact that analysis has become the major scholarly supra-methodology. Analysis proceeds through division into simpler components whose interactions are than studied so that we may learn about the whole. Analysis, effective and dominating as it has proved in 'Western' scholarship since 'the Greeks',[10] is, however, but one of the possible methods, and displays furthermore a variety of blind spots. To begin with, the split into sub-units causes some qualitative residuum to disappear, and study in terms of constituent parts may mean reduction to something quite different in quality. Furthermore, analysis presupposes a system of subdivision into units that is partly arbitrary and formally prior to investigation. Yet it is selective and has a bearing on the results. Any protestation of scientific objectivity is therefore particularly suspect here. It was argued in disciplines as far removed as psychology (Gestalt School) and physics (notably D. Bohm) that rather than the parts determining the whole, it is the whole that determines the parts. The critics of strict analytical methodology have recently been particularly active in the social sciences and psychology. Here the phenomenological tradition has challenged the analytical and quantifying positivistic tendencies, claiming the uniqueness and wholeness of human experience and consciousness as a necessary starting-point of a methodology of the 'human sciences'.[11] It may be well to remember that Kuhn's analysis referred to above seems particularly vulnerable when transferred to those fields of study.

The third type of general epistemological problem relates to types of knowledge different from, and possibly superior to, those formerly accepted as the medium of scholarly work. Polanyi's discussion of 'tacit knowledge' as the implicit yet necessary component of research or Baldamus's 'double fitting' and 'categories of pragmatic knowledge' can stand as good examples of such 'unofficial practices' of scholarship.[12] Intuitive knowledge and attempts to explain 'the spark' Popper declared to be the starting-point of scholarly advance, and then neatly left out of his earlier methodological discussion, will also come in here.[13] Lévi-Strauss's insistence on unconscious layers of cognition and Bohm's 'implicate orders' of nature, the uncoding of which must form the real subject-matter of scholarship, will clash here with the good Anglo-Saxon empiricist tradition that dismisses such issues as mystical rubbish. The approach to human behaviour and thought as to a direct response to socialization or reinforcement as well as total cultural relativism are confronted by the claim of innate capacities specific to the human mind, e.g. the linguistics of Chomsky. Again epistemology leads us to issues of human nature and to the basic axis of subject–object relations.

The issue of subject–object relations seems to provide a major unifying conceptual focus for the contemporary problems of knowledge about knowledge. Its historical roots seem to lie in the philosophical reflections of the beginning of modern sciences in the work of Descartes, Leibniz, Hume, and Kant. The first quarter of the twentieth century saw a powerful explosion of neo-

Kantian thought, especially in Germany, Austria, and Russia. Logical positivism, phenomenology, and existentialism alike have their beginnings in that development. The Kantian revival (which at its radical wing should be no doubt called neo-Cartesian) was all but destroyed in the thirties by Nazism and the Soviet purge; state-manufactured truth did not leave scope for epistemological doubt. Yet half a century later Anglo-Saxon empiricism and pragmatism seem step by step to be giving way to similar concerns and solutions. The crux of all this lies in focusing on subject–object interaction as the basis of comprehension in contrast to the idealist assertion of the absolute primacy of the subject or the strict materialist assertion of the absolute primacy of the object. It is in the rapid cross-disciplinary spread of the use of the concept of models that the methodological acknowledgement of the basic axis of subject–object relations finds its major expression. Models can on the other hand be understood only against a more general theoretical background, i.e. the ways of understanding postulated for the basic issues mentioned above. The work of the general systems theory group (von Bertalanffy, Simon, Koestler, *et al.*), attempting to define the character of the whole–part relation as well as a general hierarchical order of nature, may serve as an example of such a theoretical background associated with the use of models.

Models as Explanatory Devices

As with many 'new' concepts, the use of the term model is still somewhat of a fashion if not a gimmick. It looks scientific, illuminating, 'with it'. Yet, as time passes by, the concept has not blurred. If anything, its use has grown in an increasing variety of disciplines. Such persistence seems to result from the particular relation of the concept of model to the epistemological concerns of the permanent scientific revolution and to the subject–object relations axis of knowledge.

The extensive use of the term has been partly related to the simple fact that 'models' mean different things to different people. In further discussion we shall proceed first to peel the semantic onion to arrive at the hard core(s) of the concept of model which plays such an outstanding role in contemporary scholarly work.

To begin with, one has to dispose of two meanings of the word *model* which are only indirectly related to the concept discussed, namely the meanings 'ideal' and 'design'. The terminological residium of the word has been used in two major senses, (a) as an exploratory device of scholarship, (b) as a preconception, colouring cognition and comprehension of reality, an archetype, a pattern of thought. We shall discuss the first and return to the second later. The exploratory models can be divided into three major categories.

1 *A Physical Model* – a material representation of an object effected either by keeping all its features of interest intact, while changing the scale (icon or scale model), or alternatively by changing the medium while 'attempting to reproduce as faithfully as possible in some new medium the structure or web of relationship in the 'original'[15] (analog model).

2 *A Logical Model* – a closed set of interrelated entities or definitions which satisfy a number of axioms of formal logic.[16] In such a closed and fully formalized system there will be no definition of entities apart from the axioms accepted, and no definition of axioms but in terms of the entities used.

3 *An Analytical Model* which brings us to the 'hard core' of a concept of crucial significance in contemporary scholarship. The analytical model differs from the physical one by its symbolic form (i.e. language or mathematics) and by the necessarily theoretical framework involved. At the same time it differs from the logical models by its necessary relation to, or representation of, reality, in terms of which its validity can be judged. The analytical models 'carry over from logic the idea of interpretation of a deductive system'[17] while at the same time being rooted in the reality studied by their use. This places them metaphorically 'in between' the other two categories.

Analytical models can be defined as closed systems which provide a meaningfully selective and symbolic representation of reality. A system assumes mutual dependence of components by which change in some produces a necessary and predictable change in the others. The model serves as a purposeful simplification by selecting or isolating a small number of interdependencies under consideration. It is designed in a way that assumes constant properties and repetitiveness of the system. It therefore reproduces on a theoretical plane the conditions of an ideal laboratory in natural sciences. Selection of properties in a model presupposes both some underlying theory of the nature of the reality studied and an explicit definition of the study's purpose. As a result, in accordance with Black's celebrated dictum, 'only by being unfaithful in *some* respects can a model represent its original'.[18] The symbolic representation of reality gives it a generalized and abstract expression and the possibility of logical and mathematical manipulation. Yet models are both inferred from reality and reapplied to it through human action. An analytical model as a meaningfully simplified statement of interdependence may carry furthermore some surplus meaning and may be suggestive, either by analogy to, or transfer from, another and better-known field of knowledge.

The character of the analytical model, and especially its selective and simplifying aspects, determine a variety of problems and limitations in its use. The first problem is how much to simplify. The formulation of a relevant model (especially a model that is mathematical in form) may be particularly difficult. The greatest of the dangers seems, however, to lie in the implicit tendency to reify models, i.e. to approach them as reality and not as a simplified and purposefully biased representation. In the words of yet another celebrated statement 'the price of employment of models is eternal vigilance'.[19] So is it, of course, with all scholarship.

The basic *function* of analytical models, which explains their extraordinary significance in contemporary scholarship, is their use as the major bridge between the language of theory and that of empirically collected data, between the general and the unique, between the 'subject' and the 'object'.

To quote a recent discussion 'the commonly accepted position is that science contains two distinct languages or ways to define concepts', i.e. the theoretical and the operational. Furthermore 'there appears to be no purely logical way to bridge the gap between the languages. Concepts of one language are associated with those of the other mainly by convention or agreement between scholars.'[20] Thus the Cartesian/Kantian problem of the relation between the theoretical and the real is still with us.[21] The issue is particularly serious when laboratory controls or 'randomization' are impossible. A usual analytical procedure will be to carry out the exploration of relevant interrelations on analytical models in which the subject-matter is simplified to 'essentials', i.e. stripped of those details which are assumed to be incidental or irrelevant, to make possible 'an overview of the essential characteristics of a domain'.[22] Thus generalization can be expressed in spite of the fragmentation of the actual experience. The qualitative permanence, relative simplicity, and isolation of the system accepted as a model, makes it theoretical and 'unrealistic' as against the unique and unlimitedly complex web of interrelations in reality. Yet the realistic connotations of the analytical model allow its use in inferences about empirical data. Furthermore, the formalization of the model permits its interdisciplinary use, in whole or in part, and opens possibilities for logical manipulation and for utilization of mathematical techniques. Causal thinking can here provide examples of broadly used models that are fruitful despite the critique by empirical philosophers, the growth of probabilistic statistical studies, and the fact that it 'belongs completely on a theoretical level and the causal laws can never be demonstrated empirically'.[23]

In a broader sense models offer a partial solution to the subject–object relations dilemma. The unbridgeable break between the limited and selective consciousness of the subject and the unlimited complexity and 'richness' of the object is negotiated by purposeful simplification and by transformation of the object of study inside consciousness itself. The problem of subject–object relations is of course not 'solved' but only transferred from a relation between the student and his data to a relation between, on the one hand, consciousness and models, and, on the other hand, models and empirical data. Some additional illumination is, however, gained by that stratagem. The crux of the matter seems here to be the 'isomorphism' between the model and the field of application, which enables one to evaluate the 'fit' of the model in each particular case while at the same time providing for the possibility of deductive and generalized logical manipulation. It furthermore pre-assumes a process of inquiry in which the model's approximation to the objects of study improves through the mutual impact of accumulation of knowledge and sophistication of models and their use.

III. THEORY AND THE CATEGORIES OF ANALYTICAL
MODELS

In some treatments the term model is used synonymously with theory or even with any general proposition. Such overwhelming broadness does not seem to be very useful and blunts the selective capacity of such conceptualization. Theory as a concept seems to be broader, more self-sustaining, and of a deeper epistemological significance than that of model. The analytical model seems to rest on some broader theoretical definitions of the character of the field of study, of the relative significance of its components, and of the question asked. In that sense, and in contrast to a theory, the terms 'true' and 'false' cannot usefully be employed in the evaluation of models, while 'appropriate', 'stimulating', and 'significant' will probably do for both.[24] General theory in its broader sense is furthermore charged with the task of recognition and separation of qualitatively specific levels of reality and types of interdependence that are of strategic value in terms of comprehension. (See, for example, the paper below by Arthur Koestler.) On the other hand, models are used to concretize, clarify, and check more general theory. Theory seems, therefore, to provide a concept of more general range and epistemological depth, analytical models acting as its subordinate and partial exposition.

Various categorization systems for analytical models have been proposed. The division of models into descriptive, i.e. expressing internal structure, and predictive, i.e. defining possible results of a determining impact, can here provide an example. (In accord with the tendencies of contemporary scholarly thought, the analytical models tend to focus on dynamics rather than on statics, on interdependence of 'events' rather than that of 'things'.)[25] The extent of information expected about the character of the process studied may provide a further diversification between the causal models and the 'black boxes' of a restricted input–output analysis, in which the 'interior' of the 'black boxes' is disregarded. Most interesting and important, however, seems to be the categorization of analytical models in accordance with (i) the type of causality assumed and (ii) the type of formalization used.

A typology based on the character of the causality assumed will begin with a division between models of *linear causation* and systems of *mutual causation*. Models of linear causation assume a simple scheme in which some factors, by influencing a known set of properties, produce a predictable response. A clear division between factors (cause) and responses (effects) is accepted, negotiated by the properties of the model (the following simple diagram may help to express such interdependence). Any reverse influence of the response on its determinants is not considered, and the possible mutual impact of the factors is treated as nonexistent.

A monistic model of linear causation as against a multifactorial one will have the additional property of assuming only one operating factor, from the knowledge of which all the possible changes in the system can be deduced. The relative simplicity and clarity of the monistic models made them play a positive role both in the solution of partial problems and in breaking new paths of thought. On the other hand, those particular types of simplification for the purpose of analysis are in particular danger of reification.

Linear causation model

SYSTEM OF PROPERTIES

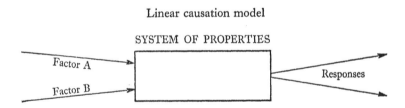

Systems of mutual causation assume and represent a more complex interactive quality of reality in which feedback plays a major role. Such a model presents a 'system' in which the division into causes and effects is transcended and a structure of simultaneous and highly interdependent relations is assumed. Models of mutual causation may therefore be considered of a higher order (in terms of complexity and the extent of their self-articulation) than models of linear causation. The models of mutual causation can be in turn divided into *equilibrium models* and *models of cumulative change*. Equilibrium models assume a negative feedback which controls deviance within certain limits and therefore stabilizes the character of the system and its components. The issue of stability of the equilibrium, i.e. of the strength of the deviance-controlling negative feedback, will here be one of the consequent issues. In the context of biology and the social sciences such self-adjusting systems have been assumed as 'perpetuating their own structure and neutralizing determining environmental pressures'[26] while a constant circulation of energy (and 'information') takes place. Technologies of industrial control and biological organisms provide extensive examples of such a system of interaction and have displayed a powerful influence on model-building.

Systems with positive feedbacks have remained less popular and less well known, though understanding of their importance has grown recently in a variety of disciplines. The cumulative nature of many processes ('vicious circles', 'circular causations') is particularly important for better understanding of structural change, i.e. changes leading to the creation of a different system of interdependencies and for the explanation of the qualitative jumps and sudden breaks in continuity.[27] Qualitative changes and runaway processes destructuring the existing system of interdependencies have been analysed in those terms. Again, the strength of the feedback and the thresholds of structural change will here be of major importance. (It is, by the way, simplistic to assign equilibrium systems to the study of statics while claiming models of cumulative change for dynamics. Equilibrium models assume on the whole *non-structural* changes and can be used also to assess conditions in which structural change will occur, i.e. the system will give way. They cannot, however, illuminate the character of such a structural process. It should also be remembered that simultaneous changes do not imply mutual causality if the size of the change of one variable is independent of the size of the change in another, or if change in both is caused by a third factor.)[28]

The typology of formalizations used provides another important division of analytical models. The models can be divided first into those using language, and those using mathematical formulae as their major media of expression. The rapid spread of the use of computers has created additional powerful pressures for the 'mathematization of conceptual thought'. The mathematical models can be deterministic or probabilistic (stochastic) in form, with the use of the second rapidly spreading as a result of the advances in contemporary statistics and in empirical studies. A serious conceptual issue is here provided by the so-called non-pictorial models in contemporary physics.[29] The models typical of nineteenth-century physics represented as a rule an integration of mathematical formalization and pictorial content and drew some illumination by analogy to more familiar systems. The contemporary models of quantum physics seem to be rapidly losing their representational pictorial content. The questions of how far such phenomena still lie inside the conceptual province of model-building as usually accepted, as well as of the epistemological and social results of types of knowledge, which are by definition inaccessible to laymen, must here be left open for further studies.

One can also proceed here to explore the other end of synchronic cultural diversities by comparing contemporary scholarly models with the myths of tribal societies as different forms of 'analogical thought'.[30] Needham's *magnum opus* on Chinese scholarship can provide a major framework for such a comparative exploration along synchronic lines.[31]

The criteria for selection of analytical models as explanatory devices are heterogeneous and can be grasped once again only within the framework of subject–object relations. Formal definitions of use tend to stress practical instrumentality, 'truth content', and at times also social acceptability and/or facilitation of creativity as the reasons for their adoption. Predictability, especially in pragmatic use, is at times acclaimed as the only criterion of substance. The evidence of scholars themselves strongly contradicts such a narrow interpretation.[32] To begin with, models are used not only to predict but also to secure coherent comprehension, to 'make sense' of experience in more general terms. The importance of that aspect seems far in excess of any pragmatic uses such knowledge could possibly provide. Models are used, therefore, not only to comprehend a structure or to estimate the future, but also to retrodict, i.e. to illuminate the past. To a degree surprising to laymen, models have been, furthermore, selected by what can be described as aesthetic criteria, e.g. symmetry or neatness. Pragmatic use, the wish to comprehend, and such aesthetic preferences have moreover to be considered within socially defined frames of reference, and this determines both the avenues of social acceptability and the paths of rebellion. People do 'make their own destiny' but they do not make it as they please. They face a ready-made world of material conditions, of power relations, and of cultural structures. Furthermore, they act and comprehend in terms of a cognition that is limiting in ways that are selective and consequential.

IV. MODELS AS PRECONCEPTIONS

Specific and selective cognition and comprehension means simply being human, or at least being human in terms of a given pattern of consciousness and social organization. No explanation can be understood outside such a human frame of reference. Even the primary issue of what do we mean by explaining things makes this clear. If indeed to explain is 'to reduce a situation to elements and correlations with which we are so familiar that we accept them as a matter of course so that curiosity rests',[33] then it is our preconceptions that determine when such transformation is considered sufficient.

The predominant images and concepts seem to have their definite intersubjective and extra-theoretical 'truth content', elements of which emerge from beneath the formally unlimited flexibility of conceptualization. As the analysts know, some data are 'stubborn'. In this sense, knowledge is doubtlessly isomorphic with the cognized reality with the 'fit' constantly re-established and tightened up by both pragmatic knowledge and scholarly inquiry. Yet at the same time no extension of simple induction of facts will suffice to explain cognition and comprehension. Once again, it is the framework of subject–object relations that cannot be disregarded without severe distortion in our understanding of the process of knowledge. Consider, for example, the reason for the overwhelming tendency for monistic patterns of comprehension, in which full understanding is achieved by tracing the phenomena studied to one major factor approached as a 'prime mover'. Such an image may form a useful analytical simplification, but its broad spread and its unquestioned acceptance as a correct and total image of reality seem to need further explanation.

The explanation may lie in the nature of the object of study, i.e. in the 'monistic' nature of the world. It may lie alternatively in the characteristics of the human mind. By such an explanation the pressure of an unlimitedly complex reality on a limited capacity to comprehend the world produces anxiety resolved only by the adoption of simple schemes of comprehension. It may also reflect social pressures for total centralization and bureaucratization, expressed in the distorting mirror of ideologies. It does in fact probably reflect a complex interrelation between a variety of such factors.

The term 'model' has been used to depict alternatively a conscious analytical device, or a preconception which selects, determines, and colours our cognition or comprehension of the nature of the object. In terms of the latter one can speak of perception through given models (or archetypes) in both scholarly and pragmatic knowledge. The specific physiological make-up of human sensory organs and the human brain seems to provide us with such a major selector of stimuli, images, and types of generalization. In J. Z. Young's words, 'Homeostats have no means for recording an "unbiased" view of reality.' His comparison of the operation of the octopus and human brain may be used as a good example of physiologically determined different cognitive worlds.[34] Furthermore, not only the capacities of the human mind but also the characteristics of social structure have their influence on cognition of reality. Issues of subject–object relations cannot be limited to the interaction of a single mind with external reality. Human beings are social, and the impact of a whole cultural apparatus – communication, reification, socialization, and control – must be part and parcel of any study of cognition.[35] Man displays unique ability to create and transfer complex symbolic systems which are the essence of human culture. These provide us with explicit and ready-made images, categories, and symbolic models of reality which then influence our comprehension, cognition, and action. The sociology of knowledge has attempted to define the nature of these influences on our minds.

A major problem of preconditioned and structured human consciousness seems to lie, however, with those parts of cognition and comprehension that appear to be neither simply 'reflections' of intersubjective reality nor sheer resultants of human physiology, nor again factors which can be self-evidently related to conscious theorizing or to social pressures to conform. Those seem to be the entities described by Black as the 'submerged models operating in authors' minds';[36] McLuhan's 'linear thinking' postulated as typical of the 'typographical man' of the sixteenth to nineteenth centuries (as opposed to the 'loose-knot' comprehension in the time of mass communication) may act here as an example.[37]

Bronowski's historiography of sciences, already referred to, and Piaget's typical stages of child development provide such examples in terms of development sequences.[38] All these tendencies will probably have to be explained in terms of interrelation between the basic characteristics of human nature and the way society is structured, though such an explanation will have to be much more complex than that which the contemporary sociology of knowledge tends to express. Eliade's explanation of the difference between the cognition typical of 'archaic' and 'modern' man in terms of different ways of solving dilemmas of time, order, suffering, and death can here be used as an example. The explanations of Lévi-Strauss, Carl Young, and M. Scheler of the preconditioning of mind in terms of group subconsciousness are relevant here. Chomsky's discussion of the innate qualities of the human mind approaches the issue from a different angle.[39] Whatever the explanation and whatever the weight we give to societal influence as against the inborn influence of the individual mind, patterned preconditioning of human cognition and comprehension must mean also the existence of 'submerged models' – unconscious or not fully conscious and yet influencing profoundly the process of our thought. Furthermore, analysis of human thought and action will have to consider not only the human capacity for 'rational judgement' but also 'irrational' components of thought, and these will have to find expression in any relevant model-building. Indeed, a generation earlier, Pareto attempted to define empirically as 'residiums' those types of human preference and action that cannot simply be treated in terms of pure logic or as the shortest cut to the declared aims.[40]

Some relation between model as an explanatory device and model as a preconditioned (or even programmed) pattern of thought exists without doubt. Yet the actual character of this relation is anything but clear, mainly as a result of the ambiguities surrounding the use of models in the latter sense. Concepts created by man have proved much easier to tackle than the issue of the investigators' own biases, lurking at the back of their minds.

In the few existing discussions 'submerged models' have assumed radically different identities and significance. At times they were treated as lower in rank than those explicitly stated, i.e. as 'half-baked', partial, or 'emerging' models of an explanatory type. The scholar's work would, therefore, consist of the clarification and tightening-up of the logical structure of the 'submerged models' with the aim of turning them into explanatory devices. On the other hand, models as explanatory devices have at times been approached as subordinate to 'deeper' preconceptions with the relevance and fruitfulness of the first determined by the second. The task of scholarship here is consequently seen in breaking the codes of the deeper layers of human consciousness in the attempt to reach types of knowledge more profound than those represented by explanatory devices of the more explicit type. Construction of models of model-selection can possibly form here an important subsequent stage to guide us through the perplexities of simultaneous and conflicting models referring to the same reality. Thorne's discussion below of definite systems generating infinite solutions may have some broader relevance here. A systematic analysis of the mutual interdependence of both types of model will have to await further developments in the study of human comprehension and of subject–object relations.

V. MODELS AND SOCIETY

'Between consciousness and existence stand meanings and designs and communications which other men have passed on, first in human speech itself and later by the management of symbols. Those received and manipulated interpretations decisively influence such consciousness as men have of their existence.'[41] Models are firmly rooted in this territory, which ranges between consciousness and 'existence', and derive their significance from this fact. This relation operates both ways. On the one hand, 'existence' is cognized through models. On the other hand, the explanatory model adopted not only represents selected aspects of reality, but also shapes it, i.e. has bearings not only on human comprehension but on human actions. Indeed, in the philosophy and theory of the sciences the very split between ontology and epistemology is rapidly growing narrower. Bohm's as well as

Bauman's and Brittan's treatment of knowledge as a 'subtle order of being' may be one of the major messages of our generation.[42] Furthermore, models play a crucial role in mobilizing, triggering off, focusing, and controlling human energy. It is in terms of 'new models' that policies are nowadays described by scholars, governments, and the press alike.[43] Models seem, therefore, to influence profoundly our consciousness and consequently our life and action. Not surprisingly they reflect the two poles of human cultural history – creativity versus formalization and control. Men live in 'second-hand worlds' determined by the cultural apparatus of socialization and of mass media, which have provided them with ready-made symbols and concepts. Gramsci's idea of 'egemonia' as against domination of men by means of coercion is deeply relevant here. Egemonia means control of men through the control and manipulation of symbolic schemes which determine human cognition. It is this insight that has grown so powerful in the mass society of our time and has made Marcuse's *One-dimensional Man* into the Bible of a whole generation of students. Reified models and language operate as determinants of cognition and as codes of behaviour defining the degrees of freedom of the individual. Control of the mass media, and mass production of models 'sold' to the masses, have become a major form of the domination of men by men. At the same time, the main scholarly elites of model-producers retreat step by step into a world of their own creation, the complexity of which makes for a seclusion greater than that of a Trappist monastery.

And yet, on the other hand, models represent time and time again the height of human creativity, liberation, and imagination. Much of the struggle for human liberation has been shaped by 'utopias' – models of a better world, capable of mobilizing masses of people for political action.[44] In scholarship, the imagination aspect of models was made particularly clear by the comparison with metaphors. 'A memorable metaphor has the power to bring two domains together into cognitive and emotional relation by using language directly appropriate to the one as a lens to see the other . . . to see . . . in a new way.'[45] *To see in a new way*, with all its intellectual and emotional undertones, is indeed the essence of whatever we call creativity, and worship as the highest expression of the human spirit. As with all other human tools and constructions, models can be used for the sake of freedom and enslavement alike. It is up to 'us'.

NOTES AND REFERENCES

1 For further discussion see, for example, Z. Bauman's paper below. Also BERGER, P. and LUCKMANN, T. *The Social Construction of Reality*, London, Allen Lane, the Penguin Press, 1967.
2 KUHN, T. S. *The Structure of Scientific Revolutions*, Chicago, University of Chicago Press, 1962, p. 62.
3 MERTON, R. K. *Social Theory and Social Structure*, Glencoe, Ill., Free Press, 1957, p. 104.
4 JASPERS, K. 'The Axial Age of Human History', in STEIN, M. R. *et al.*, *Identity and Anxiety*, Glencoe, Ill., Free Press, 1960.
5 KUHN, op. cit., p. 163.
6 BRONOWSKI, J. *The Common Sense of Science*, London, Heinemann, 1951.
7 See HEISENBERG, W. *The Physical Principles of the Quantum Theory*, 1930. Merton, R. K., op. cit. Pt I.
   For the discussion of Gödel's theorem, see J. Pym's paper below.
8 BALDAMUS, W. in his paper below. See also his 'On Testing Hypotheses', *Discussion papers of the University of Birmingham*, E/13, 1969.
9 JASPERS, K. *Philosophy*, Chicago, Chicago University Press, 1969, Vol. I, p. 174.
10 For an interesting recent discussion, see BOLLACK, J. *Empédocle*, Paris, Editions de Minuit, 1970.
11 See, for example, NATANSON, M. *Philosophy of the Social Sciences*, New York, Random House, 1963. See also, for an interesting comment, CROWSON, R. A. 'Science and Phenomenology', *Nature*, **223**, 1969, p. 1318–19.
12 POLANYI, M. *The Tacit Dimension*, London, Routledge, 1967. BALDAMUS, W., op. cit., as well as the same authors: 'On the Category of Pragmatic Knowledge', *Discussion Papers of the University of Birmingham*, E1, 1966.
13 POPPER, K. T. *The Poverty of Historicism*, London, Routledge, 1960. On the other hand see, for an attempt to tackle the issue differently, his more recent *Of Clouds and Clocks*, Washington University, 1966.
14 See, for example, the paper by A. Koestler below, as well as his *The Ghost in the Machine*, London, Hutchinson, 1967.
15 BLACK, M. *Models and Metaphors*, Cornell University Press, 1962, p. 222.
16 See the *Encyclopedia of Philosophy*, Ed. Edwards, P. Glencoe, Ill., Free Press, vol. V, p. 354.
17 Ibid.

18 BLACK, op. cit., p. 220.
19 BRAITHWAITE, R. B. *Scientific Explanation*, Cambridge University Press, 1953, p. 93.
20 BLALOCK, H. M. *Causal Inferences in Non-experimental Research*, Chapel Hill, University of North Carolina Press, 1965, p. 6.
21 The issue is explicitly set out already in DESCARTES, R. *Meditations on the First Philosophy* written at the beginning of the sixteenth century.
22 APOSTEL, L. 'Towards the Formal Study of Models in non-formal Sciences', in FREDENTHAL, H. *The Concept and the Role of Model in Mathematics and Natural and Social Sciences*, Dordtrecht, 1961, p. 622.
23 BLALOCK, op. cit., pp. 106–15.
24 For an interesting discussion, see CHORLEY, R. J. and HAGGETT, P. *Physical and Information Models in Geography*, London, Methuen, 1967.
25 RUSSELL, B. *History of Western Philosophy*, London, Allen and Unwin, 1961, p. 87, drives in this sense a straight line from Leibniz to Einstein in the basic acceptance of events as 'the stuff of the world'.
26 BAUMAN, Z. 'Semiotics and Function of Culture', *Social Science Information*, 7(5), 1968, p. 69.
27 MILSUM, J. H. *Positive Feedback*, London, Pergamon Press, 1968, which discusses the character of positive feedback in technology, mathematics, economics, and other aspects of human behaviour.
28 Ibid., pp. 80–1. For a basic discussion of the issue of mutual causation, see MARUYAMA, M. 'Morphogenesis and Morphostasis', *Methodos*, **12**, 1960, 251–6.
29 For discussion, see the paper below by Paul Clark.
30 See, for example, M. GODELIER, 'The Origins of Mythical Thought', *New Left Review*, **69**, 1971.
31 NEEDHAM, J. *Science and Civilization in China*, Cambridge University Press, 1962.
32 See, for example, Kuhn op. cit., chs VII, IX (science), or HAMMOND, P. E. *Sociologists at Work*, New York, Basic Books, 1964.
33 LUNDBERG, C. A. in Natanson, op. cit., p. 38.
34 YOUNG, J. Z. *A Model of the Brain*, Oxford, Clarendon Press, 1964.
35 See, for example, WRIGHT MILLS, C. *Power, Politics and People*, London, Oxford University Press, 1964, Part IV.
36 BLACK, op. cit., p. 239.
37 MCLUHAN, M. *The Gutenberg Galaxy*, London, Routledge, 1962.
38 For example, PIAGET, J. *The Origin of Intelligence in the Child*, London, Routledge, 1953. The introduction discusses some more general issues of the impact of heredity on human intelligence.
39 See the papers below by J. P. Thorne and Z. Bauman; also ELIADE, M. *The Myth of the Eternal Return*, New York, Pantheon Books, 1954. LÉVI-STRAUSS, C. *The Savage Mind*, London, Weidenfeld, 1966.

CHOMSKY, N. *Language and Mind*, New York, Harcourt Brace, 1968.

40 PARETO, V. *The Mind and Society*, New York, Harcourt Brace, 1935. For an extremely interesting discussion see HENDERSON, L. J. *Pareto's General Sociology*, Russell & Russell, 1967.

41 Mills, op. cit., p. 405.

42 See the papers by Bohm, D., Bauman, Z., and Brittan, A. below The quotation comes from D. Bohm's comments on the paper by P. Clark. For a recent claim of similar nature made in one more discipline, see BATESON, G. 'The Cybernetics of Self' *Psychiatry*, **34**(1), 1971.

43 See, for example, the recent discussion of economic policies in *Le Monde Weekly*, 30 December 1970, p. 5.
For a recent discussion of the impact of models on political action, see BODDINGTON, S. 'Models, Philosophy and Action' *The Spokesman*, 1970, No. 2.

44 See the testimony of a broad range of studies, from the discussion of 'Myth' in Sorel's *Reflections on Violence* at the beginning of the century as far as the recent spirited defence of utopian socialism as the only genuine part left of socialism by Marcuse at the 1967 Dialectics of Liberation Congress in London and again at the 1968 'Praxis' Conference in Korçula.

45 Black, op. cit., p. 236.

PART ONE

Models and Disciplines

Part I: Introduction

Part I incorporates papers which, while raising a variety of general issues, belong to specific academic disciplines. Its main concern is with models of thought and/or troublespots of conceptualization specific to the disciplines in question. The list of disciplines is broad and runs from the natural sciences through psychology (experimental and clinical) and the social sciences to linguistics, theology, and pure mathematics. Works on models in other fields of study, in particular in the arts and in philosophy, were hoped for, but failed to arrive on time. Their absence is not intentional but, on the contrary, much regretted. Each paper is followed by a short comment criticizing or expanding on the points made and providing a possible 'first shot' for debate.

The division between Part I and Part II is to some extent arbitrary; a number of papers would no doubt fit both. In particular, the papers by Baldamus, Bauman, and Brittan, in Part II belong also to Part I, filling the gap where the cluster of sociology, anthropology, and social psychology would rightly belong.

Image and Symbol:
the role of models in
modern physics

PAUL M. CLARK

INTRODUCTION

The major developments in twentieth-century physics, grouped
under the general headings of quantum theory and relativity, have
provoked much discussion and re-evaluation of the subject–object
relationship in natural science and, to a lesser extent, the role of
models in the development and articulation of physical theory.
Basing itself principally on the developments of classical physics
and non-relativistic quantum theory, this paper attempts to
approach the subject–object problem from a standpoint developed
from an analysis of the nature and function of models as a basis
of explanation in physics, in different historical periods and areas
of study within the field.

Quite naturally, the first problem will be to define the term
'model', for, while it is commonly used by physicists, it is tacitly
rather than formally defined and lends itself to many uses. The
definition given here is stimulated by, and conforms with, many
examples of its current use, but it is formalized in a way that gives
it a smaller breadth of reference than the general abstract terms
'theory' and 'experiment'. Having formulated the definition, an
examination of different areas of classical and quantum physics
will attempt to fill it out and show the particular nature of the
problems posed by the development of quantum theory with respect to the subject–object relationship. Finally the problem of
plurality will be defined and discussed in the light of the previously developed ideas.

It is not uncommon to hear social and behavioural scientists speak of the natural sciences as the paragon of scientific methodology and conceptual clarity. In order that the example be instructive rather than misleading, the nature of that clarity and the price at which it is obtained should be as clearly appreciated as is possible. In the attempt to contribute to this appreciation by making this article intelligible to as wide an audience as possible, detailed mathematical and physical references have been kept to a minimum. Each general point has been made in a way that, I hope, can be grasped by those who do not have a knowledge of the details which motivate it. However, the details are important since it is on the validity of the interpretation put upon them that the general considerations stand or fall.

I. MODELS IN CLASSICAL PHYSICS

1. *Approach to the Definition*

In order to approach the definition of the term 'model' to be utilized in subsequent discussion, an examination of a particular use of the term, the 'Rutherford model' of the atom, provides a useful starting-point. The atom is pictured, according to the Rutherford model, as an impenetrable nucleus of positively charged matter surrounded, at distances very large with respect to the nuclear diameter, by small, negatively charged particles, the electrons, which move in orbits about the nucleus. The mathematical structure of Newtonian mechanics is associated with certain features of this picture in order to allow the deductive power of mathematical analysis to be employed in the development of an understanding of the atom's structure and behaviour.

In many recent descriptions of the nature of physical theories,[1] two language systems have been distinguished: an 'observation language' applied to the field of immediate perception and a theoretical language to describe intellectual constructs, which includes mathematical systems. These two languages are linked or coordinated by rules of correspondence allowing the passage between theory and experiment in the course of a scientific investigation. The 'model' of the atom given above clearly falls within the realm of the theoretical language – no reference is made to any direct observation of the atom – but contains two distinct forms of discourse; a formal language of terms and relations expressed in mathematical symbols (e.g. particle positions, momentums, masses) and an informal language of descriptive terms, (e.g. orbit, nucleus) often supplemented with diagrams, which in other situations could be employed in the observation language (e.g. to describe the solar system, of which the atom is sometimes described as a miniature replica). The abstract Newtonian concepts make possible the development of detailed conclusions about the atom (and about the properties of a large number of spatially contiguous atoms) which lead to observation statements testable by experiment. But they do not constitute the totality of what is conceptualized as the Rutherford model, the pictorial image of its existence in space being given in the informal language.

An important facet of the relationship between pictorial and symbolic elements of theoretical discourse can be illustrated by the example of Euclidean geometry. There is a long history of curiosity and debate as to the role of diagrams and constructions in the study of geometry. The statement of a theorem, in the form of either symbolic equations or sentences, is not, strictly speaking, true to the diagram drawn to illustrate or to prove it. However, the approximate representation, in a diagram, of the problem set by the theorem allows a form of intuition to be brought to bear which, by means of a construction or simple association, will stimulate the equations or sentences that constitute the proof. Anyone who has attempted to teach geometry will immediately recognize the intuitive or non-deductive nature of the construction often required to make a proof obvious: there is some hope of teaching a deductive process but with geometrical construction there only exists the hope that the pupil will acquire the art of mental experimentation by watching the teacher deal in this way with numerous examples. This function of the diagram in stimulating intuition is, it will be argued here, an important function of the informal aspect of a physical model.

2. Definition and Development of the Concept of Model

With the above considerations in mind, we wish to define the term 'model' as an intellectual construction comprising an informal pictorial description united with a formal symbolic representation which allows logical (often specifically mathematical) deduction of relations which can be translated into testable statements in the observation language. As in the example first given above, the terms of each language used in a given model are a selection of the terms available, so that the model cannot be identified with the more general term 'theory', which comprises all the terms and relations of both types of description.

A distinction between two major types of model observable at work in classical physics relates to the amount of detail contained in the pictorial description of the model as opposed to the amount of detail in the observational situation to which it relates. The first, labelled here the 'perception-smoothing' type, simplify the perceptual situation by emphasizing certain features and depressing others. The selected features then form the informal representation of the model with which the mathematical variables of the formal language are united. A good example is given by one of the fundamental successful applications of Newtonian mechanics to astronomy, the derivation of the elliptical orbit of a planet moving around the sun. From a very complex observational situation (even considering only the details known in Newton's time) a simplified representation of one isolated planet and the sun as points in space is selected. Each point is endowed with a given amount of a single quality, mass. From the mathematical representation of (1) the sun and the planet as points in Euclidean space (2) the attractive force between them as a function of their masses and the distance between them, and the application of Newton's laws of motion in mathematical form, the function of space variables which describes the orbit of the planet around the sun as an ellipse may be derived.

With the second type of model, labelled as 'perception-expanding', the informal, pictorial language gives a detailed substructure to what can be observed. The formal language attached to the substructure then may allow the prediction of large-scale effects which can be observed (or whose previous observation provided the motivation for the development of the model). The kinetic theory of gases gives a good example of this process. In thermodynamics (and in everyday observation) a given mass of gas is considered to be a continuous distribution of deformable matter. Kinetic theory gives a substructure (not observed) to the gas; it postulates that a gas is made up of a very large number of infinitesimally small particles of a given mass, which obey Newtonian mechanics. The continuous nature of the observed properties of gases, for example the uniform and constant pressure exerted by a gas on the walls of the containing vessel, is explained (intuitively and mathematically) as the average effect of an unimaginably large number of discrete processes effected by individual molecules (in the case of pressure, collisions with the walls of the vessel).

In order to describe some of the changes in the conceptual structure of physics brought about by the development of quantum theory, in terms of the concept of model, it is necessary to sketch the two particular models developed by classical physics, the particle model and the field model. Each possesses its characteristic pictorial and mathematical components.

In pictorial terms, the field model is represented as an abstraction based on our perceptual experience of the behaviour of the masses of homogeneous liquids or solids whose essential properties (density, rigidity) seem to be spread continuously throughout the sample and which seem capable of infinite subdivision. One imagines (although the molecular substructure of matter removes it as a candidate for such an experiment) that if a small subvolume of the sample on view were magnified to any scale, the subvolume and the original volume would be structurally identical. The dynamical behaviour of the field model, its motion in time, is manifested through the transmission of regions of compression and rarefaction of the medium, or regions of twisting distortion through the body of the medium, which itself does not suffer permanent displacement (e.g. sound waves in a gas). A particle model is developed as an abstraction of our perceptual experience of dots on paper or stars viewed with the naked eye. The model comprises the distribution of a number of structureless points (or sometimes very simple structures such as perfectly smooth spheres centred at these points) in a given volume of empty space. Taking a small subvolume of this model and magnifying it to the size of the original volume will produce a different, less detailed structure than the original, in direct contrast with the field model. The dynamic evolution of the model manifests itself as the motion of the point particles through space along continuous curves.

At the root of the mathematical formalism of particle theories is the labelling of the discrete points in space by vectors which are functions of a single parameter, time. The properties of the particles and the forces between them are expressed as functions of these vectors, their time derivatives, and constants representing their stable properties, such as mass or electric charge. Application of Newton's laws of motion leads in general to a coupled set of ordinary differential equations whose solutions represent the paths of motion of the system. In contrast, a field theory employs as its basic mathematical terms functions of time and the space variables labelling the volume occupied by the field. The field functions obey equations in which they and their partial derivatives with respect to space and time appear along with functions of the space variables which specify the properties of the medium, such as density or rigidity.

Although classical physics, and in particular classical mechanics, developed greatly in complexity and power during the eighteenth and nineteenth centuries, the models that physicists applied to the analysis of physical systems comprised a coupling of mathematical and pictorial descriptions which conformed to the following restrictions (at least until the advent of Maxwell's theory of electromagnetism and the discovery of the electron):

1 Each physical system is described by only one form of model: either a particle model or a field model.

2 The possibility exists of correlating each basic variable of the model, in its mathematical form, with an operational definition given in the observation language.

3 The time-evolution of the model is a unique function of its initial conditions, i.e. the models exhibit causal dynamical behaviour.

4 The possibility exists of consistently holding the 'realist' position with respect to the ontological status of the model (this point will be elaborated upon below, p. 34, point 1).

The perplexities caused by these latter developments and their effect on the status of physical models will be discussed below.

3. *Philosophical Considerations in the Use of Models in Classical Physics*

(a) *General consequences*

Let us try to sketch some of the general features impressed on the intellectual activity of physics by the use of models. Firstly, in approaching the observational situation, some such simplification as is effected by the development of a perception-smoothing model as a starting-point for analysis is always necessary; the perceptual field is (1) too complex to be described *in toto*, and (2) without significance unless analysed with reference to some conceptual scheme by means of which distinctions can be made and communicated. Even in the case of the perception-enriching model, the pre-existing perceptual field has been put into relief by application of a group of concepts which proved inadequate in some way. Prosecuting the analysis of a physical system by means of a model comprising a small number of variables or features makes feasible the development (through logical or mathematical deduction) of testable conclusions. Simplicity of conception has both practical and aesthetic attractions for physicists.

Second, both the informal and formal aspects of a model make distinct contributions to the development of a physical theory. Generally speaking, the mathematical description allows the consequences of the model to be developed through long chains of deductive reasoning which would be extremely difficult, if not impossible, to follow through without the use of formal mathematical methods. While it is not the case that intuition plays no part in mathematical development and while any number of examples can be found of intuitive leaps being made during the mathematical investigation of a physical problem, this intuition is of a very specific type which causes some physicists to feel, on occasion, that the mathematical analysis has not given a complete understanding of the structure and behaviour of the physical system in question.[2] It is one, but not the only, form, of intuition brought into play in attacking physical problems. The pictorial description in a model stimulates another form of intuition; for example, the formation of analogies and associations between physically very distinct systems or observable situations based on pictorial resemblances. Supposing one model to have an associated mathematical structure whose deductive consequences or rules of operation are well developed, its pictorial resemblance to a different physical context may cause a physicist to transplant it into the new problem to see how the deductive consequences agree with experiments. The pictorial representation can function in a similar way to the diagram in a geometrical exercise to stimulate associations, conjectures, or what is referred to as a 'physical insight' in probing for an understanding of the system's behaviour.

(b) *Ontological status of models*

The problem of the ontological status of models is posed by asking whether either of the following two positions can be consistently held:

1 The simplification (or substructure) given to the observational field by analysing a model of it describes an independently existent essence of the physical system.

2 The model describes an ideal, heuristic representation which guides the physical inquiry but whose importance and validity rest solely on the agreement of the deduced consequences with experiment. This position has as a consequence the belief that, as a result of analysis using that model, nothing has been learned about the structure of nature that could be described as independently existent.

The former position contains an element of 'intuitive reasonableness' in the core of significance of the element of the physical world under examination being reflected in the central concepts of the explanatory model. From the point of view of the second alternative, it is difficult from any position other than a purely rationalist one (in the sense of 'the clear and distinct idea', mathematical structures especially, having necessary truth) to justify the efficacy of a particular model in producing the verified conclusion, especially in the perception-expanding case where no appeal to immediate sensory knowledge is possible. This point of view also questions the proper objectives of scientific inquiry itself. The development of models conforming to the second point of view described above can be likened to the production of elaborate calculating apparati which generate numbers to be correlated with laboratory observations. Such activity can regard as irrelevant the development of the understanding of either the progressively refined constituents of nature (or, more generally, some form of basic structure of the natural world, if breaking it into constituents ceases to be a useful mode of description) which has long been considered one of the aims of science.[3]

Support of one side or the other of this issue opposed some of the most renowned physicists of the nineteenth century. At the time of their introduction, both the Newtonian model of planetary motion and the molecular substructure of gases were considered to reflect the essential natures of the objects they represented. But the development of Maxwell's theory of electromagnetism (1865), interpreted in a similar fashion, led to postulating the existence of a continuous medium (the ether) to support the transmission of electromagnetic waves (analogous to the part air plays as a supporting medium for sound-wave propagation by transmitting pressure variations through space). This medium was constrained by the known facts to have the most intuitively improbable physical properties and all experimental attempts to detect its presence failed. Yet the wave nature of electromagnetic radiation, of which light and radio waves are examples, is an unquestionable fact. Maxwell himself took the medium as an imaginary, heuristic device, which allowed him to conceptualize wave motion, without granting it objective reality.[4] This is one of a number of examples[5] which illustrate the increasing tendency of late nineteenth-century physicists to dissociate the models with which their predictions were made from any possibility of reflecting the essential 'building-blocks' of the universe due to their presence as central concepts of physical theory. This tendency was developed before the advent of quantum theory, which is considered by some of its founders to show definitively the futility of any unlimited aspirations in the realist direction.

II. MODELS AND QUANTUM PHYSICS

4. *Description of the Model in Quantum Mechanics*

The basic features of a physical model, illustrated with examples from classical physics, have been discussed in some detail with the objective of being able to describe, without becoming involved in mathematical formalism, what changes the advent of quantum theory has wrought on the objectives and methods of study in physics, as reflected in changes in the form of models employed. With respect to the informal, pictorial features, no new forms of description have been generated. The images we use are still those of discrete, localizable particle and continuous field (although in the particle case the range of properties accorded to these basic entities is much wider than the single feature, mass, associated with the Newtonian particle).

Indeed, it has been repeatedly stressed by Niels Bohr[6] that these concepts, abstracted from everyday life in the course of the development of classical physics, provide the only possible basis of unambiguous communication between physicists.[7] In contrast, the formal mathematical structure to be united with these descriptive forms has changed. Two forms of change have occurred; (1) new mathematical concepts have been united with old pictorial concepts and (2) old mathematical and pictorial terms have been united in new ways. In the most general case, the distinction between formalisms appropriate to particle or field models has disappeared.[8] The most commonly used formalism, the Schrödinger representation, associates the particle properties (position and momentum) of a given physical system with the linear operators of a partial differential equation[9] into which is also fed information as to their interaction with (1) each other and (2) the boundaries of the system. Solving this equation yields a function of space and time variables, which resembles a classical field function in form, whose value at any point in space and time is related to the probability that, on repeated observation of the same system, a particle will be found there. In special cases,[10] the equations simplify so that the wave and particle models (classical pictures and mathematics)[11] may be separately envisaged for the system. Of primary significance here are the facts that (1) they must both be applied in the course of the analysis and (2) their fundamental concepts are related by mathematical equations which allow no intuitive translation of wave concepts into particle concepts or vice versa.

This fusion of particle and field pictures into a single mathematical formalism arose as a solution to the impasse created by the acceptance of the fact that any attempt to give a classical particle-model substructure to the atom[12] was either blatantly self-contradictory or led, on analysis, to unsubstantiated conclusions. Experiments done on a great variety of physical systems suggested that, in the atomic realm, both wave and particle pictures must be employed on the same physical system within the context of a single analysis in order to develop conclusions consistent with the empirical data. But the conclusions of this quantum-mechanical analysis are inherently statistical in character, in direct contrast with classical mechanical predictions which concern the time-evolution of a single system. Although the quantum model is considered a representation of a single physical system, its predictions concern only the distribution of possible results with (1) repeated operation of the same system, or (2) simultaneous operation of a large number of equivalent systems.

5. *Ideal Ontological Characterization of the Quantum Model*

The fact that a large number of equivalent physical systems will generate the same distribution of outcomes from a given experimental procedure gives strong support to the belief in the existence of some basic natural structure as a cause of this regularity. But the failure of all attempts to produce a single, adequate pictorial description of subatomic nature coupled with the success of the quantum model with its duality of pictorial representations gives impetus to the view given as (2) on page 34, which will be labelled the 'idealist ontological position', with respect to the quantum model. In classical physics, although it is useful to apply both continuum and particle models to the same empirical object,[13] the two models are kept quite distinct (in a manner to be discussed in more detail in Part III) so that the spatial characteristics of one of them could be considered as descriptive of the spatial features of the object. But when both field and particle pictures must be applied in order to develop a coherent model, then any assumptions of ontological reality (the view expressed in (1), p. 34) seem impossible and ontological ideality seems inevitable. One consistent explanation of this development might be resumed in the following points:

1 Models are always idealizations and their ontological significance must never be considered as ultimately decided.

2 At the level of direct human perception, we act on the belief that the models we construct accurately reflect the properties of the 'objects' of the external world. We are reinforced in this attitude by the coherence[14] that obtains between our expectations (or theorizing) and our perceptual experience (or experimentation).

3 The same belief with respect to the perception-expanding

model of the kinetic theory of gases leads to many consistent conclusions and some inconsistent ones.

4 At the level of atomic substructure the attempt to apply either of the models of classical physics, separately, leads to lack of coherence between predictions and results.

5 At a given level of structure the ontological realist position can only be held with regard to one of the two contradictory classical models.

6 Thus the unity effected by the quantum-theoretical model allows the correct prediction of experimental results (which often appear on a size scale directly available to human perception) at the price of losing (through the necessity of applying both wave and particle images to the same individual system) any possibility of believing that these images are anything else but heuristic devices to allow creative thought to proceed into areas where their representative function has ceased to be credible.

Borrowing Kantian terminology, wave and particle function as antinomic forms of pictorial representation. In the Kantian antinomies, the acceptance of the proofs of the existence of antinomic forms of our knowledge of space, time, and material objects implies the conclusion that all our awareness of the world is only of its appearance to us, not its real existence: in modern physics the acceptance of the necessity of antinomic forms of pictorial representation makes impossible the belief that the appearance of subatomic constituents of nature is actually described by these forms. Any synthesis that has been achieved in quantum-theoretic models has been of a mathematical, not a pictorially descriptive, kind. It should be emphasized, however, that this synthesis has been extremely fruitful in bringing for the first time mathematical order and predictability to a large range of physical phenomena. Its unquestionable success is the principal stimulus to the development of as clear an analysis and articulation of its meaning as is possible.

6. *The Crucial Change – Ontological or Epistemological?*

In most discussions of the significance of wave–particle duality and its reflection in the Heisenberg uncertainty relations, the central core of the illustrations or arguments is epistemological in character, focusing on the subject–object relationship or the interaction of object and measuring instrument. The object whose properties are to be measured is depicted in either wave or particle form, the operation of the measuring instruments is described, and the irreducible measure of disturbance inflicted on the object in the act of measuring it invoked to show that our capacity to discover the values of the property-variables possessed by a micro-object is limited by the coarseness of the means with which we are forced to operate in any measuring situation.

In the original development of the epistemological position a series of imaginary experiments were postulated by the opponents of quantum theory; the vindication of the position came through the exposition of a detailed mechanical analysis of the measuring process, using classical mechanics for particle properties, classical optics for the wave properties and equations, mathematically simple but intuitively opaque, to relate the pictures and properties of particles and waves. It was always concluded that the irreducible disturbing effect of a measurement limited its possible accuracy in a way consistent with Heisenberg's uncertainty principle. Furthermore, in the course of these analyses it became clear that, in each experimental situation posed, to measure one of the two mutually exclusives aspects (wave or particle) of an atomic system required a mechanical situation (i.e. layout of measuring equipment) which ruled out (in mechanical terms, i.e. that a given piece of equipment cannot be both rigidly fastened and totally free to move at the same time) the possibility of observing the other aspect.[15] Thus no contradictory situation could be experimentally exhibited, which was considered to mean that the theory was self-consistent. Although this position has now been raised to the rank of a principle, its validity seems to rest on the lack of success, to date, of constructing a tenable counterproposal.

While this approach to the subject-object situation in quantum theory has many adherents, and has the advantage of pictorial vividness, it can lead inquiry into blind alleys and, on occasion, make a travesty of the language supposedly being employed in unambiguous communication. In envisaging a real microphysical object in interaction with a measuring instrument, one finds oneself having to talk of an object whose properties at a given point in space and time depend upon (and can be manipulated by) the nature of the measuring instruments with which it will interact at a later time and a different (sometimes quite distant) point in space. This situation in turn has led to explanations using such improbable ideas as the following:

1 The mathematical representation of a system changes when the result of the experiment is registered in the conscious mind of the observer.[16]

2 A particle moves from point A to point B in space but cannot be conceived as having followed any determinate path in space between the two points.[17]

Consideration (1) above leads to the involvement of the physicist's eyes and brain cells as part of the apparatus,[18] which only increases the confusion. Point (2) makes the descriptive language descend into meaninglessness, since as long as a particle exists, its motion must describe a path in space.

By shifting the central point of concern from the relation between micro-objects, conceived in particular classical forms, and measuring instruments, to the validity or consistency of adopting a realist ontological position with respect to a given model, one ends up saying less (at the present stage of development) about microphysical reality, but perhaps to good effect. Central concepts in this approach would be consistency and coherence. Consistency, or lack of it, would be applied to the formal aspects of the model and its application to the mathematical structures or the rules of correspondence: coherence, a term describing a less easily formalized order, would refer (1) to the relation between descriptive elements which unite to form a visualizable picture in space, and (2) to the order perceived over a large number of cycles of theoretical prediction and experiment in which the model predicts new experimental behaviour which is found, and experiment suggests properties of the model shown by subsequent calculation to be true.

A consistent model possessed of both forms of coherence could be given the realist ontological status, as are both the particle and the field model in separate areas of large-scale nature. The attempt to apply either of them separately to the microphysical domain leads to lack of coherence between theory and experiment. While the quantum-mechanical model possesses consistency and is coherent in the second meaning given above, it lacks pictorial coherence (because of the simultaneous application of mutually exclusive pictorial descriptions to one physical system). Thus with this model, one must accept the ontological idealist interpretation. Disintegration of coherence of descriptions with changes in the scale of observation or application, has examples in everyday life which provide useful metaphors for this facet of the quantum-mechanical model.[19]

One methodology suggested by the ontological characterization of the quantum situation bases itself on the axiomatic formulations of modern mathematics. Given that (1) the descriptive images lose their representative significance in the microphysical domain and (2) the unity or consistency possessed by the quantum model is of a strictly mathematical kind, the impulse is then to regard and to develop quantum theory as an axiomatic system, in the mathematical sense, and proceed to test the deduced theorems against empirical evidence via formal rules of correspondence. While this is a legitimate avenue of approach and is aesthetically pleasing to many mathematically minded physicists, it has drawbacks which argue against its being established as the only proper methodology of modern physics. One of the concerns of this paper has been to give adequate attention to the part that the pictorial aspects of a model play in guiding a physicist's intuition to make associations and logical jumps in the course of his research. This intuitive guide is lost in a purely axiomatic methodology, being replaced by the ethereal form of intuition possessed by mathematicians, remarkable in itself, but not *necessarily* appropriate to the probing of a physical situation.

Generally speaking, while one gains in precision and orderliness in an axiomatic treatment, one loses in abstractness and in opacity when it comes to judging the relevance of a given axiomatic development to a particular range of physical problems. Therefore this method should be complemented by an approach which attempts to develop new physical concepts whose application to microphysical situations would be possessed of both forms of coherence outlined above.[20]

III. PLURALISM AND REDUCTIONISM FROM THE
PHYSICIST'S VIEWPOINT

7. *Pluralism in Classical Physics*

A focus of attention of the seminar to which this paper was
originally given was directed to questions such as the following:

1 Is it necessary or desirable to have a number of mutually
   exclusive models with which to analyse a given area of subject-
   matter?

2 Should it be a prime object of concern to reduce the statements and insights of various model analyses to those of one
   principal model?

3 Are there criteria which can be set up to decide when (a) a
   plurality is necessary or (b) a reduction can be effected?

4 What kind of synthesis can be made of the information given
   by a plurality of models focused on a given area of study?

These questions will be collectively referred to as the problem of
plurality, although these concerns, especially question (2), have
been discussed with reference to psychology as the problem of
reductionism. This section proposes to look at these questions in
the light of the preceding discussion in order (a) to consider what
distinctions can be given to the general notion of plurality and
(b) to examine the position taken by contemporary physics with
respect to the questions raised above.

From the discussion in Part I of this paper, it is clear that a
plurality of models has been present in physics since the eighteenth
century at least. It has been a source of speculation among philosophers concerned with the natural sciences; one of the Kantian
antinomies is directly motivated by the fact that Newton's laws
provide the basis of the dynamical description of either discrete or
continuous systems. This fact contributed to the conclusions that
(1) in general, human knowledge of nature refers to the appearance
of nature to human knowing faculties, as opposed to knowledge
of the essential reality of nature, the thing-in-itself, and more
specifically (2) nature appears in the two forms of the continuous

and the discrete owing to these being the two forms of representation set in the human cognitive faculty.

However, in the development of classical physics one can discern a regulating principle in the uses of these two forms of model which keeps to a minimum the perplexity of their simultaneous existence. At the level of formalism, we have already referred to the different mathematical structures used in the two models. Of more interest, however, are the different scales of size to which the different models are kept in their application to a single area of study. The hypothesis of a molecular substructure of gases is a good example. At the level of unaided visual observation, a given quantity of a simple gas can be considered a continuous substance, usefully characterized in static situations by any two of the three measurable quantities, volume, pressure, and temperature. In the absence of external disturbances (i.e. insulated from heat sources, protected against radiation) the sample of gas will preserve indefinitely a given set of values of these variables and in gradual transformations these variables change according to a very simple law. For many purposes, the theory of gases developed on these ideas is perfectly adequate and useful. One point at which it breaks down concerns the explanation of the behaviour, observed under a microscope, of tiny dust or smoke particles suspended in a mass of gas in a static (equilibrium) condition. The erratic, impulsive motion of these particles (called Brownian motion and clear perceptual evidence of some time-evolution or motion in the gas) is incomprehensible from the point of view of a static, continuous, surrounding medium. Replacing the continuum with an immense number of molecules of extremely small size obeying Newtonian mechanics and moving with very high speeds allows a satisfactory explanation of Brownian motion to be deduced, but makes the ideas of equilibrium and static pressure inappropriate, and the whole concept of temperature irrelevant. The large-scale variables regain meaning as the scale of observation becomes coarse enough to blur the details of the motions of individual molecules, so that only stable average properties result.

It is the study of the kinetic theory of gases and more generally statistical mechanics which has given a detailed mathematical description and foundation to this process of obtaining large-scale (macroscopic) properties from the combination of statistics with molecular dynamics. However, the continuum and molecular models of a gas remain distinct, operating with mutually exclusive basic terms and applying different areas of mathematics. Change of scale of size coordinates their conception and use. An evocative analogy might be given by the way in which the dots of ink in a wire-service newspaper photograph only combine to make a coherent picture when one is observing from such a distance that the dots lose their individuality. The detail of the picture can be seen to be related to the average distribution of the dots but as a picture it would be analysed (or described) in terms totally unrelated to, and not translatable into, terms basic to the description of dots; the two sets of concepts apply on different scales of size. In some sense we can comprehend how a picture is formed from dots although one can only perceive one situation, dots or picture, and cannot catch the transition in process: an analogous form of comprehension, backed up by a mathematical exposition, operates to form the connection between the macroscopic (continuous) and microscopic (particle) descriptions of matter. (The loss of significance of picture-descriptive terms on close approach to the photograph is a metaphor, referred to on page 41, of the situation described there with respect to classical concepts in a quantum situation.)

Looking at the questions that constitute the problem of pluralism in the light of this example, the following conclusions can be drawn: (1) A plurality of models is desirable in some areas of classical physics, owing to the different uses to which the applications of these models can be put; (2) the basic concepts of the two models are not always directly translatable into one another, but mathematical connections are made between them; (3) a clear indication that the continuum model was inadequate was given by the appearance of a phenomenon in basic contradiction with one of its central conceptions, that of equilibrium, while the complexity of the molecular model (10^{23} variables at least) makes it totally unsuitable for practical purposes; (4) the difference in size scale of application makes the plurality comprehensible, and statistical methods produce the connection between the models.

8. *Pluralism in Quantum Physics*

The quantum-mechanical model, as described in Part II, employs in general a plurality of pictorial representations within a single model, which separates in simple situations into the two classical models mathematically related and restricted. In direct contrast to the classical situation, these two pictures or models operate at the same scale of structural size. The clearest articulation of the nature and necessity of this plurality has been Niels Bohr's enunciation of the principle of complementarity. The first thesis of this doctrine claims that any clear, unambiguous communication between physicists must be made in terms of the concepts of classical physics: waves, particles, and their associated properties, constitute the only language available for such communication. The second thesis states that all attempts to make a coherent, causally connected description of subatomic phenomena with one of the two classical deterministic models have failed. Taken together they imply that the plurality of descriptive representations embodied in the quantum–mechanical model (along with the statistical form of prediction it gives) become necessary. The two representations are (1) mutually exclusive, in that neither can be thought of as being derived from the other (as a gas continuum is 'derived' from its molecular substructure) and (2) 'complementary' in the sense that both are required (they complement or complete each other) as components of a model whose predictions are consistent with experiment.

From this point of view (the current orthodoxy among physicists), plurality is necessary in quantum theory and reduction should not be contemplated. It should be noted, however, that the credibility of both theses rests on the fact that the converse has not been achieved as yet; impossibility in principle has not been proved.[21] Therefore, there is no legitimate ground to assert that a single, new model, with its mathematical formalism and pictorial content, with respect to which the realist ontological position might be tenable (and which might provide a standpoint from which the complementary function of wave and particle pictures in the present quantum theory would be *understood* as well as *accepted*) cannot in principle be developed.

NOTES AND REFERENCES

1 For example, SELLARS, W. 'The Language of Theories', in *Current Issues in the Philosophy of Science.* Ed. Feigl and Maxwell, New York, Rinehart and Winston, 1961, pp. 57–77.
2 For an example of this position see:
  (a) KAC, M. 1966 Brandeis Lectures, Gordon and Breach, 1968, p. 302.
  (b) BOHM, D. and BUB, J. *Rev. Mod. Phys.* **38**,(3), 1966, p. 457.
3 See reference 2b and the paper by Professor D. Bohm in this volume.
4 BLACK, M. *Models and Metaphors*, Cornell University Press, 1962, pp. 226, 227.
5 The question of the status of the Gibbs Ensemble in statistical mechanics or the 'radiation oscillators' of the electromagnetic field are two other roughly contemporaneous examples.
6 BOHR, N., *Atoms and Human Knowledge*. Reprinted in *Atomic Physics and Human Knowledge*, New York, Science Editions, 1966, p. 83.
7 Whether this proposition is capable of proof is debatable; that it is accepted and acted upon by the community of physicists is important.
8 This in contrast to the classical situation, described on pages 31–2, where each model has its distinctive formal and informal structures.
9 The form of equation usually associated with a classical field model, as described on pages 31–2.
10 The case of non-interacting particles is envisaged here, where the equations separate into a number of simple wave equations, so that waves in 3-dimensional space may be envisaged.
11 The Heisenberg uncertainty principle must be added to the formalism of classical mechanics in order to limit the degree of precision with which the Newtonian concepts of position and momentum may be applied.
12 For instance the Rutherford model discussed in the introduction.
13 For example the Debye model and lattice dynamics in the classical theory of solids.
14 See the discussion of point 2, second para. p. 41, for an elaboration of the idea of 'coherence'.
15 BOHR, N. *Phys. Rev.* **48**, 696, 1935.
   WATSON, W. H., *Understanding Physics Today*, Cambridge University Press, 1967, Ch. IV.
16 HEELAN, P. A., *Quantum Theory and Objectivity*, The Hague, Martinus Nijhoff, 1965, pp. 92–3.
17 For example, LANDAU, L. D., and LIFSHITZ, E. M., *Quantum Mechanics*, London, Pergamon Press, 1959, pp. 1–5.
18 von NEUMANN, J. *Mathematical Foundations of Quantum Mechanics*, Princeton University Press, 1955, pp. 418–19.
19 One such example is given on p. 44.

20 See Reference 3.
21 MESSIAH, A., *Quantum Mechanics*, North Holland Publishing Company, 1967, p.150

Comment

D. BOHM

This paper contains what is, in my view, a good discussion of the main ways in which models are used in physics, along with an analysis of the principal points tending to lead to disagreement among physicists concerning the significance of such models. In these comments, I should like to go further, and to indicate some of the ways in which our thinking goes beyond the notion of a model. I hope thereby to give some further notion of what may be the limitations in the use of models, as well as of the advantages that models confer in situations in which they are appropriate.

One can usefully call attention here to certain domains of experience and activity (e.g. psychological) in which our thinking is not considered *merely* as an image, model, or representation of reality. Rather, it *is* an inseparable aspect of the very reality that is under discussion.

But such inseparability of thinking from the whole of reality is, of course, common, in every phase of life, including research in the physical sciences. To see this, one has only to consider the *significance* of our thought. The key root here is *sign*. That is, our thought is like a sign, in that it *is* something real (e.g. a physical and chemical process in the nervous system) which points to broader aspects of reality. Such 'pointing' is not only at static objects. Rather, it extends on to indicate actions and movements. For example, a red traffic signal indicates the action of stopping, while 'Look!' may indicate the action of giving attention to what is further pointed out by the speaker.

Going along similar lines, we note that any human activity, including scientific research, involves knowledge of *skills*. That is to say, what has been learned contains an important non-verbal, non-conceptual aspect, which enables us to orient and direct our actual contact with reality in a concrete way. In addition, there is a more subtle sort of skill, which includes the ability coherently to relate verbal and conceptual thought to concrete action. Then there is a yet more subtle sort of skill, which enables a person to organize his thoughts and his usage of language relevantly and coherently. Though this skill involves the *handling* of words, it is in itself as non-verbal as is, for example, the skill involved in any physical activity.

It would not be consistent to separate skill in organizing, developing, and using knowledge from the content of knowledge. These are, after all, merely two aspects of one movement, each of which could not exist without the other. So in considering Paul Clark's discussion of ontology versus epistemology, I would like to propose a broader point of view; i.e. *that knowledge is itself a subtle order of being.* As such, knowledge, includes a *functional* aspect (largely non-verbal) and a *reflective* aspect (which can, in the main, be put in correspondence with a verbal expression). In the simplest case, this reflective aspect is just an *image.* But when it reflects necessary and contingent features of movement and function, it is then a model. In abstract scientific thought, there is a very extensive development of this reflective aspect (described very well by Paul Clark) which mediates between perception and ultimate action to which this perception may give rise.

In a certain sense, any verbal (or mathematical) structure can function as a model (though perhaps only in a rudimentary way). Thus, to the extent that different words (or symbols) correspond to different things, they are providing a model of the *differences* (and similarities) in the context under discussion. When the model is intended to have a sensory content (e.g. visual, tactile, or auditory) then, as Paul Clark has indicated, all the power of our sensorimotor skills can be brought to bear on organizing the model, and seeing its full significance. (This is roughly what is meant, in fact, by saying that the model is 'intuitive'.) On the other hand, just because our ability to relate our concepts to our sensorimotor skills is limited, a model can act as a dangerous and undesirable limitation in our thought.

What is called for here is thus neither the total rejection of models nor uncritical dependence on them. One has to be alert and aware, so that one can see on each occasion whether a model is called for, and whether certain models are getting in the way of freedom of thought. One also has to develop new models, by being attentive to new aspects of sensorimotor experience, which have thus far not yet been put into concepts and words. In this way, one can perhaps avoid dogmatic restrictions in thought, such as are in the commonly held view that continuous fields and discrete particles exhaust *all* the possibilities for intuitive models in physics.

Finally, I would like to emphasize once again that I regard the division between ontology and epistemology as one of limited relevance. More deeply, one has, I think, to regard *knowing* as an aspect of *being*. Perhaps I shall have more to say on this in later papers.

Analogy versus Analysis: biochemistry as a mode of biological explanation[1]

FREDERIC R. JEVONS

In this paper are set out two different views of how chemistry can be applied to biology. These views depend on different general principles which may be called *analogy* and *analysis* (these names having at least the virtue of intense alliteration). By analogy is here meant the comparison of living systems to models made from non-biological constituents. Analysis is taken in its most literal sense, to mean dividing things into spatially smaller pieces.

The choice offered by these two alternatives is whether to make models to imitate living organisms, or to start with real living organisms and take them to pieces. To put it crudely, should the biochemist fill his test tubes with reagents from his shelf in attempts to simulate the phenomena of life, or with the mashed-up debris of living things? The issue is a big one, and its implications extend to experimental biology in general.

MODELS OF LIVING SYSTEMS

Model-making is recognized as an important general procedure in science. Of course, the models need not always be physically constructed with sticks, string, sealing-wax, and the like; they may be theoretical models – idealizations of a situation for purposes of calculation, for instance. The particular kind of model that first springs to mind in connection with biochemistry is the non-living model used as an analogue to a living system, and the discussion here is restricted to this particular type of model and this particular type of analogy.

Since the rise of human societies, men have used analogies to try to bridge the gulf between living and non-living; but they have not always drawn the analogies in the direction which nowadays seems obvious to most people – arguing from non-living to living, that is. The principle behind the use of analogies as explanations is the old one that, to advance knowledge, one must proceed from the known to the unknown. To give satisfaction as an explanation, a model must seem easier to understand than the situation it sets out to clarify. In antiquity and in the Middle Ages, life seemed no more mysterious than inorganic nature – if anything less so, being closer to the thinker's immediate experience. Accordingly, it seemed at least as appropriate to explain the non-living in terms of the living as the other way round. The fall of heavy bodies was explained as due to their tendency to return to their 'natural' position below, as though they were homesick animals; and metals were thought of as 'growing' under the earth.

To the twentieth century, such explanations seem crude and essentially anthropomorphic. Are analogies in the reverse direction more acceptable?

It was in the seventeenth century that conditions became such as to make it obvious to argue from non-living to living. The decisive change was the development of mechanics – notably the formulation of laws of dynamics, such as Galileo's mathematical treatment of the motion of falling bodies. Inanimate matter and its motion now seemed wonderfully comprehensible and the incentive to explain the phenomena of life in terms of them became correspondingly irresistible.

The most influential attempt to do so was made by Descartes. His book *On Man* (published in 1662 but written thirty years earlier) has been called the first book dedicated to physiology as such; but a very peculiar physiology it was that it contained. It described a theoretical model of a man, constructed on the principles used by contemporary machines – 'clocks, artificial fountains, mills and other machines which, though made by man, yet have the power of moving in various ways'. Muscles were supposed to work by being inflated with a fluid from the brain via the nerves, making them shorter and wider. Nerves were pictured as containing tiny threads running from sense-organs to brain. On being moved by external stimuli, the threads were supposed to operate appropriate valves so that the nervous fluid was directed into the right muscles for suitable movements to occur. By means of a sufficiently elaborate series of interconnections in the brain, the machine could be 'programmed' for an elaborate series of reflex actions.

Descartes proposed that a mechanism of this type could account for all the movements of animals. (He did allow a proviso in the case of man, but not of animals, for the power of mind to direct those movements – a minority – under direct voluntary control.) The animal machines were compared to the water-actuated statues in the grottoes of the royal gardens, which could be set into various kinds of motion by appropriate arrangements of the tubes leading water to them. 'External objects acting on the sense-organs, and thereby leading to diverse movements, according to the disposition of the parts in the brain, are like strangers entering one of these grottoes and thereby setting the statues into unthinking motion. For they cannot enter without treading on certain flag-stones so disposed that if, for instant, they approach a bathing Diana, they make her hide behind reeds; if they try to follow her, they are approached by a Neptune who menaces them with his trident; if they go some other direction, they bring out a marine monster which spews water in their faces; or similar things, according to the whim of the engineers who constructed the statues.'

Descartes was not the first to think along these lines, but it was he who gave momentum to the craze of 'mechanism' in biology – explaining the phenomena of life by effects observed in non-living systems. To him, as to later generations, this approach held the great attraction of a unified picture embracing both living and non-living nature. Unfortunately, Cartesian mechanist theory rode with rough-shod unconcern over the details of biological fact. Inevitably, it brought on itself the reaction of eighteenth-century 'vitalism', in the form of protests that living organisms must be looked at as they really are, not as they conceivably might be. Nineteenth-century materialism, however, again found itself strongly attracted by the Cartesian approach to physiology. 'Can ye make a model of it?' Lord Kelvin, the physicist, is supposed to have said, epitomizing a view common among Victorian scientists. 'For if ye can, ye understand it, and if ye canna, ye dinna!'

Many different kinds of model have suggested themselves, and fashion in this respect has changed with the times. Where the seventeenth century thought in terms of simple mechanical devices, the nineteenth preferred heat engines. Nowadays, computers are in favour. These are essentially physical models; more closely relevant to the topic of this paper are chemical ones, which take the form of *in vitro* reactions with overall results similar to *in vivo* ones, and hence in some measure imitating them.

THE LIMITATIONS OF ANALOGY

Models are genuinely useful in so far as they represent theories about certain aspects of the functioning of living things, testable on material from living things. But it is not possible to get information about living organisms merely by studying artificial models. Simple and obvious though this fact may seem when so baldly stated, it can be obscured by the overenthusiasm and paternal pride of the model-makers. If this happens, misdirection of effort may result.

The trouble with the Cartesian or any similar approach to physiology is not that the details of the models may not be right; even if they are wrong they may, like any theory, suggest useful experiments. The real fault lies in the basic assumption of the intellectual procedure: that a biological process is in some way 'explained' when a model to imitate it has been thought of or constructed. Genuine explanation, with an increase in knowledge and understanding of life, is not achieved until the imitation has been critically compared with the biological reality. Quite recently, in mid-twentieth century, there has been talk of 'synthesis under physiological conditions', meaning the artificial synthesis of natural products under conditions of temperature and pH not beyond the physiological range. But physiological conditions are not, after all, defined only by temperature and pH. Syntheses in living organisms may (and usually do) proceed via intermediates quite different from those used in such artificial syntheses. Studies of this type show what *could* happen in living organisms, not what *does* happen.

Apart from their value in teaching as expository devices, analogies to models have furthered science most, perhaps, by stimulating the study of the models themselves and of the non-biological materials used in their construction. The great structure of modern organic chemistry is itself a most striking monument to such a stimulus at work. The name 'organic chemistry' is a verbal fossil which recalls the history of the subject. Originally, it meant the chemistry of organized, living beings. Not until mid-nineteenth century did it come explicitly to refer to carbon compounds rather than to natural products. (Biochemistry is thus the ancestor of organic chemistry, rather than the other way round as is sometimes supposed.) Although the study of artificial carbon compounds soon acquired justifications of its own, in terms both of theoretical interest and of practical utility, it gained impetus originally from the desire to copy in the test tube the compounds and reactions of life.

ANALOGIES APPLIED TO BIOLOGICAL OXIDATIONS

Both the strength and the limitations of the approach to biochemistry via analogies are well illustrated in the study of biological oxidations.

Of all the analogies that have ever been drawn between non-living and living, Lavoisier's comparison of burning and breathing was perhaps the most strikingly successful. 'Respiration is a combustion', he wrote in 1783, 'slow it is true but otherwise perfectly similar to that of charcoal.' The similar dependence on air of the two processes had been shown a century before. Lavoisier, however, went much further by comparing them quantitatively, not only with respect to the carbon dioxide produced but also (in collaboration with the physicist Laplace) with respect to the heat evolved. What gives this work its importance is not the analogy itself, the idea of the similarity, but the critical comparison of the two processes, both subjected to direct experiment. But for this, Lavoisier could not be regarded as having laid the foundations for the study of metabolism, in terms both of material change and of energy transformation.

The obvious weakness of the comparison was the great disparity in the temperatures at which the two processes take place. Apart from invoking the general notion of catalysis, scientists long remained at a loss how to account for this. In the later part of the nineteenth century, chemists became intrigued by the oxidizing powers of peroxides at ordinary temperatures, and studied them in model systems. This work added a good deal to our knowledge of peroxides, but not much to our knowledge of the major oxidation mechanisms of living cells.

A different kind of model turned out eventually to be more profitable. This kind was based on the catalytic effect of heavy metals on oxidations by molecular oxygen. Finely divided platinum and palladium act in this way, 'activating' hydrogen atoms in organic substances to make them combine with oxygen. This effect was, during the second decade of this century, made the basis of a theory of biological oxidation which was widely accepted as the best available.

During the early nineteen-twenties, Warburg in Germany found better model systems. The catalysts here were certain charcoals, such as that obtained by charring blood. These contain a good many substances besides carbon; Warburg tracked their catalytic activity down to iron combined with something nitrogenous. They were better models in that they corresponded more closely to the biological systems in their behaviour and properties – notably in their rather similar susceptibilities to poisons such as cyanide in low concentrations. 'Who could believe that this was only by chance in agreement with the behaviour of cell respiration?' enthused Warburg. His conclusion was that iron-containing catalysts operate during oxidation by cells. Fortunately, his intuition carried him where logic could not (possibilities other than iron were not ruled out); his guess was later confirmed by the discovery of cytochromes.

Analogies to model systems, then, have played some part in bringing us our present knowledge of biological oxidations. Progressive refinements of the models, making them more and more faithful to the originals by more and more detailed checking and critical comparison, eventually led to a valuable hint about the participation of iron. It is worth remembering, however, that cytochromes were not actually discovered except by direct approach to living organisms. Their discovery was due to spectroscopic observations on a variety of cells, followed by work on their isolation.

BIOCHEMISTRY AS THE LOGICAL EXTRAPOLATION OF
DISSECTION

An alternative and attractive way of viewing biochemistry is as the ultimate extension of biological analysis in terms of constituent parts. In this aspect, it appears as a sort of submicroscopic anatomy. The classical anatomists cut up bodies to describe the parts of which they are made in so far as they are visible to the naked eye. Microscopy revealed a whole new world of structure and organization smaller than this and, when the technique had developed sufficiently, cells became the focus of interest. With the advance of chemistry, it gradually became possible to tackle biological architecture even on the molecular scale. The grand strategy remains the same: a better understanding of living things in terms of their constituent parts. The tactics, however – the choice of techniques to apply – depend on the order of size of the parts being examined. For gross anatomy, the scalpel is appropriate, for cellular structure the microscope; for parts as small as molecules, the relevant techniques are those we call chemical – hence 'biochemistry' or 'molecular biology'. Seen in this light, biochemistry is the logical extrapolation of dissection.

Merely to determine structure, however, is far from the summit of the ambitions of biochemists. They are interested not only in what the constituents of living things are like, but also in what they do – in the way that chemical processes underlie the more obvious vital manifestations. The continuous change which is one of the most striking characteristics of life rests on unceasing chemical activity inside living organisms. Biochemistry thus continues another classical tradition of biology in linking form with function. Life, after all, is a matter of keeping events going, not only of maintaining structures; and biochemists seek to elucidate events as well as structures by isolation.

By and large, then, while the techniques of biochemistry are chemical, its problems are the basic ones of biology. Chemistry is its means, biology its end. It is the extreme extension of that approach to the phenomena of life which seeks to explain them in terms of the subunits of which living organisms are composed.

THE OBJECTIONS TO ANALYSIS

All this sounds like an admirable programme for biochemistry. Explanation in terms of smaller parts is a kind of explanation which the human mind finds particularly satisfying, and it has proved time and time again to be particularly fruitful in practice. Unfortunately, however, this approach is not without its snags. A time-honoured criticism by biologists of chemical operations, since the seventeenth century at least, has been that they are destructive. The implication of the word 'organism' must not be forgotten; a living organism is organized, and its organization is a very important and characteristic thing about it. A method that has to destroy the organization before it can set to work cannot, therefore, claim to give a good explanation of life. To put it crudely, one cannot find out much about a rat by mashing it up, because there is then no rat left to find out about. The spatial and functional relationships between the parts are as important as the properties of the parts themselves.

The point is not merely that, by destroying the relationships, the chance is lost of finding out what they were. There is the possibility that the behaviour of the parts themselves may now differ significantly from their natural behaviour. In the organism, the parts interact and influence each other in specific and delicate ways, and what they do depends on how they fit into the living machinery. Isolated, they may be made to do something different. Even supposing the parts not to have been substantially altered during isolation, the functional properties they can be made to display in the laboratory can be expected to include, besides those of physiological importance, others that are not called into play during life. How is one to tell which of the potentialities revealed by test-tube events correspond to actual biological events? It may even be possible to assemble a number of test-tube events into a series which fits together in an apparently convincing way but nevertheless bears little resemblance to any metabolic pathway operating inside cells. If one took a sledge-hammer to a washing-machine, it is conceivable that from the pieces one might construct a working toy train – but that should not be taken as evidence that a toy train was going round and round inside the intact washing-machine.

Circumspection is called for, then, before an effect observed *in vitro* is interpreted in terms of an *in vivo* process. To take one type of case that is very familiar in biochemistry: the fact that an enzyme catalyses a certain reaction in the test tube does not mean that the same reaction goes on in the living organism from which the enzyme came. Even if the enzyme has not been functionally altered during isolation, it may act on some other substrate *in vivo*. Catalysis by enzymes may be remarkably specific by comparison with other kinds of catalysis, but it is not absolutely specific; a given enzyme is usually capable of acting on a range of substrates united by some chemical resemblance – sometimes a narrow range defined by a close resemblance, sometimes a broader range. Any particular substrate tested *in vitro* may be an unnatural one which the enzyme does not encounter except through the machinations of biochemists. An enzyme, it might be said, engages in incidental hobbies when given the chance, as well as the significant work it does during normal life. To build up a picture of the functioning of intact organisms, the hobbies must be distinguished from the work.

Sometimes this is easy, when the substrate is an obviously artificial one, such as the synthetic dyes which some oxido-reduction enzymes can reduce. In other cases the answer is far from obvious. Given a number of substrates, among which it is not clear which is natural and which is not, the efficiencies with which the enzyme acts on them form no basis on which to judge; the enzyme may be more adept at its hobby than at its work – plenty of such cases are known. Even if a substrate can be shown to be present in the same tissue or cell as the enzyme, this is no guarantee that it will normally be acted on. An inhibitor may prevent the enzyme from working, or physical access of enzyme and substrate to each other may be impeded by the membranes of subcellular structure like mitochondria – for a cell is not just a bag in which enzymes and substrates mix indiscriminately. Nor can it be assumed that a series of enzyme-catalysed reactions is physiological because they fit together neatly into some plausible functional pattern or metabolic pathway; that would be like taking the satisfactory working of the toy train as evidence that it pre-existed in the washing-machine.

What grounds are there, then, for confidence that a picture of the metabolic machinery can ever be built on convincing foundations? Perhaps one can point to two main ways of tackling the general problem. One is investigation of events at levels of organization intermediate between intact organisms and molecules in free solution; the other relies on the use of isotopes.

MEETING THE OBJECTIONS

1. *Intermediate Levels to Bridge the Gap*

The disparity in degree of organization between intact organisms and purified substances is great; much has to be destroyed in passing from one to the other. But the gulf between them no longer yawns as impassably as it used to, because studies can now be made at a whole series of intermediate levels of organization.

The organization of living beings falls into a series of levels arranged in the form of a hierarchy, as in organizations such as the civil service or the army, each level embracing the members of lower levels in characteristic 'organizing relations'. For the present purpose, five main steps in the hierarchy may be distinguished. After the whole organism come organs such as liver and kidney; then come tissues and cells, then subcellular particles, and finally molecules free in solution.

Biochemical processes can be investigated with preparations representing any of these steps. To do biochemical work, it is not necessary always to destroy all levels of organization above the molecular. Quite on the contrary, it is necessary sometimes to proceed less violently – just as, to find out about the inner work-ings of a washing-machine, it would be necessary to lay aside the sledge-hammer and dismantle the machinery gently stage by stage.

In the case of intact organisms, biochemical study might take the form of feeding experiments – analysing the diet, or adding special substances to it, and finding out what is excreted. At the organ level, the corresponding experiments can be done by perfusing an excised organ with blood or with an isotonic salt solution; test substances can be added to this solution, and the emerging liquid analysed to see what transformations have taken place. Tissue activity can be studied by suspending thin slices in an appropriate salt solution; the cells in such slices metabolize for some time in a manner approaching the normal. Micro-organisms offer the advantage, as experimental material, that they can be grown as homogeneous cell populations, with no level of organization above the cellular. For studies at the subcellular level, cells can be broken and the subcellular particles can be separated by differential centrifuging, taking precautions to keep them reasonably intact functionally. Finally, the individual units of catalytic machinery, enzymes and their cofactors, can be obtained in free solution.

The levels of the hierarchy form a continuous series with an impressive degree of coherence. There are no abrupt breaks – no gaps of more than about one order of magnitude. Very roughly, 10^{-7} cm (10 Å) can be taken as representative of the molecular order of magnitude; the dimensions of subcellular particles are in the region 10^{-6} to 10^{-4} cm; cells at around 10^{-3} cm (10 μ) and larger are not much smaller than macroscopically visible structures on the millimetre scale.

The continuity of the hierarchy offers hope that by systematic, stage-by-stage comparisons the gap between molecules and large animals can be bridged, data at the molecular and whole-organism levels being brought into valid correlation. The task of bridging across intermediate levels is perhaps the major challenge facing contemporary biochemistry. It forms a sort of leitmotiv running through much current research. Thus it shows itself as the effort to relate vitamin activity for whole animals to cofactor activity for enzymes. In the case of chemotherapy, it takes the rather similar form of relating the clinical activity of drugs to their chemical properties. For muscle, there have been ingenious attempts to picture the molecular events that underlie visible contraction. Last, but far from least, there is the large problem of how the molecular structure of nucleic acids can determine macroscopic hereditary characters.

2. *Isotopic Espionage*

The other main way to study metabolic machinery is to resort to a sort of biochemical espionage, sending spies into the cells to report on what cannot be seen from outside. The biochemical spies are isotopic tracers. It was a crucial development in biochemistry when isotopic methods were introduced around the time of the Second World War, for they provided the first reasonably general way of following chemical changes without disrupting organization.

The concept of isotopes is now widely familiar. Chemically the same because of their identical electronic make-ups, two isotopes of an element differ in that their atoms have nuclei of different mass. The main natural isotope of carbon, for instance, is ^{12}C, meaning that its nucleus has a mass twelve times that of a hydrogen atom. The nucleus of ^{14}C has a mass fourteen times that of a hydrogen atom, but at the same time it has the same complement of six electrons as ^{12}C, so that it forms the same series of chemical compounds.

Isotopes can be distinguished by physical properties. In the case of ^{14}C, detection and estimation are easy because this isotope is radioactive – the nucleus decomposes, giving off β-particles which can be measured in terms of counts per minute in a radioactivity counter. The same applies to ^{32}P, a radioactive isotope which, because of the importance of phosphate compounds, is very useful in biochemical research. (Normal phosphorus is ^{31}P.) In the case of stable, non-radioactive isotopes, estimation depends on the difference of mass. The most important stable isotopes used in biochemistry are ^{2}H, heavy hydrogen or deuterium, with twice the mass of ordinary hydrogen; and ^{15}N, heavier by one unit than the most abundant natural isotope, ^{14}N.

Being chemically the same but physically distinguishable, isotopes can be used as tracers to trace metabolic pathways. The abnormal isotope can be administered in the form of an isotopically labelled compound, which may be a normal metabolite except in the isotopic respect. Later, by finding out in what substances the isotope is now present, the metabolic transformations undergone by the original compound can be detected. The isotope label thus traces the paths from precursors to products. The important point is that intact metabolic machinery can be used to bring about the transformations under study. It may be necessary to disrupt the system at the end of the experiment to find where the isotope has got to, but the processes by which it got there went on under physiological conditions.

Isotopes can thus discharge their function of biochemical espionage in a rather subtle way. Introduced into organisms under the cloak of their normal electronic shells, the abnormal nuclei mingle unobtrusively with the chemical population and spy out chemical activities without disturbing them by disrupting the natural organization of the machinery that brings them about. Masquerading as normal metabolites, the isotopically labelled molecules get into normal metabolic pathways and set the abnormal atoms as markers along it.

The isotopic tracer method is applicable to most fields of intermediary metabolism. Most of the important metabolic pathways involving carbon, nitrogen, or phosphorus atoms have by now been mapped, at least in outline, by the use of suitable isotopes.

A DATED CONTROVERSY – 'MECHANISM' VERSUS 'VITALISM'
THE ORGANIZATION HIERARCHY

The old question of 'mechanism' versus 'vitalism' is still dutifully trotted out in the first or last chapters of a large number of books on various aspects of biology – an amazingly large number, for in the context of modern thought it requires a degree of historical imagination to understand the importance this issue assumed. Why it aroused a good deal of passion is easy enough to see, for mutual misunderstanding has always been good at that; but it is harder to appreciate how it came for so long to be regarded as the central issue of biological theory.

Can biology be explained in terms of physics and chemistry, or must some other, 'higher', agency be postulated to account for the phenomena of life? This, or something similar, is a form in which the question was often put up for debate. As it happens, definitions of the subject-matter of physics and chemistry do not normally contain any explicit limitation to non-living material and forces. Pedantically, therefore, the question can be denied meaning anyway. On a common-sense level, however, its implication is clear enough. Are living and non-living things governed by the same basic laws or not? Are they fundamentally similar or fundamentally different?

The obvious answer is that they are similar in some ways and different in others. Whether the similarities or the differences are to be rated more significant is an issue of something less than crucial importance. It hardly seems meaty enough to account for all the fuss that went on during sizeable portions of the nineteenth and twentieth centuries (though it might have made an acceptable main course for a disputation among medieval scholastics).

The whole debate becomes largely superfluous if the problem is viewed in terms of living things as organisms – complex entities made up of parts organized in a hierarchical series of levels of organization. Parts organized into a whole organism do not behave in the same way as parts separate or disorganized; and different modes of organization can lead to different behaviour. Now living things are organized in characteristic ways, as is obvious even to the most superficial observer. Inevitably, therefore, they behave in characteristic ways. Their parts may be just the same as the parts of other things (and it has long been agreed that they are); but the laws governing the parts do not give the laws governing the organized whole. Qualitatively new kinds of phenomena can emerge at higher levels of organization. A motor-car can apparently violate the physical law of gravity by climbing uphill. None of its parts can, nor can all its parts together unless properly organized – the organized whole behaves differently from its parts isolated or disorganized.

For this reason, it is absurd to suppose that all the laws of life can be fished out of solutions – liquids containing no level of organization above the molecular. Work on component parts is essential in studying organized wholes – otherwise, understanding can be no more than superficial in the most literal sense of the word; but it is not enough to study only the parts themselves, to the exclusion of the organizing relations between them. To find out about these specific spatial and functional relations, which turn a collection of components into an organism, the parts, the whole, and intermediate levels of organization must all be investigated. It is the hierarchy which reconciles the claims of the analytical approach with the rejoinder that intact organisms are the biological reality to be explained. The organization hierarchy, forming as it does a bridge between parts and whole, is thus one of the really vital, central concepts of biology.

Mechanism and vitalism each took many forms – they were highly personal faiths which appeared in almost as many different manifestations as there were people who thought about them. This is not the place to attempt a complete exposé of all the heads of these many-headed monsters. There are three points, however, which deserve mention because of their relevance to topics already treated in this paper. The first concerns the adequacy of models as a means of explanation, the second the continuity of the organization hierarchy, and the third the importance of not neglecting levels of organization above the molecular.

The weaknesses of biological explanation by means of non-biological models have been pointed out above, but in the context of the mechanism–vitalism controversy there was a limited sense in which a biological effect could be said to be 'explained' by imitating it with a non-living model. Vitalists were at their most unfortunate, perhaps, in those excursions in which they postulated vital principles under various names whose intervention was assumed because inanimate forces did not seem adequate to explain some biological phenomena. While this was the point at issue, it was quite relevant to attempt to simulate the phenomena with non-living systems; to show how a process *could* happen in living organisms was enough to refute this 'argument from inadequacy'. When mechanists managed to do this, however, they were not always careful enough to avoid the pitfalls of success. The dangers of thinking in terms of models are, first, that the models tend to become invested with an aura of biological reality to which they have no claim; second, that energies tend to be diverted into the study of models instead of the direct study of living organisms and their parts. Vitalists were in a much stronger position when they issued valuable reminders that the proper study of biology is life – how it *does* work, not how it *could*.

The threat of divorce between chemistry and biology would never have become as serious as it did had the continuity of the organization hierarchy always stood out as clearly as it does today. By the beginning of the present century, biological analysis proceeded down to the level of cells; these were regarded as the units of life (and the cellular level of organization is, of course, a particularly important one for biology). Chemistry dealt with atoms and small molecules. Between the entities with which the two sciences typically concerned themselves lay an apparently ominous gap of several orders of magnitude, which could be bridged only in a very unsatisfactory way by vague talk of the 'colloidal state of protoplasm'. More recently, however, a pincer movement has converged from above and below on this gap. From above have come increases in microscopic resolution, for instance, notably by electron microscopy; from below, chemical methods have taken larger and larger molecules more effectively into their grasp. It is no accident that biochemical interest is now focused specially on that critical region of the hierarchy where macro-molecules merge into subcellular particles.

Model systems of chemical interest normally take the form of reactions proceeding in free solution or the gas phase – in general, in systems with no level of organization above the molecular. Because of this, mechanism in its chemical aspect was often criticized for ignoring the higher levels – for seeing in living things only a mass of substances and no architecture. Insistence on the importance of this architecture was another valuable reminder that came from vitalists. Though it led some of them into an obstruc-tionist resistance to analysis, others made timely contributions by keeping the higher levels of organization in the public eye.

In many vitalist attacks on the application of chemical methods to living things, however, a fundamental flaw was to deny the chemical approach any stake in levels above the molecular. It was taken to apply to 'disorganized' systems only. If this were so, it would not apply to manmade machines any more than to intact living organisms. The absurd position would be reached of deny-ing the applicability of chemistry to motor-cars because they differ from any of the substances composing them in being able to climb uphill. ('Mechanism' in its physical sense clearly implied organization; it is paradoxical that in the chemical context it should have been taken to deny organization.)

There is no point in arbitrarily splitting the organization hier-archy into precisely delimited spheres of influence belonging to various sciences. The hierarchy is an extensive one – it can use-fully be considered to go as far down as atoms and subatomic particles and as far up as societies of living individuals. It thus extends further than the range with which any single branch of science normally wants to concern itself. But to attempt, on grounds such as this, to restrict particular sciences to particular ranges of the hierarchy is misguided. Although a science of itself finds its own characteristic range, there is no need to imprison it there. Chemistry, for instance, characteristically operates at the levels of atoms and molecules; but there is considerable profit, and no logical inconsistency, in allowing it to penetrate below the atomic level to arm itself with electronic theories of valency and reaction mechanisms, and above the molecular level to learn from experience in chemical factories or living organisms.

Biochemistry does not ignore organization, as it has been accused of doing – it merely selects a certain range of levels as its normal and proper subject-matter. In general, it chooses to take the atomic and subatomic levels as given. The molecular level is its own special and characteristic concern. This does not mean, however, that it must neglect higher levels; quite on the contrary, it must take account of all levels up to that of whole organisms. The study of life in molecular terms embraces the relations between molecules just as much as the properties of the molecules in themselves.

NOTE

1 This paper is based on chapter 5 of F. R. Jevons, *The Biochemical Approach to Life*, London, Allen and Unwin, 2nd edition, 1968. In that book, the ideas discussed here are illustrated by examples from recent biochemistry.

© *Frederic R. Jevons 1972*

Comment

A. J. CAIN

I agree completely with Professor Jevons's thesis and illustrations. There are two main activities in science, explaining and explaining away; the verb 'to explain', without qualification, is usually used for both. Explaining, in science, means demonstrating a particular relationship between a phenomenon and the existing body of knowledge (both fact and theory). Merely suggesting it as highly probable is not demonstrating it, and is explaining away (unless steps are taken to verify it). We all have to do it much of the time, since life is short and no man can be a primary authority on everything; we therefore take a great deal on trust. The more intelligent and sensible a man, the more likely will be his explainings away.

Where analysis is possible (and Professor Jevons has happily illustrated its difficulties) the result should be a demonstration – that the release of energy in a cell, for example, *is* mediated by certain reactions of certain compounds, and not by others. He is concerned with biochemical analysis; but the analysis of the reactions of a whole population should proceed in the same sort of way, with mark–release–recapture methods corresponding to the use of isotopes.

Where, however, analysis is hardly applicable, only simulation by models can be used. The direct investigation in the wild of natural selection, mutation, migration, and chance effects in small populations, is beginning to be sufficiently advanced (and is so well supported by laboratory work) to give us reasonable confidence that we understand in principle how gene-frequencies come to alter in a population, and therefore that we understand the

68

basis of evolution. Any theory of long-term evolution in a particular group (the ammonites, or dinosaurs, for example) must be consonant with our knowledge of population genetics. But all we have is the fossils, something of their probable ecology (from the beds they are found in), and their relative, and perhaps absolute, chronology. Even when we investigate a group richly represented at the present day but poor in fossils (birds, for example) we are little better off. We have to look at what has actually occurred in the evolution of such a group, as far as it can be inferred with any probability from the available material, living or fossil, consult our knowledge of population genetics, and work the two up into the most coherent story possible. If others, working independently on very different groups, come to much the same conclusions about long-term processes in evolution, we feel all the more confident. In the rare examples of groups with a really good fossil history (horses, crocodiles, some groups of South American mammals, for example) the course of evolution can be determined with reasonable certainty, but there can still be – and often has been in the past – uncertainty about the mechanism and its relation to findings on living forms.

In all such cases, one can only set up models on various assumptions and see how far they agree with the facts. The only test is whether what works (i.e. gives a coherent account) with one sort of organism is found to apply to other and very different ones, making allowance for the differences if our knowledge of population genetics suggests that they should affect the processes that actually took place. The evolutionary biologist is therefore very much in the position of the historian or archaeologist, and R. G. Collingwood's delightful exposé of what he called the inductive method in 'Who killed John Doe?' and subsequent sections of his essay on historical evidence,[1] is applicable to all of them.

This sort of activity certainly has its dangers. There is a classic example in Darwin's own work.[2] That great anatomist Richard Owen, rightly regarded by Darwin as an authority, introduced that well-known object the pentadactyl limb into theoretical biology in a lecture he gave to the Royal Institution and published in 1849. He pointed out that the wing of the bat, the trowel of the mole, the fin of the dugong, the running leg of the horse, and the delicately manipulative hand of man were all based on the same anatomical plan, although the functions were so different. He further pointed out that there was no necessity for five digits inside the flipper of a dugong, nor for the complex apparatus of scapula, humerus, radius, ulna etc., which was unnecessary for the running of the horse, although the single hoof was obviously adaptive, as was the fusion of the radius and ulna, so that the hoof should not suddenly slip and overturn. The general shape of these very varied forelimbs was clearly adaptive, usually to different modes of locomotion, but the basic plan was not; and as no engineer would restrict himself by taking a single plan and modifying it in one direction into a locomotive engine, in another into a balloon or tunnelling machinery, it was clear that the basic plan showed the superhuman ingenuity of the Creator. In short, what was adaptive to special needs was adaptive through the benevolence of the Creator; what was not was there for the edification of man.

Darwin took over the whole of this, quite explicitly, in the *Origin of Species*, but changed the interpretation. What he also could see was adaptive he explained as adaptive through the action of natural selection. What he, like Owen, could not see was adaptive, he explained away as ancestral. And this was explaining away, because he made no effort to find out whether the features of the plan common to various forms were adaptive or not – admittedly not too easy to do for some of them, but hardly difficult for the horse in the London of 1859.

It is now more apparent than it was in Darwin's day that there is no clear antithesis between ancestral and adaptive. What has been retained for hundreds of thousands of generations in millions of individuals against all the disturbing factors of mutation and recombination, is much more likely to be selected for than not, even if we cannot see what advantage it is on a very superficial examination. The same style of explaining away still goes on, however, both in evolutionary studies generally where 'historical' factors are invoked, and in population genetics. At one time every genetic character that could be demonstrated to be, or seemed likely to be, acted on by selection was believed to be so. Any that had no obvious selective advantage was explained away as merely a sideproduct (a pleiotropic effect) of the gene concerned, which was really selected for some other character mediated by it. If the character had a somewhat odd distribution in wild populations, not clearly correlated with the most obvious features of the environment, it was usually regarded as non-adaptive, and its distribution was put down to chance (genetic drift), an explaining-away very popular in the USA and disposing of the necessity to do any further investigation. More popular nowadays are coadapted genotypes – the character is bound up with the rest of the genetic constitution and therefore varies with it. In nearly all cases (not quite all) these are explainings-away, of different degrees of probability. Where they have actually led to further research, they are, of course, perfectly respectable.

REFERENCES

1 COLLINGWOOD, R. G. 1946. *The Idea of History*, Oxford: Clarendon Press. Oxford Paperbacks, 1961.
2 CAIN, A. J. 1964. 'The perfection of animals', *Viewpoints in Biology*, **3**, 36–63.

Model-building in
Probability and Statistics

JOSEPH GANI

Man's ability to develop conceptual models of reality has proved of immense value in establishing his mastery over the environment. Starting in early childhood, every individual appears to construct for himself an internalized model of the world, however fragmentary; foresight, and the capacity to plan and predict, are based upon his manipulation of the components of this model. Usually, the thought processes involved occur without conscious effort or difficulty, but when a serious discrepancy arises between the model and hard facts, the individual is forced to recognize the falseness of his conceptual construct. This acceptance, and the subsequent modifications of the model, often give rise to severe emotional disturbances.

Such model-building activities, though beginning in early childhood, continue throughout each individual's life. The Swiss psychologist Jean Piaget has been concerned in his researches with the growth of internalized models among children;[1, 2] at a more practical level, John Holt has given an intuitive account of the learning process in children.[3] It may therefore be useful, before discussing mathematical-type models, to describe briefly some of Piaget's work on children's understanding of the real world.

CONCEPTUAL MODELS

Piaget argues that a child is at work creating a model of his surroundings from his very birth. The persistence and continuity of objects (even when they are moving), and the recurrence of certain events in his life, are noted fairly early. A rudimentary internal model of his environment is constructed, which the child enriches from experience throughout his life.

An elementary understanding of spatial relations is arrived at within the child's first eighteen months of life. He will learn by trial and error the positions of particular objects, and their inter-relation. He will also grasp the basis of a sequence of events in time, as well as their recurrence; he may, for example, expect to be burped after feeding-time. After a while, he will recognize certain objects and persons, and expect them to persist despite movement and alterations in particular details. The recurrence of certain patterns in time may lead him to the concept of cause and effect. By the age of eighteen months, the child has achieved a certain purposive behaviour which indicates the development of a structured internalized model of the world around him.

Between eighteen months and five years, experimentation, play, and sheer curiosity increase the child's understanding of relation-ships in both space and time. This is the stage at which the child develops patterns of intuitive thought, though many of his con-cepts remain vague and illogical. It is characteristic of this period that length may be confused with movement, or time with speed, or apparent visual size with volume. From about the ages of five up to eight, the structural concepts of the child's model of the world begin to stabilize. This is the period when schemes of rational thinking become established, and chains of reasoning are developed which eventually lead to the logic of mathematics and the sciences. By the age of eight, children are capable of dealing with experimental situations in much the same way as adults do, though full capacity for abstract reasoning is not usually reached until the ages of eleven to fourteen.

While it is clearly not possible for a layman in the field to give a critical evaluation of Piaget's research, the experimental nature of his studies carries some conviction, and the main outline of his findings leads to a consistent theory of how children create a working model of the universe. An example of the methods which he uses to reach his conclusions may help to understand the chil-dren's approach to conceptual thinking. In the first experiment, children between the ages of five and a half and eight and a half are presented with lengths of wire AB and CD tacked to a board; a cardboard strip may be used for measuring lengths.

They are told that the beads α, β threaded onto the wires represent trams travelling along tramway routes AB and CD respectively. The experimenter moves β and asks the child to move α by an equal *distance*, this being very carefully explained. Three stages of understanding emerge in the children's response.

Figure 1

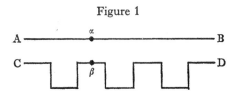

At the first conceptual stage, children between the ages of five and a half and six feel that if the beads are opposite each other, as in *Figure 1*, they have travelled the same distance. At the second stage, between the ages of six and seven, discussion with the experimenter enables the child to distinguish between the concept of distance travelled and the positions of points of arrival. However, suggestions that the cardboard strip be used for measuring are disregarded. At the final stage, between seven and eight and a half, the child actually measures, at first hesitantly but later with greater assurance, to establish whether distances travelled by α and β are the same.

This progression clearly shows that, in constructing his conceptual model, one of the child's most important steps is the realization of what is relevant in a problem. At the beginning, the child's conception of distance travelled appears to refer merely to progress along the direction from left to right. Only later does he grasp that distance travelled refers to the total length of path, and later still that the cardboard can be used to measure distances along such paths. This notion of relevance recurs in the more sophisticated mathematical models which we shall discuss later.

In another experiment, Piaget discusses the growth of the concept *conservation of volume* among young children.

Two vessels of identical size A and B contain the same quantity of coloured liquid. The contents of A are poured into C, a broad but shallow dish, while those of B are poured into a tall narrow jar D. In each case the child is asked whether the quantity of

Figure 2

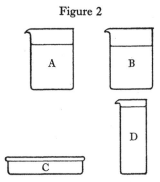

liquid in C or D is the same as that in A, and this is carefully explained.

Once again, in the first stage, children aged about five always take for granted that the quantity of liquid in A and C or D is different. There is no understanding of a volume which remains constant independently of the change of form. At the second stage, around the age of six, children hesitate between the impact of visual appearances and the dawning concept of conservation of volume. Some try to allow for the varying cross-sections of the vessels, but are not able to reach any clear conclusions. At the final stage, between the ages of seven and eight, children are able to give correct answers directly, often pointing out that the same quantity of liquid has only been poured from one vessel into another.

Piaget's books contain several similar experiments, on which his conclusions are founded; of particular interest are his accounts of children's ideas of number. The growth of children's understanding of numerical relations appears to run parallel to their grasp of logic. It is in the context of these internalized models of the world that I propose to consider mathematical model-building. Mathematical models can be regarded as a specialized extension of that psychological process which consists in creating internalized models of the world. It is the remarkable success of mathematical models in scientific explanation and prediction which reinforces the value we set upon them.

MATHEMATICAL MODELS

The advantage of introducing mathematics into a conceptual model is that the relations between analytic components of the model are now defined far more precisely. A highly developed calculus becomes available, which allows prompt and complex logical deductions to be made; in addition computational results can be rapidly derived from the basic assumptions. These results, both logical and computational, can be checked against reality; if they are verified to a reasonable degree of accuracy, the mathematical model is held to 'explain' reality. It would be fruitless to become involved in a philosophical discussion of precisely what we mean by such explanations; it is my personal belief that the main function of a model, whether conceptual or mathematical, is predictive. In this paper, I put forward the viewpoint that a model is simply a functional construct, which enables one to make accurate predictions. Perhaps the best way to illustrate this is to discuss in some detail examples of simulation, deterministic, probabilistic, and statistical models.

Simulation Models

We are all familiar with architectural and engineering models, scale models of ships, aeroplanes, and buildings. The function of these concrete models is to simulate in miniature the objects which they represent, so as to allow one to imagine more realistically the problems that may arise in their construction. Thus, in laying out a new town, it may be necessary to provide an architectural model of the design of streets and buildings. In studying the behaviour of ships in certain types of water waves, the response of models in artificial waves created in an experimental tank may be helpful. In considering the behaviour of aeroplanes in airflows, it is often extremely helpful to set up scale models in wind tunnels, in order to subject them to conditions of turbulence which the aircraft may later encounter.

I should like to illustrate the idea of simulation models in an area in which I have worked personally: the theory of water storage in dams.[4, 5]

One way in which such water storage can be studied for a particular river system, is to construct a miniature model of the river system itself, and run a water flow through it which simulates on a smaller scale the actual water flow in the river. One could then construct a scale model of a dam, and study from the actual (scale) water flow precisely what would happen in a similar situation in the real river system. This, however, may be an unnecessarily complicated way of simulating the river and dam systems. We may use numerical models to replace the scale structure. In this case, we would use numerical relations to represent the inflow of water, the constraints of the dam, and the subsequent outflow. In precisely the same way, stresses in ships and aeroplanes can be represented by numerical rather than scale models.

Suppose that in the case of a dam, we had inflow and release rules of the following type. Let the capacity of the dam be K gallons (1 million, say), so that if the river inflow caused the content of the dam to be greater than K, then any excess over K would overflow. The release rule could be M gallons (100,000 say) to be released at fixed regular intervals, possibly once each year in the summer. Then, if at any stage just after releasing M gallons, the content of the dam were 500,000 gallons, where this is smaller than K, and the input were 50,000 gallons, the total content of the dam before release would be 550,000 $< K$ gallons. After the release, the content of the dam would be 550,000 $-$ 100,000 $=$ 450,000 gallons, and the process would then be repeated indefinitely.

Some numerical calculations can be carried out fairly easily, provided the rules of input and release are known. An electronic computer can perform these computations very rapidly and give the required outputs in a very short time. In this way, the numerical simulation of the river and dam systems avoids the complexities of building a scale model. A further step in abstraction is achieved by considering deterministic models involving algebraic equations for the river and dam systems. The main contrast between simulation and deterministic models is that, in the former, only the operating rules of the system need to be known for numerical answers to be obtained. In the latter, it is necessary to formulate the structure of the process in some detail before a theoretical solution can be found; as a result, a deterministic model often provides more profound insights into the problem than the equivalent simulation model.

Deterministic Models

Mathematical models can be represented most conveniently by a set of deterministic equations. In such equations every relevant mathematical condition or constraint has a precise effect not subject to chance variation. Relevance is often determined by the degree of accuracy to which the model is required to work. Most of us will have encountered such models in school mathematics or mechanics.

Figure 3

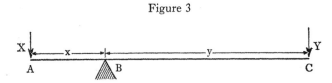

A simple illustration of a deterministic mathematical model is provided by the lever. Suppose ABC represents a lever of light-weight material with its fulcrum at B, such that two weights are balanced at its ends A and C. The length AB is equal to x feet, while the length BC is y feet; it is well established experimentally that if a weight X lb operates at the point A, then it can only be balanced by a unique weight of Y lb operating at C, so that the lever is then in equilibrium. The precise relation between Y and X, neglecting the weight of the lever itself, may be written in the form of the equation

$$Y.y = X.x;$$

if X, x, y are known, the balancing weight is then

$$Y = X.x/y.$$

This tells us that if we wish to lift the weight X lb at A using the lever in question, we must place a weight $Y = X.x/y$ lb at the point C. The equation summarizes mathematically our model for the lever; this model is only approximately accurate, as we have entirely neglected the weights of the arms AB and BC of the lever, If these were thought relevant, a more precise set of equations would need to be derived.

We can similarly use a set of deterministic equations to represent the mathematical model for the river and dam system previously discussed. If Z_t is the content of the dam at time t just after a release has been made, and X_t the inflow into the dam in the period $(t, t + 1)$, then the equation

$$Z_{t+1} = \min (Z_t + X_t, K) - \min (Z_t + X_t, M)$$

will represent the dam process. The first part of the expression indicates that if an input X_t occurs in the interval $(t, t + 1)$, then the content of the dam after this input will be the lesser of $Z_t + X_t$ and K; the second states that the release from the dam at time $t + 1$ will be the lesser of the content of the dam just before release, and M. Clearly, the mathematical equation expresses in a short precise form the conditions under which the dam system is functioning. One great advantage of such equations is: they act as a symbolic shorthand for the operating rules of the system.

Similarly, when scientists and engineers need to calculate stresses in ships' hulls or aeroplane wings, a set of algebraic or differential equations will describe the operating rules for the mathematical models used to describe these stresses. While the models themselves may be based on observation and experiment, the equations provide a shorthand description of their structure at a level of abstraction somewhat removed from the physical reality. It is this level of abstraction which permits mathematicians to note the similarities in structural equations for a variety of different mathematical models. These analogies allow the development of unifying concepts and principles which span a wide variety of apparently unrelated practical problems.

Probabilistic Models

While deterministic mathematical models provide the simplest description of natural phenomena, it is clear that many real-life processes are not deterministic but involve a large element of chance and uncertainty. This can only be allowed for mathematically by using probabilistic models, or what are sometimes referred to as 'stochastic' models, from the Greek for guessing.

We can attach a measure of chance or uncertainty to a mathematical model by considering the probabilities of the events involved in it. These probabilities will be positive numbers whose values lie between 0 and 1; if an event has practically no chance of occurring, we attach the probability 0 to it, while if it is almost certain to occur, we attach the probability 1. Without going into a detailed explanation of the meaning of intermediate values, we may regard a probability lying between 0 and 1 ($0 < p < 1$) as indicating on a numerical scale the chance that an event will occur; the larger the probability, the greater the chance that the event occurs. Precise rules have been developed for the calculus of probabilities since the sixteenth century, and probability theory has since become one of the most lively fields of mathematical research.

In the case of the dam system considered, we have so far discussed the exact inputs in particular time intervals, and the exact dam content after a release. In a stochastic model we would consider the probabilities of the events that the input X_t should be i units in the interval $(t, t + 1)$, and the dam content j units thereafter. We should then proceed to frame equations relating these probabilities; it might be assumed for example that probabilities of inputs were known from past meteorological data, and one would attempt to derive probabilities for the dam content Z_t from them. For the particular model we have discussed, these considerations lead to Markov chain equations for the probabilities of Z_t; these probabilities can be found, and will then describe the likelihoods of particular levels of the dam. Thus, instead of obtaining exact results from precise data, we would have, for known input probabilities, results in the form of probabilities of the dam content. These would allow us to describe in a much more realistic manner the way in which the dam behaves, since its level is clearly subject to chance and uncertainty. Exact mathematical statements for the dam content are replaced by probabilistic statements, reflecting the elements of uncertainty under which the dam system operates in reality.

Probabilistic models are invaluable in such diverse areas as insurance problems, biological models, the theory of traffic, the prediction of economic fluctuations, the planning of university enrolments, the relation between heights and weights of children, the analysis of experimental data, and a variety of other real-life situations. They are perhaps more complicated than deterministic mathematical models, but the fact that they take account of chance effects means that the predictions obtained from them are far more realistic than those derived from equivalent deterministic models. Associated with such probabilistic models are a variety of statistical tests now in common use; I shall attempt in the next section to describe the way in which statistical models are developed to test hypotheses based on empirical data.

Statistical Models

In statistical models one is usually concerned with whether certain empirical data fall under one of two categories for which alternative probabilistic frameworks have been constructed. Roughly speaking, whereas a probabilistic mathematical model is concerned with characterizing a certain real-life situation, statistical models are used to test whether experimental data can be said to arise from one or other of two different probabilistic models. An example, which is well known in statistical literature, is that of patients on whom two competing types of sleeping tablets are tested.

A simplified description of this experiment is as follows: Suppose that five patients, Mr Smith, Mr Jones, Mr Roberts, Mr Wilkins, and Mr Marple are to test two types of sleeping tablets. Tablet A is the Deepsleep brand, while tablet B is the Dozum brand; the hypothesis H_0 to be tested is that there is no difference at all between them. The probabilistic models assumed for the length of sleep induced by these two tablet brands are normal probability curves, though possibly with two different means. The table below indicates the lengths of sleep induced by both Deepsleep and Dozum tablets on the five patients.

The column A–B indicates the differences in the lengths of sleep induced in each patient. It is well known from mathematical statistics that, on the previous assumptions, this difference will also be normally distributed with a mean which is the difference of the mean lengths of sleep for tablet A and tablet B respectively. If we are testing the hypothesis H_0 that there is no difference

	Tablet A: Deepsleep Length of sleep hr : min	Tablet B: Dozum Length of sleep hr : min	Difference A–B Length of sleep min
Mr Smith	8:00	7:30	30
Mr Jones	8:15	8:30	−15
Mr Roberts	7:45	7:30	15
Mr Wilkins	8:45	8:40	5
Mr Marple	8:20	8:00	20

between these two, then the differences in column A–B should be normally distributed with mean 0.

This is not the place to go into the rationale of Student's t-test, used to test the hypothesis H_0 that the difference in mean sleep induced by tablets A and B is equal to zero. Suffice it to say that by fairly simple calculations one obtains for the data available the estimate $t_4 = 1\cdot5$ of the relevant statistical parameter. On the basis of statistical tables for the t distribution on 4 degrees of freedom (where these are one less than the number of patients), one discovers that this result is not significant at the 5 per cent level. That is, since the tables give the probability

$$\Pr\{\,|\,t_4\,|\geqslant 2\cdot78\} = 0\cdot05,$$

it follows that the data obtained from the five patients, leading to a value of only $t_4 = 1\cdot5$, are not sufficient to reject the hypothesis H_0 that the effects of Deepsleep and Dozum tablets cannot be distinguished. The notion of what is considered significant is fairly arbitrary, but it has become accepted in statistical literature that the 5 per cent and 1 per cent levels of significance are adequate for most situations.

We have now described in brief detail four types of mathematical model that are used to describe and analyse real-life problems. There are a variety of others, but they are similar in principle, though perhaps more complicated in detail than the ones we have outlined. These should be adequate to provide the reader with some idea of the power of mathematical models in resolving problems that can be logically analysed.

Models as Predictors

Perhaps we should now look back to draw some conclusions from the models we have considered. Some theorists would like to assign to internalized or mathematical models a reality all their own. My personal viewpoint is that they are tentative sketches whose main function is predictive: a model is merely an internalized blueprint which allows one to analyse, project, and plan in a realistic manner. As soon as the model fails to provide reasonable agreement with reality, it must be rejected or modified until it accords more accurately with the hard facts. It is one of the strengths of probabilistic models that they take realistic account of the uncertainties of real life and incorporate variability and chance effects into mathematical models.

A personal anecdote may help to illustrate this point. When I first came to live in Britain in 1965, interest rates on mortgages from Building Societies were fixed at around $6\frac{1}{2}$ per cent per annum. There have been subsequent changes almost every year, until, in 1970, the interest was $8\frac{1}{2}$ per cent per annum. If, in 1965, instead of accepting a deterministic model for which the interest rate was to remain at $6\frac{1}{2}$ per cent indefinitely, I had had the foresight to construct a stochastic model with substantial probabilities of changes in interest rising from $6\frac{1}{2}$ per cent to $8\frac{1}{2}$ per cent over five years, I would have predicted much more realistically what I was to repay my Building Society.

One of the difficulties of conceptual and mathematical models is that they tend to oversimplify the complexity of natural events, if only in order to derive solutions and reach working conclusions. Human minds seek the simplest model that will lead to realistic results or predictions. But, as the real situation is studied in greater depth, it becomes clear that the simple model needs to be modified to take account of the intricacies of nature. An example of this increase in complexity is apparent in the progress from the Newtonian model of the universe to the more sophisticated relativistic model. The Newtonian model is by no means superseded; under certain conditions, namely when the velocity of moving objects is much smaller than that of light, it is still adequate. The relativistic model is far more accurate when the velocity of the moving objects considered approaches that of light. Thus, a more complicated model may only be relevant under a particular set of conditions; it becomes important for the mathematician to know when it is necessary to rely on the simpler or the more complicated model. A similar increase in complexity is found in the passage from deterministic to stochastic mathematical models. Here again one leaves the certainties of precise cause and effect for the uncertainties of variable cause and probable effect.

Among the intellectual sins, possibly the greatest is an unwarranted reliance on models as a substitute for reality; this often leads to dire practical results. There are scientists and mathematicians for whom models appear to have a greater degree of reality than the ascertainable facts themselves; some of their mental constructs are so inflexible that they cannot pass beyond their artifices to a more accurate understanding of the real situation. In dealing with models, it is always salutary to remember that we are using an intellectual shorthand for analytic and predictive purposes; the shorthand is no substitute for reality and must not be confused with it. So long as human beings, scientists, and mathematicians treat models both conceptual and mathematical as functional constructs, blueprints to assist in the analysis and prediction of reality, no serious difficulty can arise. Only when models assume an independent reality of their own beyond this, do they become misleading and dangerous.

REFERENCES

1 PIAGET, JEAN. *La Construction du Réel chez l'Enfant*, Neuchatel, Delachaux et Niestlé, 1937.
2 PIAGET, JEAN. *The Child's Conception of Number*, London, Routledge and Kegan Paul, 1952.
3 HOLT, JOHN. *How Children Learn*, Harmondsworth, Middlesex, Penguin Books, 1970.
4 GANI, J. 'Problems in the probability theory of storage systems', *J. R. Statist. Soc.* B **19**, 181–206, 1957.
5 GANI, J. 'Recent advances in storage and flooding theory', *Adv. Appl. Prob.* **1**, 90–110, 1969.

Comment

SHULAMIT RAMON

It seems fashionable today to speak about model-building in statistics. To quote an authority on the subject; 'Twenty years ago everyone writing a theoretical paper felt obliged to mention analysis of variance. Nowadays it is either set theory for the purist, or model building for the practical man, but the ease with which we can write down simple models tends to obscure the essential difficulties of the whole subject, which appear to me not even to have been made explicit, let alone resolved' (Kendall, 1968).

This is an attempt to make explicit one of the difficulties of applying statistical models to research in psychology and sociology. Professor Gani refers in his paper to statistics as 'the model-building branch of science' and to mathematical models as 'a specialized extension of the internalized model of the world' à la Piaget (p. 75). Mathematical reasoning in the perception of reality is no doubt a possible model for the representation of relationships; doubts begin when the mathematical model is accepted as a valid representation of all spheres of reality.

The core of internalized models of the world lies in the child's growing capacity to grasp *relationships* in the world around him (Piaget, 1963).

The usefulness of a specific model of a specific sphere of reality (let alone models of 'the world') lies in its capacity to express the basic relationships characteristic of this sphere and to infuse them with meaning. The usefulness of statistical models has to be evaluated not only in terms of predictive capacity but also in terms of ability to express meaningful relationships. In Kendall's words 'Looking inside the black box means really looking and trying to

85

find out what the relationships are' (op. cit.). As a social scientist I can only concur with Professor Gani in stating that statistics can provide us with an answer to the question of whether certain empirical data fall under one of two categories for which alternative probabilistic frameworks have been constructed (p. 81). If the data seems to correspond to one category, this means that the data share the qualities recognized in that framework. In the field of sociology and psychology the only framework whose qualities are known fully as yet is the normal distribution. Unfortunately, many of the phenomena in these fields, when studied by statistical methods, do not show a normal distribution. The distributions they show come under the headings of 'non-parametric statistics' or 'distribution free', which means that we do not know their qualities as far as statistical models are concerned. Therefore, they are judged according to their (*a priori* doubtful) approximation to the normal distribution. Alternatively, they are judged according to their 'goodness of fit' to a non-parametric distribution of which we have some description but no knowledge about its qualities.

The price paid for being able to use statistics in sociology and psychology is:

1 Reducing variables to the point of choosing one of several possible operational definitions.
2 Formalizing hypotheses which permit checking only two possible relationships – one suggested by rejection of the hypothesis, one by its acceptance.
3 In some cases making the phenomenon studied quantifiable involves distorting, *a priori*, its meaning.

One may argue that models are usually a simplification of reality, and that this is therefore the case when statistical models are applied in sociology and psychology. But simplification becomes reduction when the applied model does not explain the network of relations leading to a certain end-product, when there is no knowledge as to what happens between the input and output points. My claim is that this is the point to which the use of statistics brings us in the majority of cases in research in sociology and psychology.

It is the researcher's decision whether to use statistics in a sociological or psychological study. The majority of researchers share the belief of statisticians that their method is 'the scientific method' and that prediction is the sole aim of research. This belief is stated also by Professor Gani (p. 76). In the following example I will try to amplify what happens when the statistical model is adopted fully to the study of a psychological phenomenon, even in a case where a normal distribution is employed: 'Different psychologists have championed these definitions of intelligence and much research has been addressed to these questions. However, none of this research has resulted in a clear definition of intelligence. For this reason many psychologists today have reached the point where they no longer ask "what is intelligence". They have decided that they can do a useful job in measuring intelligence without defining it. Since an intelligence test is designed to measure the "intellectual" rather than, say, temperamental or motor skills, it seems clear that the items in the test should be of an "intellectual" nature. If the psychologist is satisfied that it is an intellectual task, it is included. A test made up of such items is, by definition, an "intelligence test" ' (all quotation marks in the original) (Krech and Crutchfield, 1965, p. 573). We learn therefore that psychologists:

1 Once wanted to have a definition of intelligence.
2 The suggested definitions could not be proved statistically.
3 Therefore they no longer need such definitions.
4 Every test thought by a psychologist to consist of intellectual items (yet another undefined concept) becomes a test/expression of intelligence, when it is capable of showing a normal distribution of results in the sample to which it was administered (this last conclusion is based on the content of later sections in the same book).

As is well known, intelligence is used in the Western world as a key factor for classifying the ability of human beings to study and work and to denote changes in psychopathology. All of this is based on the façade of face validity and the belief that only statistical discriminations are valuable (i.e. scientific – objective, non-biased, standardized). True, many of the intelligence tests are standardized. They are objective in the sense that they are not the subject's creation but the psychologist's. They are biased, being the psychologist's choice based on his personal definition of the concepts of both intelligence and intellectuality.

It seems as if it is of no significance that we do not know what we are looking for, as long as we can statistically measure something. It is not being suggested that these tests are valueless, but rather that one must spell out this type of tautology and the underlying definitions used for intelligence which psychologists seem to be ashamed of since they cannot be proved statistically. It goes without saying that more research should be devoted to the nature of intelligence, by statistical or other methods.

To sum up: it is not suggested here that statistical methods and models should no longer be used in sociology and psychology. Nor do I think that by definition statistical models act to reduce social phenomena. I would suggest, rather, that statisticians for their part need a thorough acquaintance with the field of social science to which they act as consultants. Then the possibility arises of building models integrated with the field, provided that prediction as a sole aim is abandoned, as well as blind adherence to models that fit the natural sciences. For their part, social scientists must develop their own methodology – one corresponding to their theoretical models – and apply statistical techniques only when they do not involve simply the reduction of the phenomena under consideration.

REFERENCES

KENDALL, M. G. 1968. 'On the Future of Statistics – a Second Look', *J. Roy. Statist. Soc.*, A. 131, 186–204.

KRECH, D. & CRUTCHFIELD, R. S. 1965. *Elements of Psychology*, New York, Knopf.

PIAGET, J. 1963. *The Child's Conception of Space*, London, Routledge & Kegan Paul.

Models in Experimental Psychology

NEVILLE MORAY

The history of psychology as a self-consciously developing science has been marked by an obsessive concern for the scientific respectability of its theories. The reasons for this seem to be threefold. First, being recognized as a 'science' has seemed to many psychologists a sign of intellectual respectability and an indication that positivistic certitude is indeed possible in the realm of human nature. Second, the enormous range of qualitatively different phenomena has led to many different types of exploration being applied to that supposedly single topic, man's nature, and a difficulty in relating each to the others. Third, it has been characteristic of psychology that it has used theories, models, and concepts derived from other disciplines, notably physics, engineering and lately computer theory, to explain human behaviour, with the result that certain quite difficult philosophical problems have been raised, solutions to which have not yet been adequately formulated.

Although I shall examine only one kind of model in this paper, the following fable may be illuminating.

There was once a sociologist who investigated a community in which he discovered that the effect of moving people from a slum area to a new housing estate unexpectedly gave rise to an increase in delinquency. He reported that the cause of this was the lack of a stable community social framework. 'Oh, come now,' said a social psychologist, 'that's merely redescribing what happened. The *explanation* is that group norms were relaxed and new peer groups formed as a result of social learning and the search for cohesive peer-group structure.' 'Loose talk!' said a passing Skinnerian, 'we know now that social pressures are properly described by reference to the mutual schedules of reinforcement which people provide for one another, thereby shaping the acceptable patterns of behaviour in the group'. A physiological psychologist who overheard them pointed out that while reinforcement theory certainly allowed behaviour to be predicted, you couldn't in all honesty say that it explained anything; but that fortunately we were now in a position to say which nerve cells must fire in order for behaviour to be learned. But his companion (a biochemist) said that the firing of nerve cells should be discussed in terms of its *cause*, namely depolarization of cell membranes and the resulting change in concentration of sodium and potassium ions in and outside the neuron. 'But I must confess,' he added sadly, 'that I am sometimes worried by my brother-in-law who is a physicist and insists that the only proper account of ions and molecules is to be given in terms of dynamic equations relating to quantum theory.'

Moral: one man's cause is another man's description.

Psychological theorizing can be found at many of the levels of discourse mentioned in the above fable, and at several not included in it. There seems no logical reason to regard any level or type of explanation as inherently better or more correct than another in any absolute sense. The reason for choosing one kind of model, or one level of explanation, rather than another *may* be a matter of logic;[1] but it may also be determined by the interests of the investigator and the kind of theory he *likes* (much as the desire for symmetry played so great a part at certain stages of the development of theoretical physics); or again by the purpose for which the work is being done (if one knows that certain moulds can prevent blood-poisoning, an explanation is not necessary for treating people, though it may be useful to the pharmaceutical manufacturers).

There are, then, many different *kinds* of explanation used in psychology, and the logical analysis of a psychoanalytic theory will differ considerably from the similar analysis of, say, a model based on the applied mathematics of Shannon's communication theory. While I shall use the latter as an example of modelling in psychology it should not be taken as the sole, or even typical, psychological model. I do believe, however, that the conceptual problems attendant upon the use of a communication theory model are similar in many respects to problems inherent in other models.

At the heart of the problem is the logic of *analogy*. We take a model, with its concepts, its state-transition matrix, and its rules for relating to the real world, and try to map psychological phenomena (behaviour, scores, etc.) on a one-to-one basis onto the concepts of the existing model, and onto the states of the real world. If this can be done, then the state-transition matrix of the model can be used to predict the future behaviour of the system from its present state, and the future behaviour is explained by the paths in the state-transition matrix.

Looking at a specific example, consider Senders's[2] model for the monitoring of an instrument panel by a human observer. Consider an observer watching a dial, such as a speedometer, of which the reading varies in a random or quasi-random way as a function of time. The movement of the needle of the dial can be described by means of a Fourier series as a fundamental frequency plus some higher harmonies, having an upper limit W Hz beyond which frequency there are no frequencies which contribute significant power to the signal. The variation of the reading of the dial will also allow us to ascribe an amplitude A to the time function.

Shannon's information theory now says that in order to extract all information from this instrument (in the sense of being able to reconstruct its movements exactly from the observations we take) we need to sample the instrument at a rate of exactly 2W samples per second. Taking fewer samples than this means that our reconstruction must be in error, while to take more is unnecessary, *if the human observer is an ideal Shannon Information Transmission Channel.* Now, such a channel has a *limited capacity*, measured in *bits per second* of information. The amount of information as a continuous function of time, such as the output of the instrument the observer is watching, is defined as:

$$H = 2W \log_2 \left(1 + \frac{A}{N}\right) \text{ bits per second}$$

where W and A have the meanings originally given, and N is the 'noise' in the system.

If our observer is set the task of monitoring several instruments simultaneously, whose bandwidths are W_a, $W_b \ldots W_m$, he should,

by the Shannon theorem, take samples from instruments a, b, . . .
m, at intervals $\dfrac{1}{2W_a}$, $\dfrac{1}{2W_b}$, $\cdots$ $\dfrac{1}{2W_m}$ respectively, provided his
total channel capacity is not exceeded; while if it is exceeded, the
error in his performance can be predicted from the equation given
above.

Whether information theory is successful in predicting behaviour is not the question that here concerns us. (As a matter of fact it is, when appropriately used, highly successful.)

What is of interest is the logic behind the use of the model.

The original theory selects four variables N, A, W, and H, and relates them to each other. They are identified with 'noise', 'amplitude', 'bandwidth', 'information', and related by the concepts of 'channel' and 'capacity'. In this original theory each of these concepts is well defined, and there is no problem in identifying the properties of the real world with which they correspond.

In order to use the information theory as a psychological theory, we are required to map these concepts, properties, relationships, etc. onto some property of the human organism. Thus, we may say, 'let us assume that the human observer is a limited-capacity information-transmitting channel', and then see if his behaviour is appropriate. That is, we claim that, in *Figure 1*, one of the many physical objects which can play the role of the box is a human being. Others are radio receivers, telephone lines, etc.

Figure 1

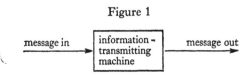

But if we are to use this model, we must also say what constitutes the message whose properties are defined by H, W, and A, and what is the 'noise', N. Since H is a variable whose value is dependent on W, A, and N we may concentrate on the latter. In the example given, the values of W and A can be directly related to the rate and extent of the excursions of the pointer of the dial which is being monitored by the observer. N presents more difficulty. We might attempt to identify it as those events in neural activity of the brain which modify the neural events representing the observation of the instrument so that it becomes distorted. Or we might keep all the concepts of our model as stimulus variables and define noise as any variation in the stimulus which is too fine for sensory discrimination to observe, i.e. that range of variation to which the observer is indifferent.

Having made the identification, we can then relate the variables one to another by the mathematical functions of the equation. That is, performance is a function of the value of H, of which the value is itself calculated by taking the logarithm to the base 2 of the ratio of the maximum amplitude to the amplitude of the noise, adding one, and multiplying the result by twice the maximum frequency present in the signal.

The final stage consists in identifying some feature of the response with the relevant variable in the equation. We now have the following situation:

A. *The World*

(i) A set of events $\{A, B, \ldots P\}$ whose values can be varied

(ii) A set of events $\{S, T, \ldots Z\}$ whose values vary when the values of $\{A, B, \ldots P\}$ vary.

B. *The Model*

(i) A set of symbols $\{a', b', \ldots p'\}$ which stand for $\{A, B, \ldots P\}$

(ii) A set of symbols $\{s'\, t', \ldots z'\}$ which stand for $\{S, T, \ldots Z\}$

(iii) A set of rules, expressed in this case as mathematical relationships, which relate $\{a', b', \ldots p'\}$ to $\{s', t', \ldots z'\}$ by means of a mathematical function Φ, such that the values of $\{s', t', \ldots z'\}$ can be deduced from the values of $\{a', b', \ldots p'\}$ by the rule $\{s', t', \ldots z'\} = \Phi\{a', b', \ldots p'\}$

We say that the model explains the observed phenomena when, for any values of $\{A, B \ldots P\}$, we put $a' = A$, $b' = B \ldots p' = P$, apply the function rule Φ to the resulting set of $\{a', b', \ldots p'\}$, obtain the values of $\{s', t', \ldots z'\}$, and find that the values of

$\{S, T, \ldots Z\}$ are identical, within the limits of accuracy obtainable, to the values of $\{s', t', \ldots z'\}$.

At first sight it would seem that we have merely redescribed what happens, rather than explaining it. But this is because we have concealed the fact that there is not one column of 'real-world' phenomena, but two. In the case of information theory as applied to psychology, we have the following:

Source Real-World Phenomena	Psychological Real-World Phenomena	The Model
Events $A, B, \ldots M$	Events $a, b, \ldots m$	Symbols $a', b', \ldots m'$
Events $S, T, \ldots Z$	Events $s, t, \ldots z$	Symbols $s', t', \ldots z'$
		Function rule Φ

We map $A \rightarrow a', B \rightarrow b'$ etc. in formulating the original theory (in this case an engineering theory), in which field the resulting functional relationship

$$\{s', t', \ldots z'\} = \Phi\{a', b', \ldots z'\}$$

is descriptive of the relation between $\{A, B, \ldots M\}$ and $\{S, T, \ldots Z\}$.

But when we find that, on mapping $\{a, b, \ldots m\}$ onto $\{a', b', \ldots m'\}$ and applying Φ, we obtain $\{s', t', \ldots z'\}$ we say that the relationship explains the phenomena, because we claim that in some sense we can identify the set of events $\{a, b, \ldots m\}$ with $\{A, B, \ldots M\}$.

Thus we find people who are supporters of the application of information theory to psychology saying such things as, 'Let us assume that the human operator in a limited-capacity channel.'

The exact nature of this identification of a set of psychological phenomena with the components of an existing theory is problematical. At its weakest it is probably analogical, at its strongest a claim for true, formal, identity. We may express the problem in the diagram (*Figure* 2 opposite).

By 'empirical identification' I mean a discovery such as the fact that nerve fibres transmit messages from one end of a cell to the other, and that therefore the brain must be regarded as an information-transmission channel. There are formidable difficulties in performing validly such empirical identification.

If the above outline of the nature of a large class of psychological

Figure 2

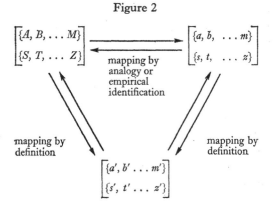

models is correct, we can see where the most severe difficulties lie. They are:

1 The construction of an adequate taxonomy of psychological phenomena which allows states $\{a, b, \ldots m; s, t, \ldots z\}$ to be distinguished and identified unequivocally when they occur.

2 The construction of unequivocal mapping rules which allow the transformations $a \rightarrow a'$, $b \rightarrow b' \ldots m \rightarrow m'$ and $s' \rightarrow s$, $t' \rightarrow t, \ldots z' \rightarrow z$ to be carried out.

3 The justification for identifying a with A, b with B, etc.

In some areas of psychology, such as that commonly if misleadingly[3] called experimental psychology, these difficulties are relatively small, although by no means trivial. In others, they are more difficult. It is common, for example, to find research in social and personality psychology which has been adequately carried out in every way confronted with the criticism, 'Oh, but surely you don't think that *that* is how to measure X, however consistent your data may be.' (X would commonly be such a thing as political or religious belief.) Here we have a failure in operational definition, the first of the above three difficulties. Difficulties in the mapping rules are seen where the cut-off point on a measuring scale is to some extent arbitrary, such as deciding where 'high' intelligence becomes 'normal' intelligence.

An example of the third difficulty is the concept of 'tension' or 'force', and we may usefully discuss this at greater length.

It is obvious why the concepts of psychological forces, or tensions, have arisen. Quite apart from the use of the term in clinical or technical language, most people have had the subjective experience of being unable to control their own thoughts, dreams, wishes, behaviour, etc. to a greater or lesser degree. The classical example of a psychological model using the concept of 'force' is of course Freud's account of the way in which the instincts affect the psychological life of men and women.

It is clear, however, that the use of 'force' is only weakly analogical, and it is largely due to this fact that the theory is so notoriously weak predictively. In physics, 'force' is precisely defined by the relationship:

$$\text{force} = \text{mass} \times \text{acceleration} \qquad F = MA$$

where acceleration itself is defined as the second derivative of length with respect to time,

$$\text{acceleration} = (\text{length}/\text{time})/\text{time} \qquad A = LT^{-2}$$

So that, in terms of the well-defined primitive concepts of mass, length, and time, we have

$$F = MLT^{-2}$$

The importance of this, and what gives the concept of 'force' so precise an explanatory power, is that we are not merely restricted to scaling force values self-consistently, 'this force is twice that force', but we expect exact results when the value of the force is related to the value of a mass to which it is applied. For a given F and a given M a given acceleration will result.

In the application of the force concept in psychology, however, it is used in isolation. There are no precisely defined equivalents of mass and acceleration, and indeed force seems to function as a primitive concept in psychology, rather than a derived one. Its use is analogical, not a true identification, since the latter is only possible when not only force, but also equivalents of mass and acceleration, are defined.

At this point, we may come to a conclusion.

When psychological models draw on existing theories from other disciplines, their explanatory and predictive power is dependent on their success in identifying all the variables in the source theories with psychological phenomena, using scalar or vector measurements as demanded by the original *theory*.

Is such precision possible? There is not room in the present article to discuss this in detail, but let me outline where a clue may be found. In Turing's work on the nature and properties of machines he defined a machine as a set of states and the rules for changing from state to state. Formally, this can be represented as:

$$\{s, t, \ldots z\} = \Phi \{a, b, \ldots m\}$$

where $\{s, t, \ldots z\}$ and $\{a, b, \ldots m\}$ are states of the system, and some states in $\{s, t, \ldots z\}$ may be identical with some states in $\{a, b, \ldots m\}$. The function rule Φ is more properly regarded as a *set* of function rules $\{\Phi\}$, and we see that a scientific theory can be regarded as the description of a Turing machine.

McCulloch and Pitts showed that such machines could be designed to show any behaviour (phenomena) which can be defined in a finite number of words. This we may similarly translate as 'a scientific theory may be discovered which unambiguously describes any behaviour (phenomena) which can be defined in a finite number of words'. The relation between description and explanation has already been touched on earlier.

If, and only if, psychology can achieve such precision in describing and defining the phenomena with which it is concerned, can the full power of models from other disciplines be used. At present, we do not know to what extent this aim can be achieved. In some areas of psychology there have been outstanding successes, in other areas a notable and notorious sequence of overambitious failures. There are certainly some fields in which powerful predictive models of extensive generalization exist already. But I suspect that there may well be logical barriers to extending such areas indefinitely, and that in the most deeply human of human activities a man may be the best model of himself.

NOTES AND REFERENCES

1 See, e.g., WINCH, P. *Idea of a Social Science*, London, Routledge, 1958.

2 SENDERS, J. *Attention and Performance*, Vol. 1, edited by Senders, North Holland Publishing Company, 1967.

3 Misleading in the sense that other areas of psychology also use the experimental method.

© *Neville Moray 1972*

Comment

GEOFFREY PEARSON

In the field of psychology, and in the neighbouring fields of psychiatry, sociology, and anthropology, one thing in particular makes progress difficult. It is this: to set out upon a new area of investigation is not merely to begin looking at a new part of the universe external to the self. The human universe does not possess that character of objectivity which has been such a source of reassurance and comfort to natural scientists since the days of Locke and Newton. Rather, for those of us who are in the business of studying human behaviour and mentality, that reality which for the natural scientist is very solidly *out there* has more of the ring of an uncanny Berkeleian presence. That old Berkeleian mot *esse est percipi* can, of course, be put to many uses. It can be used, for example, to get knotted up in puzzles about whether the trees which I can see are here when I am not here to see them. It can also lead to the profound and compelling discovery that the processes of perception join us inextricably to that which we perceive, providing a bridge which links subject and object. This means in the sciences of man that every new exploration of the universe is an exploration of self. Whenever we probe further into new areas of knowledge, the back end of the probe is always firmly embedded in our own vital parts. Of course this is nowadays recognized as being no less true in the natural sciences and mathematics, the matter being so convincingly demonstrated that not even Euclidean geometry can be regarded as the objective natural history of external space, but only of 'space' in quotation marks – not space as it exists, but space as defined in someone's imagination; space as defined by a perceiver.

98

And yet all this seems to escape the psychology of which Neville Moray gives his account, and it is all the more surprising that it is psychology which, of all sciences, should drive a wedge between perceiver and perceived. It is to this paradox that these few remarks address themselves. I will also attempt to look briefly at how the requirements of a psychology *qua* psychology might relate to the requirements of a psychology *qua* science.

The loyalties of many psychologists seem to lie not to psychology – not the *logos* of the *psyche* – but to Science and to Method. The history of 'respectable' psychology is the history of behaviourism. And yet the behaviouristic account of action is already an abstracted version of actuality: no one can or will seriously contend that action – human or animal – is 'only' or 'nothing but' behaviour. Behaviourism, nevertheless, obtains its validity from being an 'as if' assumption – 'Let's proceed *as if* action is merely behaviour, as if action is *out there* in the world of objects' – the pay-off from this assumption being that it renders up a version of action which is altogether more manageable, permitting more precision and scope in the specification and manipulation of certain variables. In brief, it is a model.

Psychology, then, has attached itself to one particular type of modelling activity – itself only an abstract, partial version of what science is about – and has proceeded as though model were actuality, abstract were concrete, *action were behaviour*, justifying this through the claim that psychology thereby becomes more scientific, despite the fact of being encapsulated within one particular scientific procedure, one abstract version of science. The validity of this type of model is surrendered if its impoverished form is not continually fed back into and compared against concrete actuality. When this is not done 'model' becomes 'System of Thought'. The behaviouristic account is valid for its purposes. The abstract, however, is not real: Senders's accounts of air-pilot eye movements which are cited by Moray are no more instances of concrete human action than is salivation in harnessed dogs allowable as 'behaviour' (Merleau-Ponty, 1965) and to begin from such premises will by necessity yield up a restricted vision of human action. Abstraction and the procedures of experimental design are (or should be) processes whereby men tie down their universe; it usurps its function when it is abstraction which ties down man.

There are certain very cogent objections which must be raised against the application of positivistic scientific method to the study of man. Primarily, psychology studies those factors which determine man's behaviour, but any study that accounts for those determinants only, as it were, from the outside will neglect *man as determiner* and how these determinations will be perceived. Determinants of human action do not impinge on behaviour in the direct fashion that, say, heat is transmitted or energy transferred from one object to another in collision. Rather, it impinges via the mediation of that person's experience, this experience influencing the effect on his organismic response, thereby determining the determination. All this should be abundantly clear to any student of psychology and with it that the idea of objectivity or constancy of determining variables becomes spurious and the application of a scientific method which assumes such objectivity questionable.

Without question the objection will be raised here that I am knocking down a straw man of my own making, that psychology has changed since its happy-go-lucky behaviourist days, that excesses have been corrected and techniques refined. It must be contended, however, that *in so far as its methodological base* is concerned psychology has *not* changed and still adheres to mechanistic–positivistic–behaviouristic assumptions. Indeed, Moray writes that the human being is only 'one of the many physical objects' which can fit the Shannon–Weaver model. Human beings do, of course, have a material presence, but it seems hardly appropriate to refer to them simply as *physical* objects although, of course, the requirements of the model demand this.

The question remains as to what would constitute an alternative psychology and what status that alternative psychology might aspire to. The fact that the nature of my argument here is currently fashionable lends itself easily to the idea that we are on the verge of a 'revolution' or 'breakthrough'. On the contrary, it is a simple matter to criticize psychology but far more difficult to see what might be put in its place. Certainly, unless there is developed a rigorous alternative psychology, grounded in the concreteness of human experience, 'humanistic psychology' will remain merely as an objector, skirmishing on the periphery and suceeding only occasionally in reminding the psychologist of the actualities of his subject-matter (see Jourard, 1968; Bugental, 1967; Bannister, 1966). It is possible that this is the role in which a humanistic psychology is most effective; it is even possible that while the basis of intersubjectivity in psychology is arbitrary and illusory it is an illusion necessary to the development of an understanding of man.

Moray's final recommendation is to the possibility of man as a model of himself. It is a blunt challenge to a task which, when it has been occasionally attempted, has resulted in inglorious defeat. It is, however, a meaningful challenge, although one that must be prefaced in a rigorous re-examination of the conceptual substructure of psychology.[1] It is a great pity, and it signifies the extent of the disease process within psychology, that more weight is not given by experimental psychologists to these fundamental objections to the idea of a psychology. What is really required from psychology is not a further refinement of its technical apparatus, but – to echo the words of von Bertalanffy (1967) – a new conception of man, a clean break with its Newtonian inheritance. If one wished to one might characterize psychology as essentially a *romantic* activity, madly in love with the idea of itself as a science. What is sad is that the science which psychology still woos is long dead some forty years.

NOTE

1 I have in mind such problems as the relationship between the constraints of experimental design and the form of emergent theory (cf. Matson, 1968), taking this beyond the superficial study of experimenter effects (Rosenthal and Rosnow, 1969); the justification for operationalism within psychology; the relative merits of the intelligibility of theory as opposed to its predictive power; the *validity* of analogical thinking within psychology in contrast to Moray's preoccupation with its logic; the whole vexed issue of the feasibility of a monadic conception of action, involving the relation of psychologistic forms of thought to sociology and the linguistic and historical traditions which underlie the reification of mental process (Cf. Sarbin and Juhasz, 1967); and, finally, a *proper* recognition (Krech, 1969) of the mind–body problem.

REFERENCES

BANNISTER, D. 'Psychology as an Exercise in Paradox', *Brit. Psychol. Soc. Bull.*, **19**, 63, 21–26, 1966.
BERTALANFFY, L. VON *Robots, Men and Minds*, New York, Braziller, 1967.
BUGENTAL, J. F. T. *Challenges of Humanistic Psychology*, N.Y., McGraw-Hill, 1967.
JOURARD, S. M. *Disclosing Man to Himself*, N.Y., van Nostrand, 1968.
KRECH, D. 'Does Behavior Really Need a Brain?', In: American Psychological Association, *William James: unfinished business*, A.P.A., 1969.
MATSON, F. W. *The Broken Image*, N.Y., Braziller, 1968.
MERLEAU-PONTY, M. *The Structure of Behaviour*, London, Methuen, 1965.
ROSENTHAL, R. and R. L. ROSNOW (eds.) *Artifact in Behavioral Research*, N.Y., Academic Press, 1969.
SARBIN, T. R. and J. B. JUHASZ 'The Historical Background of the Concept of Hallucination', *J. Hist. Behav. Sci.*, **3** (4), 339–358, 1967.

Man and his Shadow: models of normality and non-normality

SHULAMIT RAMON

A number of dictionaries contain no definition of psychic normality. Yet the term normal is used in every description of a psychological phenomenon. Definitions, when found, consist of descriptions such as 'average' or 'optimum level of well being'.[1] Whether defined or not, normality is used as a base for evaluation of overt human behaviour. Such a definition acts as a class criterion of the normal or non-normal, either exclusively or inclusively. On the surface it seems relatively easy, almost unrehearsed, for a layman to conclude whether a certain behaviour is normal or not. Some specific details of behaviour act as signs, the appearance of which usually indicates non-normality. The appearance of these details leads one to exclude from one's evaluation all other existing details of behaviour and personality. This exclusion is achieved by denying either the existence of the other details or else the significance usually attached to them. Furthermore, the identifying detail acts as the carrier of a personality which is constructed around it. For example: 'He is a thief' means, factually, that he has taken somebody else's property. It also means that he has broken the law / he will be punished / he is a criminal / he may become a prisoner / only non-normal people steal / he was born like that / something is wrong with him / he is wicked / he must be poor / he is very clever / he is ugly and frightening. We already know so much about this person from the single act of theft that there is no need to see him or to hear him out.

Three major features emerge from the above statement:

1 The identifying detail.

103

2 The inclusion / exclusion of qualities on the basis of this single detail.
3 Moral judgements.

Given these three elements, the categorization of behaviour is complete. They act as a diagnostic unit, each reinforcing the others. Whence comes the overpowering need for this categorization? Why must it be so undifferentiating? An answer to these questions relates to more than one level of consciousness and to interpersonal as well as intrapersonal relationships. At the level of everyday consciousness this categorization acts as an interpretation of human behaviour.[2] The need to interpret differences that we perceive between human beings is based on the very fact of living in the same world, which involves an endless process of decisions about our future actions, thoughts, and feelings. The interpretation of experience – and of the other's observed behaviour as part of our experience – validates our past decisions and at the same time traces a path for future ones.[3] Our conception of interaction with others also serves as a basis for the interpretation of their behaviour. We assume that, as human beings, we are more alike than different in our behaviour and experience. We act and interpret on the assumption that we know ourselves and therefore understand the other in terms of our own behaviour and motives.[4]

Living in a specific society narrows the sphere of common experience and makes it more homogeneous, since we share (to differing degrees) the same set of values and act within a similar social framework. All this is 'taken for granted'[5] as part of the process of internalized socialization. 'Taking for granted' is the root of our security about our own place in relation to others. But it also implies a denial, from the beginning, of the multiplicity of systems of life and values. The categorization of behaviour in terms of a dichotomy is used in every society. This universality reflects both the need to orient oneself in the world of others and the need to attribute meaning to behaviour and is emphasized by the anxiety evoked when these needs are not fulfilled. Nevertheless, various types of behaviour are labelled as deviant and are dealt with differently in different societies. The differences reflect not only the specific way of life of each society but also the degree of coexistence of rationality and irrationality in that society.

Rationality is defined here as the employing of logical processes from valid premises either in the process of choice or in the choice itself. In a broad sense it denotes a style or behaviour that is appropriate to the achievement of given goals within the limits imposed by given conditions and constraints. Decisions based on social consensus are incorporated in the definition of what is 'valid', 'appropriate', which are the preferred goals, and what are the given conditions. Therefore, irrationality will be defined socially as employing illogical processes based on invalid premises and using inappropriate behaviour for the attainment of goals.[6]

Many so-called 'primitive' societies do not fear what is termed by us irrational to the extent we do. They have managed to institutionalize periods of insanity in the life of each member (as well as accepted roles of deviancy), neither of which bear stigma. It seems somewhat paradoxical that societies with more rigid systems of life than ours (i.e. modern civilization) possess a higher level of tolerance of irrationality. It appears that there are two main reasons for this difference: (1) They have more confidence in their perception of reality than we do. This confidence is partly due to the fact that they utilize a more concrete level of conceptualization, by taking into consideration only the most repetitive elements of life and denying the independent significance of the less repetitive ones.[7] (2) We prefer rationality to be the way of experiencing and are unable to accept the duality of rationality and irrationality, while this duality serves as the foundation of other societies in which people behave differently. Though there are several possibilities of reacting to this awareness, the usual one is that of suspicion and unease. This attitude is somewhat surprising since one of the few shared human qualities is satiation with old stimuli and search for new ones. But the acceptance of new phenomena would mean that 'the taken for granted' is not so sound and solid as it should be. It would mean that on a more hidden level of consciousness we are not so sure about the similarity between ourselves and others and about the capacity for mutual understanding of behaviour and motives. It throws into doubt the absolutism of our values and the rational control of behaviour. To sum up, it would imply that we are not sure whether our experience, and the world in which we live, have an inherent and coherent meaning.

This feeling, or notion, is usually hidden beneath layers of socialization and rationalization, layers acquired very early in life and welcomed in our personal search for meaning as a reassurance of our sanity and integrity.

As individuals we differ in our ability to tolerate ambiguity. But even those of us who have a higher threshold of tolerance than most have to select meanings and to adopt some more strongly than others if our behaviour is to be consistent in our own eyes. In the field of human behaviour meanings are not selected on the basis of factual evidence. This is so because much still remains either unknown or unobserved and meaning is only deduced. The differences among societies contribute to this lack of clarity since they show that there are no absolute rules for judging which way of life is the 'true' one. The proof of a chosen meaning is so thin that for purposes of everyday life one has to attach *faith* to this meaning by denying all other possible ones.

The historical analysis put forward by Foucault[8] points to a struggle in the modern world for the supremacy of rationality over irrationality. It is only at the end of medieval times that madmen became the social scapegoats instead of lepers. These are the centuries of the slow rise of rationalism as the preferred mode of experiencing. The method used for the elimination of madmen reveals the growing fear of irrationality. They are just sent away, from city to city, without attempts at punishment or cure (the 'ship of fools'). Later, once the supremacy of rationality is established, imprisonment and deprivation of all human rights are considered as the best method of dealing with madness – i.e. in a similar manner to that in which sovereign power deals with its enemies. With the beginning of the Enlightenment the idea of the madman's human dignity, together with the possibility of transforming him into a conforming citizen, acquires converts. The insane are no longer chained, but they are required, directly and indirectly, to behave rationally. Inasmuch as they are able to meet this requirement they receive 'special' rewards, i.e. more rights, similar to those of ordinary citizens.

The motives for maintaining and reinforcing the categorization of normal versus non-normal differ for the individual, the family, and society. For an individual, the very act of judging another's behaviour as non-normal serves as a reinforcement of his own normality.[9] Since the sanctions used against non-normality are known, judgement passed on another acts as a warning for the judge. In the sphere of rationality versus irrationality, where everyone is aware (though to different degrees) of his own irrationality and has been taught to fear it, projecting it on the other is an agreed act and therefore is not labelled as a mental illness (unagreed projections are usually labelled as insanity). It means that only by the denial of the significance of important parts of one's own experience is one's sanity retained.

Some people are perturbed by the possibility of their experience receiving a conventional meaning. Being dissatisfied (for various reasons) with the usual explanations, they are ready to accept the unconventional one as truthful. By this acceptance they open themselves to several unequal alternatives of careers for life as (1) psychotherapists, (2) artists, or (3) mentally ill patients.

(1) If they still believe in the supremacy of rationality but do not deny either to themselves and/or to others the reality of irrationality they can become valuable psychotherapists. They will be able to enter the private logic of the other with sincere sympathy.

(2) They may become artists, since creativity means discovering, or infusing, a meaning that was not attached before to a certain phenomenon, i.e. an unconventional meaning. The artist has the capacity and readiness to perceive the new meaning and to try to communicate it to others. On the one hand, in distinction to the psychotherapist, he is not bothered by the question of rationality versus irrationality because his private understanding is the ultimate criterion. On the other hand, he differs from the mentally ill in two major respects. The first is his ability to *organize*, in his unique way, his experience. The second is his non-surrender to suffering.

(3) To become mentally ill signifies that every meaning is questioned, nothing is taken for granted, and in the most acute periods only feelings of nothingness prevail. Rationality and irrationality are interwoven, with no clear boundaries. One's suffering becomes the all-embracing feature, the only element which does not lose its painful grasp on the person. This is seen clearly in cases where no stigmatizing social reaction has occurred – e.g. in medieval saints and in those undergoing initiation rites

involving isolation and visions. In reporting their history such individuals describe some moments of revelation, but intense suffering is felt most of the time.[10]

Is it drift, self-determination, or a long-standing ego impairment which makes one cross the border and become mentally ill? The answer is far from clear on the common-sense level as well as on the professional one (to which we will turn later). This is so because of the uniqueness of each person, on the one hand, and the number of factors which have to be considered, on the other. The one element that plays a major role according to common sense as well as to all theories is anxiety.[11] When anxiety – as a symbolization of suffering – becomes too strong to be contained, the outcome will be an outward expression of unexpected behaviour. It has the meaning of a call for help, of despair, and some hope of change for the better. At the level of the primary group, the family, the first reaction to this cry for help is that of denial before the larger social environment. This denial can be seen as an act of self-defence. The family members know that the significance and the sanctions attached to the behaviour of one of their members will be generalized – to a lesser degree – to the whole family. The reaction inside the family will depend on the other members' needs which the patient's behaviour satisfies. When the family is relatively healthy in terms of interaction (e.g. without any strong need for a scapegoat) the reaction will be one of fear and annoyance together with attempts to understand and give help along the lines desired by the patient. In less healthy families there will be an avoidance of the meaning of the unexpected behaviour, with encouragement and sometimes even initiation of such behaviour at an unconscious level.[12] This is done in order to maintain the previous equilibrium. Some of these families will be the first to ask for hospitalization – not for psychotherapy – of their 'ill' member. As the patient plays the role of the scapegoat, his insanity is the proof of the other members' sanity and hospitalization serves as a rubber stamp for this role. The family's eager cooperation with the authorities is designed to prove that they are different from him – sane, reliable citizens.[13]

On the more general social level, if the unusual behaviour is thought to be dangerous, the first reaction is to see the patient as delinquent. If he is diagnosed as mentally ill by psychiatrists, this transfers him from one type of deviancy to another and from a prison to a mental hospital. When the person's behaviour is not dangerous to others, but only unusual, he will be transferred directly to a mental hospital as a result of a complaint. From the point of view of the inmates there are several differences between the two institutions. Inmates of a prison are expected to be healthy but somehow corrupted. On the one hand they are thought to be drifters – i.e. having weak will-power. But on the other hand some criminals seem to represent a type of hero, possessing strong will-power. Their action is feared and may be envied at the same time by those outside prison.[14] The prison system reflects this attitude – inmates are put behind bars, required to work, and subjected to harsh treatment and physical punishment. But their stay in prison is for a set time, and in the majority of Western countries they have legal rights just as before imprisonment, including all financial and family ones. Inmates of a mental hospital are supposed to be sick in mind and – to a lesser extent – in body. They are, therefore, given treatment – whether they want it or not – even when permanent negative side-effects are known to occur (e.g. from lobotomy and electroshock). They are considered all along as irresponsible (like children, the retarded, and the senile) and therefore most of their civil rights are taken away. They are hospitalized for no fixed period. As has been so clearly shown by Scheff[15] and Katz,[16] even when they succeed in bringing professionals to court, their chances of winning are extremely slight from the very beginning because their evidence is thought to be unreliable. They are not usually exposed today to harsh treatment and physical punishment, but are treated like children. Thus the threat of irrationality and ambiguity – shared by all – is minimized by attributing to those who express it the stigma of being irresponsible and weak, completely dependent on the agents of society to whom their treatment is delegated. The stigma is the one element shared by inmates of both prison and mental hospital after they leave these institutions. The price of giving up sanity, even for a short time, thus means becoming an irresponsible dependent creature. For some, it is the fulfilment of their wishes. For many, this is not the case.

Society, as opposed to the family, cannot afford to ignore insane behaviour. The threat to the ever fragile net of conformity to social norms is too great for both ruling and ruled groups to remain aloof.[17] Yet negative sanctions against insanity are employed more often against the ruled than against members of the ruling groups. Since there is no problem of face-to-face relationships, as in the case of a family, society may act more directly and brutally. Each action against any sort of deviancy strengthens the conformists in their conformity. At the social level it may be claimed that the deviants have themselves opted out. There is probably some truth in this claim. It is also claimed that deviants are given the possibility of becoming obedient citizens. This is a half truth, inasmuch as the stigma attached to any type of deviancy accompanies for a very long period those once labelled as such. The feeling of being stigmatized enhances their already existing feelings of estrangement and they are led to believe that they can be accepted as full human beings only among other deviants (in the case of prisoners), or by retreating into their private world (as in mental illness).

We have just described attitudes, needs, and processes accruing to normality at the level of individuals and groups on the plane of everyday life. We will now turn to a discussion of the issues involved in the theoretical explanation of these attitudes and processes. The requirements that a complete (and hence ideal) model should meet in order to answer the main queries concerning normality and non-normality, seem to fall into two main categories:

(*a*) sources of knowledge and method of checking on them;
(*b*) explanations of the field (e.g. processes, phenomena, results).

SOURCES OF KNOWLEDGE

The peculiarity of the field of normality, psychopathology, and deviance lies in its being related to more than one level of human experience. Therefore the attempt to understand the field has to derive from more than one type of knowledge.

(*a*) *Intellectual knowledge*
This is the most used type of knowledge in model-building in all branches of science. The same accepted rules of logical inference are relevant for the study of normality as for any other field of inquiry. Thus, intellectual knowledge is used for comparison,

differentiation, elimination and selection, definition, statement of general laws and intervening variables, and the delineation of the range of operational definitions. In the majority of studies use is made of intellectual knowledge by the procedure of positivist, mainly empirical, research. Only in the minority of cases the approach upheld by scholars is that of the deductive (mainly non-empirical) method. Though the same phenomena are studied by the two methods, the assumptions, procedures, and therefore results are very different. Objectivity of the observer and standardization of procedures are the keynotes of the positivist approach, whose adherents believe in the possibility of achieving objectivity in the study of interpersonal relationships. The coming into existence of a phenomenon is not questioned. What is questioned is the variability and characteristics of a phenomenon. Thus the existence of the categorization of normality or non-normality is not questioned. The modalities of normality are studied focusing on the standardization of methods of observation, quantification, and inference – i.e. from formalized operational definitions to hypotheses and from quantified data to statistical tests of significance.[18]

According to the deductive method of inquiry the very coming into existence of interpersonal relationships is questioned and studied, through the mind of the observer – the philosopher. Objectivity is a specified aim in only some of the schools. The degree of rigour of a study is evaluated differently according to the method of a specific school of thought. Thus inferences may be achieved not necessarily from quantified data or standardized methods, and an extreme case may provide more insight than a representative sample.

The differing conceptualizations of anxiety exemplify the different attitudes of the two above-mentioned methods. Anxiety, as an object of inquiry, entered the field of psychopathology through literature and subjective descriptions (i.e. non-scientific sources). The adherents of the deductive method speculated about its origins in relation to the human race and the individual, and in the context of history. Thus ontological insecurity and death anxiety are thought to be the two main types of anxiety, anxiety recognized as having a great motivational impact on everyone's life.[19] For the positivists, for a very long time, anxiety did not exist, being difficult to observe and measure. It came into recognition after being distinguished from fear – as a non-specified fear – and when the physiological correlates of non-specific fear were discovered. Even then, for the classical learning theorists, anxiety is synonymous with general level of drive arousal in an individual.[20] For other positivists, by now the majority, anxiety is a specific factor acting as an intervening variable between stress situation and emergency reaction. Anxiety is variously defined by scholars. Some of the definitions are compatible – e.g. non-object fear, sign of danger, and reaction to perceived threat. Some of the definitions, however, are incompatible – such as unease due to regret at doing wrong[21] – with reaction to the unexpected interruption of an expected course of behaviour.[22] The very idea of an intervening variable is problematic in a framework in which observed phenomena are clearly preferred to inferred ones.

(b) Experiential knowledge
Anxiety, as well as suffering, uncanny fear, and tragedy, are some of the terms which remain basically unclarified by an intellectual frame of reference. They may be analysed intellectually, sometimes to the point of dissection, but are not understood in their impact upon the non-logical level of human experience, or upon the logical level. The insights we get into madness and deviancy from paintings, literature, autobiographies, and from our own empathy cannot be reached by us in any other way.[23] The experiential type of knowledge is indispensable for grasping the subjective component in the field of psychopathology. This type of knowledge constitutes the only way to transcend the subjective and arrive at the level of intersubjective meaning. Is it scientific? To a certain extent it is possible to apply to information received through experiential knowledge the usual rules applying to logical inferences. But by definition the basic information will be unobservable and unobjective, unreproducible and not fully quantifiable (at best only an ordinal level may be achieved). An attempt to make this experiential knowledge observable will mean rendering it meaningless. This type of knowledge clearly does not fit the positivist method of research, and therefore was renounced by extreme positivistic scientists as unreliable, and unscientific; in fact, it is not considered by them as a source of knowledge.[24]

In my view, this type of knowledge gets its validation to a certain degree by mutual agreement and by its ability to enlighten for us hidden corners unreachable by the 'scientific' method. In the sphere of human experience, an experience which is truthfully recorded subjectively exists as much as a collection of measured data. The fact that the more frequently used scientific method is incapable of dealing with experiential knowledge indicates a disadvantage of that method rather than a refutation of the value of this type of knowledge for our understanding of normality and psychopathology.

A. Van Kaam's[25] study of the meaning of 'really fully understood' suggests a method of dealing with essentially experiential data without depriving them of their special nature, at the same time aiming towards an evaluation of consensual validation in order to arrive at a fuller understanding of the concept.

(c) Weltanschauung

This is usually perceived as an aspect of personal bias. These biases should be detached and concealed while a man acts in his role as scientist.[26] This compartmentalization can be achieved only partially, at best, because we act as integrated organisms. More than that – it is doubtful whether a detached observer will be able to grasp better than an involved one the many meanings of non-normative behaviour. In the absence of precise non-reductive means of observing phenomena in the field, the human observer remains the most important instrument. In order to be used to his fullest capacities he has to be aware of himself, and of his *Weltanschauung* among other facets of his personality – if he is to try to understand the manifold experience of others.[27]

Weltanschauung acts as a frame of reference. Thus it can be employed to generate questions and hypotheses. If the scientist is not rigid, he may change his *Weltanschauung* according to the evidence accumulated. In this case, his *Weltanschauung* is used as a working hypothesis, as well as the base of the final interpretation of his findings. To disregard the existence of *Weltanschauung* means either not to know what to question or to deny the true origin of the questions one is asking. In the main models for normality we find three major preferences regarding human aims in life: (1) the ability to function well (salient in traditional psychiatry);[28] (2) the ability to adjust to social control (found in the normative model[29] and in psychoanalysis[30] to a certain extent); (3) the achievement of personal happiness (in existential psychiatry[31] and psychoanalysis). The preference of the advocates of each model has direct bearing on the answer given to questions such as: the role of free will and responsibility, the need for social change, levels and methods of intervention, methods of research. Integration of all sources of knowledge is needed in order to obtain the fullest possible understanding of psychical normality.

Concerning intervention, it must be stressed that one of the aims of every theory existing in the field of normality/non-normality is either to enhance specific methods of intervention or to take a stand in regard to the already existing methods. The ability of a theory to advance methods of intervention has become one of the criteria for evaluation of the theory. From the philosophical standpoint, all the existing theories take for granted that a model is a reflection of concrete reality and that one can apply deductions made from a model back to that reality. Historically, this position resulted from the fact that the theorists in this field went from practice to model-building.

Before turning to the specific explanations of psychopathology, let us check the use of different sources of knowledge in the major approaches to the field. Intellectual knowledge is used in every approach, of course. But even 'the obvious' is used in different ways. On the one hand, the adherents of the medical and the normative models emphasize the use of positivist method in science – i.e. mainly deduction and quantification. On the other hand, the adherents of the existential approach and of psychoanalysis (to a lesser degree) put their emphasis on induction – though their ways of induction differ greatly.

Experiential knowledge is used primarily by the followers of the anti-normative and the existential models. They use this type of knowledge to enhance their insight into another's subjective experience. The insight thus gained is employed later in the attempt to help the other in integrating his experiences. The same process takes place in psychoanalysis. Experiential knowledge is used completely differently in the medical approach. There it becomes a technical tool for checking the appearance of empirically known evidence that indicates specific states of psychopathology. Its meaning for the person–patient is denied. Explicitly, *Weltan-schauung* is not considered as an inherent part of any model. On the contrary, its elimination is claimed. As such, *Weltanschauung* has not yet been used (its 'non-official' uses were pointed out above).

(d) Explanations of the field

A model of normality and non-normality has to take account of and attempt to explain the following issues: (1) Processes of de-cisions made concerning normality, e.g. categorization (see page 103) including diagnosis; (2) the place of individual responsi-bility and free will in phenomena of deviancy and psychopathology; (3) the relationship between rationality and irrationality in pheno-mena of accepted normality and psychopathology; (4) the role of society as a factor exercising power in the field; (5) the relative place of social-psychological and physiological (biological) factors involved in the phenomena studied. The last issue is directly con-nected with the search for causes. At the present time, we know of only a very few causes – all of them somatic – leading directly to a specific pathology. We do not have any methodological procedure for identifying empirically a group of specific factors and studying them in isolation to discover whether they produce the pheno-menon in question. The reference is to a group of factors rather than to a single factor, because we have learned so far that more than one factor influences a given phenomenon. We have evidence concerning the operation of factors, but we can only *deduce* the causality we assume to underlie it.

The issues mentioned above are, once again, interconnected. A stand taken in regard to one implies implicit attitudes towards the others. The main theories differ in many aspects, the majority of which can be deduced with reasonable exactness from their characteristic definitions of normality.

In the model of traditional psychiatry, for example, normality is defined as the absence of disease.[32] We can deduce from this definition that non-normality means illness; that a system of diagnostic categories of illnesses and methods of treating patients will be needed. Such a system and method were, in fact, developed and elaborated by scholars using this model. The concept of disease is adopted from somatic medicine and, accordingly, an ill person is irresponsible, does not act upon his free will, and is in need of being cured in a way unknown to him. The causes of illness are somatic, though the symptoms may also be psychological; therefore the treatment must be physical. The patient's subjective feelings do not count much, because they are products of the true illness and its causes. The illness is viewed as a biological process which should come to termination after a successful medical treatment. Because the patient is both irresponsible and ill, society has to take care of him for society's sake as well as his own. Thus society is allowed to enforce hospitalization for indeterminate periods. Once a patient is cured, he is capable of going back to 'normal life'.

This account, neat and simple as it sounds, does not explain on the conceptual level the processes leading to the social decision about normality, the issue of rationality and irrationality, and the ambivalence expressed by treating the patient as irresponsible and yet blameworthy for uncooperativeness. On the more practical level it does not explain the high percentage of rehospitalization, or the appearance of mental illness in a specific population and its relative absence in another.[33] Using its own method of study, traditional psychiatry has not proved, as yet, the somatic origin of the majority of mental illnesses. More is known about the effects of pharmacological treatment on mentally ill patients than about the aetiology of mental illnesses. These effects are negative as well as positive from point of view of a patient returning to his premorbid level of functioning. But the causes for these effects have not been studied because the adherents of this model deny the existence of independent psychic phenomena (which are not solely products of the somatic one) as well as of independent social phenomena which influence normality, deviance, and psychopathology. Because of shortage of space, the other existing models will not be described. I shall simply state their definitions of normality, leaving it to the reader to deduce the impact of each definition along the lines stated above. Thus, normality is defined in the normative and anti-normative models as social conformity.[34] In psychoanalysis it is defined as the domination of the conscious over the unconscious.[35] Definitions of normality hardly appear in the literature of existential psychiatry. The reasons for their rarity are twofold: (1) partly because mental illness is recognized as one mode of life among others; (2) partly because normality is viewed in this conceptual framework as a normative term, used by social groups as an instrument of discrimination between individuals, and, as such, as dangerous.[36]

Though the existing models cover a wide range of phenomena and explanations, there is not as yet, in my view, a satisfying model along the lines stated above (i.e. including the three sources of knowledge and giving a causal explanation of the main processes in the field).

Many may feel it desirable to cease using the concept of normality, but since we are selective about our experiences, and therefore need rules of selection, this concept has a functional utility. For this reason, it will retain its power, even if we deny its reality. We can aim, however, at reducing the element of rigid and indeed harsh categorization that it carries with it at present. Such a reduction can be achieved only slowly and by education towards tolerance of ambiguity in all fields of human interaction.

NOTES AND REFERENCES

1 See HARRIMAN, P. L. *The New Dictionary of Psychology*. N.Y., Philosophical Library, 1943, p. 240, and p. 3 for the definition of 'abnormal'.

2 ALLPORT, G. *The Nature of Prejudice*, N.Y., Doubleday Anchor, 1958, p. 3.

3 SULLIVAN, H. S. *The Interpersonal Theory of Psychiatry*, N.Y., Norton, 1953.

4 SCHUTZ, A. *Collected Papers. I: The Problem of Social Reality*, The Hague, Nijhoff, 1962.

5 SCHUTZ, A. *Collected Papers*. op. cit., p. 67.

6 GOULD, J. & KOLB, W. L. *Dictionary of the Social Sciences*, London, Tavistock, 1964, pp. 573–7.

7 ELIADE, M. *The Myth of The Eternal Return*, N.Y., Pantheon Books, 1965.

8 FOUCAULT, M. *Madness and Civilization*, London, Tavistock, 1967.

9 ERIKSON, K. T. 'Notes on the Sociology of Deviance' in Becker, H., *The Other Side*, Glencoe, Ill., Free Press, 1964, pp. 9–22.

10 ERIKSON, E. *Childhood and Society*, N.Y., Norton, 1950, pp. 110–15.

11 Anxiety is a very complex concept, and is variously defined, usually as unpleasant feelings, differentiated from fear by being referred to as 'non-specific fear'. I am here following Sullivan's conceptualization of anxiety as a range of unpleasant feelings. These feelings differ in their intensity and therefore in their

influence upon us. They arise out of emotional disturbances whose origin is in disturbances in interpersonal relationship. In their most acute and primary form these feelings may be regarded as uncanny emotion, characterized by feelings of awe, dread, horror, and loathing (Sullivan, p. 10). Anxiety accompanies every one of us and is focused on different content areas in different periods of one's life, as well as differing in intensity according to one's personality and specific history of interpersonal relationships (for reference see note 3, op. cit., pp. 3–12).

12 VOGEL, E., & BELL, N. 'The emotionally disturbed Child as the family Scapegoat', in BELL, N., & VOGEL, E. (eds), *A Modern Introduction to the Family*, Glencoe Ill., Free Press, 1970, pp. 382–97. See also SCOTT, R. D. & ASHWORTH, P. L. ' "Closure" at the first Schizophrenic Breakdown: a Family Study', *Brit. J. med. Psychol.*, 1967, **40**, pp. 109–45.

13 GOFFMAN, E. *Asylums*, N.Y., Doubleday Anchor, 1961.

14 GOFFMAN, E. *Where the Action Is*, London, Allen Lane the Penguin Press, 1969.

15 SCHEFF, T. *Being Mentally Ill*, Chicago, Aldine, 1966, pp. 128–68.

16 KATZ, J., GOLDSTEIN, J., & DERBHOWITZ, N. M. *Psychoanalysis, Psychiatry and Law*, N.Y., Free Press, 1967.

17 ERIKSON, K. T. 'Notes on the Sociology of Deviance', op. cit. note 9.

18 For example, see EYSENCK, H. J., & PRELL, D. B. 'The Inheritance of Neuroticism: an Experimental Study', *J. Ment. Sci.*, 1951, **97**, pp. 441–65.

19 LAING, R. D. *The Divided Self*, London, Tavistock, 1960.

20 SPENCE, K. W. 'A Theory of Emotionally Based Drive and its Relation to Performance in Simple Learning Situations', *Amer. Psyche*, 1958, **13**, 131–41.

21 MOWRER, O. H. 'The Basis of Psychopathology', in Spielberger, C. (ed), *Anxiety and Behavior*, New York, Academic Press, 1966, pp. 143–55.

22 MANDLER, G., & WATSON, D. L. 'Anxiety and the Interruption of Behavior', in Spielberger, C. (ed), *Anxiety and Behavior*, op. cit., pp. 263–87.

23 For example, see SECHEHAYE, M., *Autobiography of a Schizophrenic Girl*, N.Y., Grune & Stratton, 1951.

24 EYSENCK, H. J. *Uses and Abuses of Psychology*, Harmondsworth, Penguin Books, 1953, pp. 221–42.

25 VAN KAAM, A. *Existential Foundations of Psychology*, N.Y., Image Books, 1969, pp. 305–37.

26 NAGEL, E. *The Structure of Science*, London, Routledge and Kegan Paul, 1961, pp. 447–502.

27 For an example of how the exposition of the researcher's biases may help in shaping his study see MYRDAL, G., *A Report from a Chinese Village*, London, Heinemann, 1965, pp. 13–26.

28 For the accepted definition in psychiatry as well as for a discussion of its elements, see RELICH, F. S., 'The Concept of Health in Psychiatry', in LEIGHTON, A. H., CLAUSEN, J. A., & WILSON, R. N., *Explorations in Social Psychiatry*, N.Y., Basic Books, 1957, pp. 138–66, especially pp. 143–6.
29 CLINARD, M. (ed), *Anomie and Deviant Behavior*, Glencoe, Ill., Free Press, 1964, pp. 1–56.
30 KUBIE, L. S. 'The Fundamental Nature of the Distinction between Normality and Neurosis', *Psychoanal. Quart.* **23**, pp. 167–204, 1954.
31 LAING, R. D. *The Politics of Experience and the Bird of Paradise*, Harmondsworth, Penguin Books, 1967.
32 See note 28.
33 The type of social problems involved in mental disturbances and illnesses is exemplified in studies like those of HOLLINGSHEAD, A., & REDLICH, F., *Social Class and Mental Illness*, N.Y., Wiley, 1958, or LEIGHTON, D. C., HARDING, J. S., MACKLIN, D. B., MACMILLAN, A. M., & LEIGHTON, A. H., *The Character of Danger*, N.Y., Basic Books, 1963.
34 See note 29.
35 See note 30.
36 For the first issue, see BINSWANGER, L. *Being in the World*, New York, Torchbooks, 1963. For the second, see note 31.

Comment

JOHN D. DAVIS and MARCIA L. DAVIS

Mrs Ramon reminds us forcefully in her paper of a point that we, as clinicians, are apt to forget: psychological normality and abnormality are not qualities that reside in an individual, but are attributions made by one person about another (or about himself). To understand such attributions, it is not sufficient to refer to the characteristics of the person about whom they are made; they arise from the impact he makes on the attributor and therefore depend equally on the attributor's characteristics. Where an attribution is idiosyncratic, the idiosyncratic characteristics of the attributor must be considered; where consensus exists within a group or culture as to the circumstances in which an attribution is appropriate, the distinctive characteristics of the group or culture must be considered.

In clinical practice we act as agents of the society in which we live and take its implicit rules and values for granted; psychological abnormality, reified in persons, is a social problem, and the terms of our contract require us to deal with the problem by altering the beliefs, feelings, and behaviours of abnormal individuals so as to restore them to normality. The insights provided by Mrs Ramon widen our possibilities for action: where attributions of abnormality are idiosyncratic, we can focus our treatment on the attributor as well as on the attributee – we are beginning to do this in family therapy; where attributions of abnormality are collectively endorsed, we can attempt to deal with the problem by making abnormality permissible, by changing the consensually agreed rules for its attribution, or by abolishing normality-abnormality as an attributive category – to do so we must question

120

the implicit rules and values of our society, abandon the psychiatric hospital, and enter arenas of education, social reform, or revolution. But although recognition of the relativity of concepts of normality and abnormality frees us to choose among such courses of action, responsible choice requires a proper understanding of the social psychology and sociology of the attribution process, or perhaps its phenomenology.

In exploring this process Mrs Ramon suggests that attributions of psychological abnormality are mediated by the attributor's experience of anxiety when his (consensually agreed) constructions of experience and reality are threatened. We feel that this formulation is too limited: an attribution of abnormality may be precipitated, not by one, but by a variety of dysphoric experiences in the attributor, including fear, anger, disappointment, and embarrassment. In these cases treatment of the attributee serves primarily to alleviate the distress of the attributor. In addition, however, an attribution of abnormality may be prompted by the attributor's experience of concern, pity, or compassion – an empathic response to the suffering of the attributee; in this case treatment is aimed primarily at relieving the distress of the attributee. In practice these disparate bases for attributions of abnormality tend to be inextricably entangled, and even where an attribution of abnormality is made about the self, it is difficult to ascertain to what extent it is an echo of social condemnation by others or a pure statement of personal suffering. Thus the clinical practitioner is cast in the incompatible roles of law-enforcer and protector of public sensibilities on the one hand and of spiritual aide or secular priest on the other. The untenability of his position generally passes unrecognized.

Mrs Ramon's analysis appears to be aimed at attributions of a particular kind of abnormality – madness, insanity, or (in the trade) schizophrenia – and here, we feel, the analysis is more penetrating. The need to impose a structure on the chaos of raw experience, to attach meaning to the experienced world, to predict and control events, is imperative. Through consensual validation of our constructions we seek to solidify external reality and thereby our selves. Self-attributions of madness, we believe, attend the loss of such certainty and the experience of alienation when our constructions are felt to be arbitrary, fragile, or different from others'; attributions of madness to others may arise, as Mrs Ramon suggests, from a threat to our constructions of the world, but we would not regard such attributions as projections. More often the madman alarms us because we cannot trust him to obey our consensually agreed rules governing social interaction; by abusing the rules he deprives us of the possibility of predicting and controlling the course of our encounters with him. We fear that he may give expression in his behaviour to the impulses we deny in ourselves – this is the projection of irrationality, the shadow, of which Mrs Ramon speaks – and we may attribute madness to ourselves if we experience a loss of control over such impulses.

With regard to the formulation of theories of psychological normality and abnormality, we strongly endorse Mrs Ramon's injunction to recognize the existence of a variety of avenues to knowledge. Ultimately, however, knowledge is a construction we put on our experience and may be private or governed by rules consensually agreed within groups or cultures; thus by different sources of knowledge we refer to alternative modes of construing. Knowledge obtained from different sources is therefore disjunctive, and epistemologies are a matter of personal or social preference. In presenting the possibility of experiential knowledge, Mrs Ramon need be neither apologetic nor defiant towards scientific method; there are no God-given rules of the game. However, while no one modality of understanding is inherently more valid than another in respect of some illusory criterion of apprehending the true nature of a phenomenon, different modalities may be useful for different purposes. A consideration of such utilities would have been valuable.

Mrs Ramon reminds us, finally, that a theory of psychopathology not only has a manifest content, but also lays bare the *Weltanschauung* of the theorist. We feel that in appraising the theory it is essential to be aware of such a *Weltanschauung*, but ultimately we must accept it in silence; the ghost in the machine cannot be exorcized.

© *John D. Davis and Marcia L. Davis 1972*

Marx's Economics as a Newtonian Model

MICHAEL BARRATT BROWN

This essay will be concerned mainly with Marx's economics but it is impossible to understand him in this field except in relation to his general view of society and its development. For it was precisely Marx's relating of the political economy at any time and place to its sociology and history that distinguishes his thought from most modern economics.

I. MARX'S GENERAL THEORY

Marx's major work was concerned with 'the system of bourgeois economy', as he called it in his Preface to *A Contribution to the Critique of Political Economy* (1859), of which *Capital* (1867) was, he says, 'the continuation'.[1] In the word 'system' there is already implied what he goes on to analyse in the Preface to the Critique as the latest of several successive historical social formations. He designates these as 'so many epochs in the progress of the economic formation of society'.[2] In this Preface to the Critique, Marx provides the most succinct statement of his general theory, of the 'leading thread in my studies' as he calls it. The phrasing is extremely tight and indicates a very precise schema, which is shown in *Figure 1*. The essence of this general theory is just this, that human history can be divided into epochs in each of which it is possible to distinguish a system or social formation with an economic structure 'corresponding to a definite stage of development of (man's) material powers of production'.[3] Marx distinguishes 'the Asiatic, the ancient, the feudal and the modern bourgeois modes of production'. Between each of these systems or epochs Marx's

123

Figure 1   Marx's schema of social structure and development (Source
O. Lange, *Political Economy*, p. 33, derived from Marx, Preface to *A
Contribution to the Critique of Political Economy*)

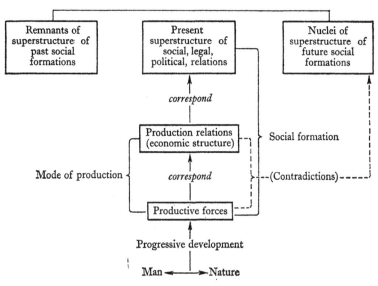

Social consciousness
(social ideas: conscious social relations and attitudes)

historical studies led him to see the transformation as a sharp
break, a period of social revolution, and from this could therefore
be predicted the revolution from the bourgeois mode of production in a capitalist society to a socialized mode of production
in a communist society.[4]

Marx envisages these epochs as stages in a progressive development just in so far as they represent stages of man's technological
advance, as we should now call it; and this undoubtedly is unilinear. He does not suggest that all societies must go through all
the stages, nor that conquest might not disturb the order, but
only that the economic structure of any society (the relations of
human beings in production) must correspond to its technical
process of production. If it does not, 'at a certain stage of their
development, the material forces of production in society come
in conflict with the existing relations of production or – what is but
a legal expression for the same thing – with the property relations

within which they had been at work before'.[5] For Marx the essential point that distinguished his general theory from that of his Hegelian predecessors was that it was out of changes from below in the material conditions of life, and not out of changes from above in the 'so-called general progress of the human mind', that 'legal relations and forms of state' were to be understood. 'The mode of production in material life', he says,[1] 'determines the general character of the social, political and spiritual processes of life.'[6]

It is only the general character that is determined and the whole mode of production is the determinant. On the other hand, the way Marx writes suggests a number of corresponding structures at different levels – as they are shown in *Figure 1*. The base of productive forces, to which the economic structure of production relations correspond – these together making up the mode of production – and above that a superstructure with corresponding definite forms of social consciousness – the whole constituting a single social formation. We may quote the crucial sentences together because we have to decide here on the meaning Marx is giving to the two words 'correspond' and 'determine' if we are to understand the essence of Marx's general theory.

'. . . In the social production which men carry on they enter into definite relations that are indispensable and independent of their will; these relations of production correspond to a definite stage of development of their material powers of production. The sum total of these relations of production constitutes the economic structure of society – the real foundation on which rise legal and political superstructures and to which correspond definite forms of social consciousness.'[7]

The line of correspondence is thus clearly upwards, but Marx does not say that each separate level is determined by the one below. If it were, change would be economically determined. For each level has to correspond with the one below and not conflict with it. The material forces of production in society are always developing and at a certain stage of their development they may come into conflict with the existing relations of production. Marx goes on: 'From forms of development of the forces of production these relations turn into their fetters. Then comes the period of social revolution. With the change of the economic foundations the entire immense superstructure is more or less rapidly transformed.'[8] It is the economic structure in Marx's view that is overturned and it is in this structure of property relations that Marx finds the generator of social change – in the struggle of classes.

This immediately raises a question. Since man is himself inside any model of the social sciences there must be room for a feedback of his consciousness into the working of the model. How then can it be the material conditions that *determine* this consciousness?

Marx goes on to provide his answer:

'The distinction should always be made between the material transformation of the economic conditions of production which can be determined with the precision of natural science, and the legal, political, religious, and aesthetic or philosophic – in short ideological – form in which men become conscious of this conflict [of the forces and relations of production, M.B.B.] and fight it out. . . .'

So Marx says 'this consciousness must rather be explained from the *contradictions* of material life, from the existing *conflicts* between the social forces of production and the relations of production' (my emphasis M.B.B.).[9] Thus, in *Figure 1*, consciousness is shown as deriving from not only the existing social formation but from the superstructure of past social formations and from what Oscar Lange, whose schema the figure reproduces, called 'the nuclei of superstructure of future social formations'.[10] This last is fed by a broken line reflecting the appearance of contradictions between the existing economic relations and the development of productive forces. Lange makes the broken line emerge from the economic structure, which suggests a much more deterministic relationship than I think Marx meant. It seems to me clear that it is from the conflict that the feedback of consciousness derives. It is by their understanding of these new forces and by their control over them that a new class of men became historically agents of social change.

Marx was, however, not prepared to leave his predictions of the future course of social change to such tenuous connections. Within his general theory and at the heart of it there is the economic structure whose transformation 'can be determined with the precision of natural science'. When Marx came to write the Preface to *Capital* he says that 'it is the ultimate aim of his work, to lay bare the economic law of motion of modern society – it can neither clear by bold leaps, nor remove by legal enactments, the obstacles offered by the successive phases of its normal development. But it can shorten and lessen the birth-pangs.'[11] These laws then are something independent of the will of individuals. 'My standpoint is one', says Marx, 'from which the evolution of the economic formation of society is viewed as a process of natural history.'[12]

The economic laws that Marx enunciated in *Capital*, 'The Law of Value', 'The Law of Property', 'The Law of Capitalist Accumulation', 'The Law of Increasing Misery', 'The Law of the Declining Rate of Profit', 'The Law of Wages' – all these are manmade and not 'laws of nature', but they are not consciously manmade. When production comes to be socialized, when 'the extraneous objective forces that have hitherto governed history pass under the control of man himself, only from that time will man himself, with full consciousness, make his own history'.[13] In the meantime Marx is describing a self-regulating system and 'it is a question of these laws themselves, of these tendencies, working with iron necessity towards inevitable results'.[14] Between the different levels of interconnected structures in Marx's schema of society, then, the necessary conditions are not deterministic. Inside the economic structure the laws are much more mechanically applied.

In his general theory Marx seems to be reflecting Darwin's thought. Just as species cannot survive unless adapted to their environment, so societies cannot develop without adapting the relations of production to the forces of production. In his model of the economic structure Marx seems to be following Newtonian concepts. Two examples may suffice, both taken from *Capital*, Volume 1. 'In the form of society now under consideration, the behaviour of men in the social process of production is purely atomic.'[15] 'As the heavenly bodies, once thrown into a certain definite motion, always repeat this, so it is with social production. . . .'[16] Of course, Marx was perfectly aware that he was abstracting from reality. 'In the analysis of economic forms, moreover, neither microscopes nor chemical reagents are of use. The force of abstraction must replace both.'[17] And the whole of Marx's major work is devoted to the elucidation of what can in one sense be described as a Newtonian model. In another sense of course the speed at which it runs down is expected to be faster than that implied in the second law of thermodynamics.

It is impossible to separate what we have been calling Marx's economic model from his general theory, at least in his own thought in his day. What we do now in applying Marx's thought to our own times will depend upon the predictive power of the model; not simply on whether it is a useful aid to description, as the analogies from physics may have appeared to Marx. The Newtonian model of the physical world, it must be emphasized, although now superseded, remains an extremely powerful instrument of prediction. This has most recently been demonstrated by man's successful orbiting and landing on the moon. Marx's model, although now superseded, might still have useful powers.

Before we leave Marx's general theory and look at this economic model, it is worth putting down schematically the apparent relation between theory and model as we have been using the words. With a given theory and selected facts, a model is here used to yield predictive hypotheses. The test of the consistency or inconsistency of the predictions with events can be used to modify the theory and the selection of facts. The predictions themselves may, of course, alter some of the facts. The usefulness of the model depends on its fruitfulness in yielding hypotheses which prove to be consistent with events. In the third section of this paper we shall test Marx's economic model for fruitfulness and consistency with events. Now we need to look more closely at it.

II. MARX'S ECONOMIC MODEL OF THE CAPITALIST SYSTEM

Enough has already been said about Marx's general theory of society for it to be clear that he feeds into his economic model a quite specific set of socio-economic assumptions. Given the historical and sociological assumptions, the economic development seems to him inevitable. For the bourgeois or capitalist economy these assumptions include the following: production is for the market, incomes are unequal, large sums of capital are accumulated (free from real estate), the means of production are in relatively few hands, labour is itself a commodity to be bought and sold (free from feudal ties, etc.) and a class of capitalists exist who are motivated, or rather driven, to make money in a particular way. It is this last which gives Marx the driving force of his model and the title of his work, the drive to capital accumulation. This is the most necessary and central feature of the capitalist system, what makes it indeed a *capitalist* system.

Marx's method of work was to proceed from historical studies to greater and greater abstraction in the revelation of essential laws of development and variation.[18] 'My results have been won by means of a wholly empirical analysis based on a conscientious critical study of political economy,'[19] is how he opens his first economic work. Thus the *Contribution to the Critique of Political Economy* (1859) and *Capital* itself (1867) followed after the historical studies in the *Grundrisse* (the ground plan of *The Critique of Political Economy*) which Marx composed in 1857–8. Marx's method of presentation, however, was to proceed from the abstract to the concrete. Thus at every stage in *Capital* the analysis is presented in its bare essentials and then clothed with factual material; and the first and most difficult theoretical chapters of *Capital* precede the historical exposition in the last hundred pages of Volume I.

We therefore find the essential workings of Marx's economic model laid out in the early chapters on the basis of certain historical assumptions about society. He first analyses the nature of the commodity, as something having both value in use and a market or exchange value, and then considers the exchange of commodities in the market through the medium of money. 'The circulation of commodities,' he says, 'is the starting point of capital.'[20] Into the life of a precapitalist economy Marx asks us to imagine commodity exchange developing, the market becoming ever wider and money becoming capital, not landed property or stored up treasure, but a new kind of wealth. This new wealth arises from the historical emergence of manufacturing production in a society already divided into a relatively small number of owners and a large number of labourers. But now the capital–labour relationship replaces in importance the land–labour relationship, and merchant capital is soon replaced by industrial capital. In other words capital is most profitably employed in setting men to work for wages to produce commodities for sale on the market. Labourers can find employment and a living only by going to work for the owners of capital. The two essential elements in Marx's model have been established – wage labourers and capitalists. They are set in an 'antagonistic struggle' in which 'victory goes necessarily to the capitalist. The capitalist can live longer without the worker than the worker without the capitalist.'[21]

The capitalist's money is not hoarded, not used to buy goods, nor to buy labour to produce goods for the capitalist's own use; it is used to produce goods for the market. Labour is a commodity to be bought on the market to produce more commodities to be sold on the market, the object of the whole exercise being for the capitalist to end up with more money than he started with. Otherwise it is pointless. Marx sums up the position for the labourer and for the capitalist in two simple formulae:

1 The labourer must sell his labour or some other Commodity to get Money to buy Commodities with which to live, i.e. C-M-C.
2 The capitalist uses his Money to buy Commodities, including labour, to make more Money, i.e. M-C-M'.

Marx is not concerned with the motivation of individual capitalists. 'We shall see first,' he says, 'how the capitalist by means of capital exercises his governing power over labour; then, however, we shall see the governing power of capital over the capitalist himself.'[22] The reason for this latter development is the competition between the capitalists. This is a further crucial assumption in Marx's model. Each capitalist must make sure that his products sell and sell at a profit. Each will try to widen his market and reduce his costs. Moreover, since the process of production is a lengthy one, the capitalist will at any time have money laid out and will be forced to continue producing and reinvesting his profits to recoup what he has originally laid out. If his business is prospering he may sell up and retire. What he cannot do in a competitive system is to pass on his losses, by raising his prices as a merchant may, or by lowering his payments to labour beyond a certain point or he will lose his customers in the first case and his labour in the second. He is thus driven to reduce costs by improving his machinery and widening the market for his product.

The detail of the argument is not important for our purpose. What matters is to understand how Marx has set up his economic model. The historically and sociologically determined elements – wage labourers and capitalists – are not the same as labour and capital. That is the 'fetishism', as Marx calls it,[23] of commodity exchange which conceals the owner behind the thing that is offered on the market. But the capitalists and wage labourers are forced to act like atoms or heavenly bodies in determinate ways according to the laws of the system. Newton did not question how the solar system began but postulated a first cause. Marx, of course, questioned the origins of the capitalist system, as we have seen, but for the purposes of his economic model he starts from given elements with a certain essential nature that he has identified. Like Newton who isolated the *mass* of the heavenly bodies as the one aspect of their structure which he needs to know, so Marx isolated, as the essential elements of his system, those contained in the commodity sold on the market; on the one hand, the necessity of the labourer to offer his labour for sale as a commodity and, on the other, the necessity of the capitalist to accumulate. From these elements Marx derived the 'law of wages' and the 'law of capitalist accumulation'. Given these elements then their trajectory is determined, and calculations can be made similar to those which Newton made of velocity, acceleration, and force, to predict the results in time and space.

The whole working of Marx's model is contained within one law – the law of value – which is reminiscent of the law of the conservation of motion in the Newtonian system. There are in effect no leaks. Now, whereas Marx's 'law of wages' and 'law of capitalist accumulation' are quite specific to Marx's model, arising as they do from his socio-economic analysis, the law of value can readily be rewritten in terms of equilibrium analysis. In a market economy without any major element of state planning, the law of value is the equilibrating tendency of the forces at work at certain levels of prices (or exchange ratios of commodities), at certain levels of activity (or quantities of goods produced) and with a certain mixture of resources. Marx writes of individual capitalists:

'Since these meet one another only as owners of commodities, and every one seeks to sell his commodity as dearly as possible (being apparently guided in the regulation of his production by his own arbitrary will), the internal law enforces itself merely by means of their competition, by their mutual pressure upon each other, by means of which the various deviations are balanced. Only as an internal law, and from the point of view of the individual agents as blind law, does the law of value exert its influence here and maintain the social equilibrium of production in the turmoil of its accidental fluctuations.'[24]

For Marx this equilibrium lies behind the surface equilibrium of market prices which reflect only short-term supply and demand. In the long run commodities will be exchanged according to the proportion of any society's labour that is incorporated in them at the current average levels of productivity. Of course, this is only an abstract concept – involving what Marx calls 'socially necessary labour-time', being that required 'to produce an article under the normal conditions of production and with the average degrees of skill and intensity prevalent at the time (i.e. using modern machinery)'.[25] This is the basis of Marx's labour theory of value and has been widely disparaged for example by Joan Robinson[26] as a metaphysical concept. To talk of the labourer not receiving the 'true value' of his product, she says, was a source of inspiration for a whole historical movement but of no scientific value. Subsequently, in the form of 'dated labour'[27] and computer shadow prices,[28] Marx's concept of socially necessary labour-time has come into its own to provide not only an explanation of exchange ratios or prices, but a measure of them for use in conscious regulation of a socialized economy.

This is to go beyond what Marx directly envisaged, but it serves to emphasize that the labour content of commodities is for Marx what the mass of a body is for Newton. This is why Marx starts *Capital* with his analysis of commodities as a 'form of value in general' – that is, 'the reduction of all kinds of actual labour to their common character of being human labour generally, of being the expenditure of human labour power'.[29]

Once this is given, Marx can embark upon examining the trajectory of the bodies containing varying proportions of general labour, that is the circulation of commodities. In a static equilibrium, or what Marx calls simple commodity production, commodities are exchanged for money to buy other commodities (C-M-C). The commodities in both cases have exchange value but the second group have greater use value than the first. Production is for consumption. The equilibrium for simple commodity production to continue is that the amount of social labour that is used up in production balances the amount of social labour that is used up in consumption. Even though money is used for exchange and goods are brought to the market 'on spec', and not bartered, whatever is produced is sold. This cannot be guaranteed but it is the limiting term of the law of value. If too much of any particular product appears, or too little, this is soon rectified when producers can switch easily from one line of production to another.

What Marx insists on is that the extension of the capitalist system all over the world and the rising organic composition of capital (i.e. the proportion of machines to labour power – what Marx calls Constant to Variable Capital or C/V) constantly creates a reserve army of labour, that is of men unemployed in

Figure 2   Simplified diagram of Marx's model of economic activity

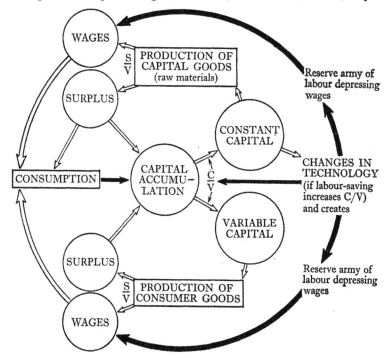

partial or general crises of reproduction.[30] It is this which acts always to depress real wages and, taken together with the attempts of capitalists to maintain and increase the surplus for accumulation (Marx's Surplus to Variable Capital or S/V), this which leads to crisis and breakdown in the system. For it to be worth the capitalist's while to lay out capital, the goods he produces must be sold at a profit, but it is to the workers themselves whose wages are being depressed that the goods have to be sold.

We can attempt to show the working of Marx's economic model in a simplified diagram. Capital accumulation is the dynamo of the system. The white arrows indicate flows of the capital laid out. The black arrows represent forces working upon the capitalists at the centre: consumption of goods makes it worth while for the capitalists to lay out their capital on production both of consumer goods and of capital goods. Changes in technology work both on the organic composition of capital (C/V) and on the rate of surplus (S/V) tending to reduce the powers of consumption which alone make the capital accumalation meaningful since profit $= \dfrac{S}{C+V}$.

Finally, to complete Marx's economic model, we must add the tendency of capital accumulation to take place in fewer and fewer hands and for technological advance to mean that production occurs in larger and larger plants. The small self-employed producer is wiped out and then the small company too.

III. TESTS TO BE APPLIED TO MARX'S GENERAL THEORY
    AND ECONOMIC MODEL

It is not intended here to attempt a proper evaluation either of Marx's general theory or of his economic model; but only to suggest tests that might be applied to them. It is not a simple question of establishing whether either is true or false in any easily demonstrated manner. Nor are the two necessarily susceptible of similar tests, since one is a general theory of social change and the other a model of the economy of a particular society. But they are both of the type that Professor Popper has designated as 'historicist',[31] in that they attempt to reveal laws of motion of whole societies. This is an exercise which Popper regards as one that cannot be validated because it cannot be falsified. The predictions themselves are bound to influence the outcome of what is predicted. Man's future knowledge cannot be predicted, so other long-run predictions are pointless. All the social scientist can do is to limit himself to a piecemeal social-engineering type of prediction, limited to precise and currently knowable social conditions, where tests of false or true can be usefully applied as in the physical sciences.[32]

If Popper had been criticizing Marx's rather deterministic economic model only, then the logical test he applies, viz, that Marx proved too much since he himself was inside the model, would be appropriate. But Popper makes it abundantly clear that he is criticizing Marx as a sociologist for his *general* theory of social change, however hedged around it may be with phrases about tendencies and trends. The same test of falsifiability is to be applied to both. Yet, as E. H. Carr has pointed out in a critique of Popper, Popper concedes in a parenthesis that in a 'plurality of interpretations some of them may be distinguished by their *fertility* – a point of some importance'.[33] To which Carr adds: 'It is not *a* point of some importance: it is *the* point, which proves that "historicism" is not so poor after all.'[34]

We shall not then necessarily expect to be able to apply the same tests to Marx's general theory or to his economic model which can be applied to theories and models in the physical sciences or in a narrowly conceived economic science. We may still test them by their fruitfulness. And we shall not be put off by Popper's disparagement of prophesies which are only partly correct, or are made more or less likely by the very act of foretelling.[35] A distinguished historian recently wrote, 'By foreseeing the future we alter it and then falsify our prophecies. Marx does this by correctly predicting what would happen to capitalism if it continued on its actual line.'[36] This must seem reassuring to the Marxists, and the writer gives many telling examples of the fruitfulness of Marx's general theory in yielding what another historian has called 'guiding insights'.[37] But in what sense can we say that Marx did *correctly* predict what would happen to capitalism? Even if long-term prophesies can only guide us to see after the event where matters turned out differently from what was foreseen, this capacity they give us for 'retrodiction'[38] may be as good a test of the usefulness of a prophecy as its successful predictiveness.

Fruitfulness, successful predictiveness, the possibility of retrodiction – can then all supply tests to be applied to Marx's general theory as we have understood it. The tests to be applied to his economic model could be of the same sort, but here it is possible that we might take into account two other tests – first its contribution to the tools of thought available to man in understanding the world, and secondly, the energy which it generates in men to make great social changes. In applying such tests we should be very close to Marx's dialectical materialism. For, as we have seen, what he was insisting on was not that the growth of technology, of man's control over his environment, determines everything else but that the models we build of the world in which we make technology the determining factor help us most in understanding social change and thus in making changes.

'In the study of economic categories as in the case of every historical and social science, it must be borne in mind that as in reality so in our mind the subject, in this case modern bourgeois society, is given and that the categories are therefore but forms of expression, manifestations of existence and frequently but one-sided aspects of this subject, this definite society.'[39]

It is thus the categories that we have to test.

We shall examine first the tests that may be applied to Marx's general theory. Its predictive usefulness is widely supposed to have been undermined by the appearance of the first communist revolution in the least industrially advanced, rather than in the most industrially advanced land. That such a revolution occurred in Russia and subsequently in other *under*developed lands raises important problems for Marxists. But retrodiction is rather more favourable for Marx. On his view we should not have expected a socialist economic structure to emerge from a rather backward industrial economy; and no such socialist structure has emerged. An industrial revolution, not a socialist revolution, was carried out by Stalin, and all except the devotees of the Soviet Union should recognize that this is what Marx would have expected.

The fact that the less-developed countries have not all followed the more developed on the capitalist road of development but some have stagnated in underdevelopment from which non-capitalist solutions seem the only way out would not have surprised Marx either. He expected India to follow where Europe had led once the railway and electric telegraph had begun what he called the process of 'regeneration', but its conclusion was subject to 'throwing off the English yoke'.[40]

Marx evidently expected most countries to have to go through the same 'stages' of social formation as they developed their technological forces. But since the main point for Marx was the developing of human consciousness and the growing conflict between technical forces of production and existing property relations, he would not be surprised at the world-wide eruption of rising expectations. For what modern communications have permitted men everywhere to do is to compare their actual condition with that of the most advanced – their poverty with the capacity of man to circle and land on the moon.

But what of Marx's insistence on the importance of economic class in social change? Since a class is defined as a self-conscious group of men with a certain special relationship to the productive forces, a revolutionary class is one that has a special relationship to the new productive forces and is therefore opposed to and must struggle with the ruling class related to the old forces. Thus the industrial working class, which becomes increasingly skilled, united, and self-conscious under the pressures of capitalist development, is for Marx the revolutionary class. Although in the *Communist Manifesto*, Marx and Engels assume that a 'portion of the bourgeoisie goes over to the proletariat and in particular, a portion of the bourgeois ideologists who have raised themselves to the level of comprehending theoretically the historical movement as a whole',[41] they saw no future for any other class. Fractions of the middle class would be driven one by one into the proletariat or into the 'social scum' whose 'conditions of life prepare it far more for the part of the bribed tool of reactionary intrigue'.[42] Has this happened? Certainly the self-employed middle class has been almost eliminated in most advanced industrial countries and what remains has often 'become the tool of reactionary intrigue'. But what of Burnham's managerial class[43] and Wright Mills's intellectuals?[44]

Marx already foresaw, through the growth of joint stock companies and the concentration of capital, 'the transformation of the actually functioning capitalist into a mere manager, an administrator of other peoples' capital, and of the owners of capital into mere owners, mere money capitalists . . .' reproducing 'a new aristocracy of finance, a new sort of parasites in the shape of promoters, speculators and mere nominal directors'.[45] He assumed, however, that the competitive drive of the system, requiring perpetual capital accumulation, would affect the managing capitalist just as much as the owning capitalist. This was the ground of the argument between C. A. R. Crosland and myself in the early 1960s[46] and all the evidence of merger and take-over in recent years has tended to support my defence of Marx's assumption.[47]

The question of the role of the intellectual is much harder to answer. Are they (we) just a portion of the bourgeois ideologists 'who go over to the proletarians' or have they (we) a revolutionary role in our own right? In most of the underdeveloped countries there has been no proletariat to revolt. In the case of the Russian revolution, the Communist Party became not simply the vanguard but the substitute or 'caretaker', as E. H. Carr has called it, for the few proletarians. The extremely rapid growth in the number of intellectuals in the Soviet Union was required by the infrastructure of industrialization at a late stage in the first industrial revolution. They were needed to provide the bureaucracy of the state, and, as more and more of them have thought to play a truly revolutionary socialist role, their repression by the state and Party organs has apparently been intensified, if we may judge by the cases of Solzhenitsyn, Daniel, Volpin, and others. Even in the state bureaucracy, and here what follows is as true of the capitalist state as of the Soviet state, the role of the state's servants – in medicine, teaching, child care, welfare, literature, and the arts too, as well as in social and economic planning – becomes increasingly ambiguous, as simultaneously servants of the state and quite literally 'social workers'.

In Marx's day the state's functions were limited to law and order – the protection of bourgeois property at home and overseas. Marx simply did not envisage this kind of 'Welfare State' being either possible under capitalism or necessary under socialism. We should be able to test the emergence of a truly socialist society, as Marx would have expected to see it, by its allocation of resources for people to spend for themselves, without direct state control. This is the real meaning of Marx's concept of alienation – the separation of use and value in the process of exchange – which socialism would correct. He did not envisage the emergence of a great number of intellectuals for whom work was an end in itself before the arrival of a socialist state. It is a point of much importance that they have a new and special relationship to the means of production – not as owners or managers, nor as direct production workers. Machines increasingly take the place of production workers as we enter the second industrial revolution. The key men and women are those who design and use the machines, who prepare the computer 'software' and analyse its results, who teach our children and help us to survive in the complexities of modern society. Are they any less proletarians than Marx's industrial proletariat? They own little or no property. They are increasingly at odds with the system of private ownership that frustrates their efforts. They are often as alienated by the market from the results of their work and its social meaning as ever their grandparents were. Today, indeed, the major social decisions are even more remote in the giant multinational company; the growth path of the whole economy being now determined by a tiny number of directors of competing giants whose drive for capital accumulation still determines where and when and how society's capital resources will be laid out. What the new proletarians are *not* is impoverished.

If, then, Marx's general theory continues to provide a fruitful source of conceptual relationships for understanding social change, his economic model was quite evidently misconceived. Of the five main predictions which Marx made from his economic model two were proved right, two wrong, and one remains in doubt.

1 The centralization of capital has taken place and continues indeed more rapidly today than ever;
2 The polarization on a world scale of wealth and poverty has certainly occurred, or at least the gap between rich and poor has certainly widened and the process shows no sign of being reversed;
3 The rate of profit has *not* declined for reasons mainly that Marx himself put forward as counteracting forces, but for other reasons also, which we shall examine;
4 The proportion of workers unemployed – Marx's reserve army of labour – has *not* steadily increased, at least inside the

advanced capitalist countries, as capitalism has developed, nor the insecurity, misery, and impoverishment that goes with unemployment, and if Marx meant to include falling real wages in his prediction of an 'accumulation of misery', this has not occurred either;[48]

5 The cyclical crises of the capitalist system did certainly become more and more severe up to 1929 and 1937, but they have since then certainly been moderated. The results of the next stage of the development of the productive forces in the second industrial revolution, with its strong labour-saving effects, have still to be seen.

The reason for the non-fulfilment of the last three predictions is, of course, to be found in the new role of the state in advanced capitalist economies, and especially in the vast increase in state expenditures. That Marx did not anticipate this was inevitable, given his self-regulating economic model in which the state had no role except the protection of property at home and overseas. It is often argued that Marx underestimated the role of the trade unions in raising their wages relative to the capitalists' surplus.[49] It was Marx's view that 'this resolved itself into the respective power of the combatants';[50] and in 1865 he did not believe that the trade unions would overcome the labour-saving effects of new machinery in constantly undermining the trade unions' power through the influence of the 'industrial reserve army of labour'. Thus there was no force inside the model capable of modifying it. Only the intervention of the state from outside the model could do that.

It is worth devoting a final word to the intervention of the state in capitalist economies, because this might be regarded as a counter-acting force which offsets rather than one which actually modifies the working of Marx's economic model. In that case the increasing tendency in the model to instability would require ever-increasing state intervention. If, on the other hand, the state's intervention profoundly modified the model, then no increase in this intervention would be needed once it was established. The economic intervention of the state has been of six main types:

1 Assistance with labour mobility – Labour Exchanges, housing, re-training, redundancy payments, public sector finance;

2 Support for the incomes of the poor – in sickness, unemployment, and old age;
3 Some redistributive taxation of higher incomes (which has had, however, little or no effect on the distribution of property-ownership);[51]
4 Keynesian management of aggregate demand through monetary and fiscal policies to maintain near-full employment;
5 Support for private industry, through loans and grants, for large-scale investment for research and for development of declining areas;
6 State spending on arms and on the economic infrastructure of education, transport and communications, fuel and power, etc.

American Marxists have for long argued in relation to the falling rate of profit that the capitalists' surplus must be taken to include a high proportion of unproductive expenditure – advertising, packaging, and selling costs as well as the arms bill.[52] Since 1963 the share of the military in total state spending in the USA has been considerably raised. Even before then, the state's share of GNP was accounting for more than half the surplus. What is more important, it was steadily growing over four decades, with major increases after 1947. In Britain the share of the national product passing through the state's hands has grown even faster since the Second World War, to over half of GNP – a share almost twice that in the USA.

Similar figures could be obtained for other advanced capitalist countries. There is no doubting the facts of the rising share of the state in what Marxists would call the economic surplus. And yet there are still great areas of poverty in all capitalist countries, including both Britain and the United States, and there are levels of unemployment varying between 2·5 per cent and 7·5 per cent of the employed population. These obstinate facts, which even a rising share of state spending have been unable to prevent, are hard to explain except on some polarizing model of a Marxian sort. So long as capital accumulation in a competitive market is the driving force of the economy, wealth and poverty, it seems, will continue to develop at opposite poles and the state will be hard put to it to offset these tendencies.

We may conclude that the Newtonian self-regulating model of

the economy which Marx constructed and from which he predicted the ultimate collapse, stagnation, and breakdown of capitalism as an economic system was misconceived. State intervention
could, and to a major extent did, correct its more self-destroying
tendencies. The warning that the model gives us, however, of the
effects of its uncontrolled operation are of more than academic
interest, at a time when the labour-saving effects of automated
production are becoming more marked, and governments in both
the USA and UK have been returned to power on programmes
designed to curb state spending. As automation in industry
advances, James Meade, the Professor of Political Economy at
Cambridge, has drawn the awful prospect for us of what he calls
'The Brave New Capitalists' Paradise':

> 'There would be a limited number of exceedingly wealthy
> property owners; the proportion of the working population
> required to man the extremely profitable automated industries
> would be small; wage rates would thus be depressed; there
> would have to be a large expansion of the production of the
> labour-intensive goods and services which were in high demand
> by the few multi-multi-multi-millionaires; we would be back
> in a super-world of an immiserized proletariat and of butlers,
> footmen, kitchen maids and other hangers-on.'[53]

Meade's argument is conducted in terms of marginal economic
theory, but here the language is Marx's.

We may round this essay off by considering briefly one final
test which we suggested earlier might be applied to Marx's
general theory and economic model – the test of the human
energy generated by them. We cannot live without some organizing
conceptual model of the world. A model of class struggle may seem
to many to be an unattractive one. It has certainly proved an
energizing one, as the power of communist movements the world
over bears witness. It is the fear, moreover, of the gathering danger
of slump and stagnation, if appropriate economic relations are not
found to correspond to changing technology, that forces us to
experiment with new models of democratic planning to replace
the self-regulating market for competitive capital accumulation
as the organizing force in the economy.

NOTES AND REFERENCES

1 MARX, K. Preface to the first edition of *Capital*.
2 MARX, K. Preface to *A Contribution to the Critique of Political Economy*, 1859.
3 Ibid.
4 This is spelled out in Marx's *Critique of the Gotha Programme*, 1875.
5 MARX, K. Preface to *A Contribution to the Critique of Political Economy*, 1859.
6 Ibid.
7 Ibid.
8 Ibid.
9 Ibid.
10 LANGE, O. *Political Economy*, London, Pergamon, 1963, p. 33.
11 MARX, K. Preface to the first edition of *Capital*.
12 Ibid.
13 ENGELS, F. *Anti-Dühring*. London, Lawrence and Wishart, 1955, ed. pp. 392–3.
14 MARX, K. Preface to *Capital*, first edition.
15 MARX, K. *Capital*, vol. I, ch. 2.
16 Ibid. ch. XXV, Section 3.
17 MARX, K. *Capital*, Preface to first edition.
18 See MARX, K. *Capital*, Preface to second edition.
19 MARX, K. *Economic and Philosophic Manuscripts of 1844*.
20 MARX, K. *Capital*, vol. I, ch. 4.
21 MARX, K. *Economic and Philosophic Manuscripts of 1844*, Section 1.
22 Ibid.
23 MARX, K. *Capital*, vol. I, ch. 1, Section 4.
24 MARX, K. *Capital*, vol. III, ch. 51.
25 MARX, K. *Capital*, vol. I, ch. 1, Section 1.
26 ROBINSON, J. *Economic Philosophy*, Chicago, Aldine; London, Watts, 1962, p. 37.
27 SRAFFA, P. *Production of Commodities by Means of Commodities*, New York, Cambridge University Press, 1960, ch. 6.
28 ŚIK, O. *Plan and Market Under Socialism*. White Plains, NY, International Arts & Sciences Press, 1967, Part III.
29 MARX, K. *Capital*, vol. I, ch. 1, Section 3.
30 MARX, K. *Capital*, vol. 1, ch. 25, Section 3.
31 POPPER, K. *The Poverty of Historicism*, London, Routledge & Kegan Paul, 1957.
32 Ibid., Preface and p. 58 ff.
33 POPPER, K. op. cit. p. 130 ff.
34 CARR, E. H. *What is History?* 1961 (Harmondsworth, Penguin, 1964), p. 101.
35 POPPER, K. op. cit. p. 151.
36 KIERNAN, V. 'Notes on Marxism in 1968', *Socialist Register*, London, Merlin, 1968, p. 204.

37 I owe the phrase to Royden Harrison.
38 I owe this phrase also to Royden Harrison.
39 MARX, K. *Introduction to the Critique of Political Economy*, Section 3 on The Method of Political Economy.
40 MARX, K. 'The Future Results of the British Rule in India', *New York Daily Tribune* 8 Aug. 1853, in Marx and Engels, *On Colonialism*, F.L.P.H., London, Lawrence and Wishart, 1960.
41 MARX, K. and ENGELS, F. *Communist Manifesto*, 1848, Section 1.
42 Ibid.
43 BURNHAM, J. *The Managerial Revolution*, London, Putnam, 1941.
44 WRIGHT MILLS, C. *The Causes of World War Three?* New York, Ballantine, 1960. Part IV, The Role of the Intellectuals.
45 MARX, K. *Capital*, vol. II, ch. 27, 'The Role of Credit'.
46 CROSLAND, C. A. R. *The Conservative Enemy*, London, Cape; New York, Shocken, 1962, ch. V and M. BARRATT BROWN 'Mr. Crosland's Enemy', *New Left Review*, No 19, April 1963.
47 See BARRATT BROWN M., 'The Controllers of British Industry', in K. Coates (ed.) *Can the Workers Run Industry?* London, Sphere, 1968, p. 36 ff.
48 MEEK, R. L. *Economics and Ideology*, London, Chapman & Hall, 1967, p. 113 ff., for a discussion of what Marx meant by 'Increasing Misery'.
49 MEEK, R. L. op. cit. p. 118 ff.
50 MARX, K. *Value, Price and Profit*, 1865, Section XIV.
51 See MEADE, J. E. *Efficiency, Equality and the Ownership of Property*, London, Allen & Unwin, 1964, Table 1, p. 27.
52 BARAN, P. and SWEEZY, P. M. *Monopoly Capital*, New York, Monthly Review Press, 1966, pp. 176 and 389.
53 MEADE, J. E. op. cit., p. 33.

Comment

TEODOR SHANIN

Newton's closed systems of physical determinism served as the nineteenth-century basic prototype of successful scholarship. In the biological and social sciences it was linked with evolutionary theories in which change was explained monistically, i.e. by tracing its various aspects to one major factor – a prime mover. Eclecticism was seen as the only alternative to monism and was rejected by the major minds of those times. Marxian dialectical materialism represented a highly sophisticated form of monistic thought, in which the feedback of the 'resultants' on the 'determinant' was acknowledged and discussed.

In the twentieth century determinist theories rapidly fell into disfavour. Models of this type are however both used and useful, subject to understanding of their limitations. Their validity and relevance are related to the theories they came to represent. In our case, both the heuristic strength and weakness of the Marxian model of economic determinism seem to have their root in its broader philosophical and sociological assumptions.

The theoretical insights and the evidence of contemporary scholarship seem to highlight a contradiction between the dialectical and materialist facets of Marxian philosophy. Through interactionist theories a number of basic principles of nineteenth-century dialectics were accepted and developed into major trends of contemporary thought. Such analysis focuses on systems of which the components display specific and irreducible articulation of their own and interact in a structure of mutual feedbacks. Each factor has to be understood therefore in its mutual interaction with others. Furthermore, all that holds true also for the relation between the observer and his data. (Dialectical analysis also accepted and sought some further qualities of reality less relevant to our discussion, e.g. change – generating internal contradictions in each system and qualitative 'leaps' resulting from quantitative changes.) Yet, the basic dialectical–interactionist assumptions make the very idea of materialist monism doubtful if not obsolete. In a well-known metaphor Marx declared his intention to put Hegelian dialectics from its head on its feet, substituting as prime mover, 'matter' for 'general spirit'. Real advance of social analysis was, no doubt, achieved this way but do not the very principles of dialectics put in doubt monism from whichever quarter? Or, in Marx's own language, do complex processes have any 'head' or 'feet' to stand on, or are those relative only, with the character and strength of the feedbacks forming the crux of the matter.

Nor can the simplistic dualism of *either* monism *or* eclecticism of theory be accepted nowadays. Monism provides an important, possibly necessary, and at times, sufficient framework for analysis. The 'richness' of reality may eventually call for multipictorial questions, however. Such questions must not stop at the eclectic listing of factors but can and should proceed to study their hierarchy of significance and structure of interaction. That provided, its preferences may be obvious.

To proceed from philosophical generalization to the social-science issues in hand, it is the division into 'base' (i.e. prime mover) and 'superstructure', with subsequent focusing on the former, which seems to underscale the discussed failures of Marxian prediction. To be sure, the illumination gained by considering the impact of the political economy on major social processes has been considerable. At the same time it was the strengths as well as the specific and relatively autonomous character of the 'superstructure' (the *political relation*, e.g. the state or the trade unions as well as the *social consciousness*, e.g. nationalist ideology or Keynesian economics) which have been mainly responsible for the unanticipated developments of capitalism. The overdeterminist tendencies of some of the Marxian interpretation and analysis are rooted in a rigid base/superstructure pre-assumption. All that may also explain why the Marxian theory initially blurred the issue of 'backward' nations, necessitating the twentieth-century revisions by Lenin, Mao, and others. Not surprisingly, even as orthodox a

Marxist as Althusser suggested recently the notion of 'overdetermination', i.e. of a meeting of interlinking, relatively autonomous factors of both 'base' and 'superstructure' as a necessary condition of social revolution. In such an analysis the acceptance of an economic prime mover, in the final resort, can be in fact painlessly dropped or treated as a declaration of faith rather than a relevant analytical method.

The impact of Marx has been fruitful, powerful, and lasting yet it was he who declared himself once 'not a Marxist'. In that spirit any interpretation of Marx in a new century should move towards critical post-Marxism. Should we not consider therefore in philosophy a new Hegelian 'triad' in which Hegel's dialectical idealism followed by Marx's dialectical materialism may reach its higher stage by outstepping monism of all kinds and 'dialecticizing' further the nineteenth-century dialectics. Or, in the social sciences, to put it visually, would it not be advantageous to try to turn the vertical representation of forces and relations of production–politics–consciousness (*Figure 1*, p. 124) horizontally, manifestly moving the stress of such a model from the order of components to their interaction and relative strength?

© *Teodor Shanin 1972*

Models inherent in History

GORDON LEFF

Historians as a profession are not given to constructing or employing models in any formal or explicit sense; where they do, it is mainly in areas bordering on other disciplines, especially economics and social studies. Most historians, if asked, would probably deny that models had anything to do with their subject. In that they would, I believe, be mistaken. As I hope to show, a historian could hardly put pen to paper without having an implicit model of what he was studying.

The reason for this apparent discrepancy between precept and practice lies in the seemingly empirical nature of history. The object of all historical study is to render a particular area of mans' past intelligible through a coherent reconstruction of what occurred. This can only be done from the records and remains which have survived. In that sense the evidence must determine the scope of any historical inquiry; and to that extent the evidence can be said to shape the writing and study of history as a limiting factor. 'No evidence no history', however, is not the same as 'the evidence is history', which it can too easily become. The sovereignty of the evidence appears the more overwhelming because the historian is entirely dependent upon it: in default of some kind of record – written, oral, physical, linguistic, or whatever – he has no recourse to other sources: he cannot observe or experiment with what no longer exists; in contrast to natural and social scientists he is entirely in the hands of what the past has bequeathed, once and for all. When we add to these disabilities the anthropomorphic terms in which history is written it seems to be little more than the common sense retrojection of the present into the past, for which the most important attributes are a knowledge of the facts, human sympathy, and, if possible, a good literary style. In such a perspective, which historians are prominent in sharing, little remains to the autonomy of history as a distinctive kind of knowledge or to the historian as the agent who fashions history from what would otherwise be an undifferentiated past.

This seems to me to be a false perspective, as I shall try to show. History cannot be systematically studied or written unless the historian observes the criteria which are peculiar to it as a body of knowledge. For that a conceptual framework is necessary, which, however empirically founded, becomes intelligible only through following the same intellectual processes of definition and inference necessary to all conceptual knowledge. That framework is provided by the historian's models, which, as mental constructs imposed upon the evidence, make the facts speak in response to his prompting and not of themselves.

I shall consider first the nature of these models and then briefly their application to historical situations.

Historical models, however diverse, share two main characteristics: they are time-bound and they are comparative. The first is peculiar to history; the second to all the human studies which have man, other than as a biological organism, for their subject. The first is expressed by the contexts in which events occur: the second by the concepts which we apply to men's activities as social beings, taken both generically – as political, economic, military, artistic, intellectual, and so on – and qualitatively, when we evaluate them by terms like progress, decline, turning-point, masterpiece, and so on. Together, the juxtaposition of the contextual with the universal forms a historical category. These can vary from being a mere epoch or period such as Middle Ages or Tudor Age to referring to a specific set of occurrences of greater or less particularity like the Renaissance or the Industrial Revolution or the Seven Years' War. What unites them all is that they are framed in terms of a period of time, which is defined in terms of its epochal characteristics. That brings us to the role of periods, their criteria and their status.

Periodization, the division of the past into spans of time of whatever duration, is to history what axioms are to the formal sciences and probability hypotheses, or laws of universal conditional form, are to the natural sciences. They bring into order a mass of happenings which of themselves have none. By distinguishing sequences of events and cutting them into shapes, the historian is able to give coherence to what would otherwise remain formless. His divisions enable the events of the past, undifferentiated in themselves, to be differentiated into intelligible groupings.

It is important to stress the word intelligible. To understand any occurrence it must be convertible into a sufficient number of terms which explain it. Since any explanation is directed to some-one else, it is a reciprocal process which logically is capable of in-finite regress, each term requiring a further term to define it, if the hearer, like a child, repeatedly asks 'why' to each of them. That does not ordinarily happen because each body of knowledge has its own conventions which set its appropriate level of explanation.

In the case of history it is provided by the conception of an epoch. A historian discussing, for example, the persecution of the Huguenots by Louis XIV will have to explain that they were Protestants in order to make the term persecution intelligible; but that does not in turn commit him to defining what Protestants were or why Catholics should regard them as inimical, or how each came to be opposed to the other, or why religious opponents should persecute one another. All of that is contained within the historian's notion of the epoch which forms his conceptual frame-work: whether he calls it the Age of Absolutism or simply the Reign of Louis XIV, it will include such conceptions as the perse-cution of religious minorities, which establish the appropriate level of explanation, in the same way as, say, nationalism and industrialism help to do so for our epoch. But unlike the categories of the generalizing sciences, periods as categories are both indi-vidual and variable, because the standpoint of history is that of difference; its events have an existential import – whether as the lives of individuals or societies – which can only be characterized, not subsumed. However much historical, like any other, discourse must rely upon general terms they are treated neither causatively nor predictively. The standing presumption of historical study is that its events are sufficiently different to need approaching through their own concatenations.[1] If the persecution of the Huguenots by Louis XIV could be explained merely by invoking the appropriate law for the persecution of religious minorities, there would be no need for their separate study. But that would be to negate the very asssumption that gives the writing or study of history its *raison d'être*, namely that Louis XIV was not just *any* king, that the Huguenots were not just *any* religious minority, that France was not just *any* country, that 1680 to 1690 was not just *any* decade, so that the events contained under the expression 'the persecution of the Huguenots' belong to their own context and no other with which they could be interchanged. It is for that reason that periods are necessary, not as immutable landmarks, but as conventional divisions which help to give history a structure.

That brings us to the second aspect, of how periods are formed. As its simplest, we can say that a period is the outcome of the need to relate generic continuity to temporal discontinuity. On the one hand, the historian is confronted with an institution like the Christian Church which has endured for two millenia; on the other hand, he is equally presented with a church sufficiently different at say AD 400, 800, 1200, and 1500 to require different contexts for its comprehension. Period, as we have said, provides that context, but it can only do so according to some organizing principle, which must be the work of the historian. That makes his choice of context, although demarcated temporally, more than merely temporal. Absolutely every event has its own context, if it is only that of different peas. Formally, context only becomes important when it involves different criteria – the case in differentiating epochs. To identify a sequence of events as a new epoch – whether the reign of a king or a phase in the life of an institution – is to type it by certain characteristics which are considered not to hold in the same way at other times. From that point of view all periodization is comparative and evaluative: it is designed to point to difference and to resume it under a common term.

Now history, beyond – or more properly because of – being the study of man's recorded past, is without inherent unity. It offers rather an irreducible number of histories according to presupposition, topic, and scale. The first of these three is central to the study of history: as one of the human studies a conception of history can never be dissociated from a conception of men; and since there is no exclusive way in which we are bound to conceive men and human affairs so there is no one way in which their history must be treated. In contrast to the natural sciences where for all practical purposes the law of gravity or the boiling point of water are that and nothing else, man's past – as his present – can be viewed from an almost unlimited number of standpoints, Christian, Marxist, liberal, as the unfolding of a divine plan, as having no plan, as the record of progress or of man's follies, vices, and stupidities, and so on, according to the scale of values adopted. These go beyond mere prejudice: they constitute the indispensable prerequisites for history of any kind. History is of its nature anthropomorphic, as the terms – despotism, barbarism, enlightenment, and so on – in which it is written clearly show. It is no more possible to write history without some initial construct of what men are than it is to write it without using words common to all men, like love, war, pride, law. The history of history is testimony to that: for every accepted historical event – a Norman Conquest or a French Revolution – there are innumerable different interpretations, ranging from its status and nature as an event to its place in the scheme of things. The reason in every case is that in the human world facts are inseparable from the evaluations put upon them: for everyone who can agree that a glass if half full there are as many for whom it is half empty. Irreducible individual difference as the constituent of human affairs is also the constituent of history. That is why it is repeatedly rewritten to new presuppositions. That holds for any branch of history. Like anyone else, the historian has a view of the world, however inchoate.

It may be little more than the received prejudices of his age. Even so, merely as a man he can hardly fail to have some conception of man's condition; and as a historian his profession makes some notion of man as a social being inescapable. Whatever the area, no study of history can avoid terms like progress, decline, justice, atrocity, ambition, idealism, dishonesty, and a range of others, all of which imply some scale of valuation. These are no less present for being implicit or frequently so obvious that dissent from them hardly arises. It does not need recourse to an explicit frame of reference to conclude that Periclean Athens was of a higher order of civilization that Visigothic Spain or that Napoleon was a greater general than Marshal Saxe. Yet the very terms 'higher' and 'greater' are part of the historian's stock-in-trade, and imply just such a system of value-judgements. Usually, however, they only become apparent when their applicability is less obvious, above all where moral judgements are concerned. It is when we debate, not so much whether Napoleon was a great general but a good thing, that dispute begins. This leads to the common mis-conception that only moral (and perhaps aesthetic) judgements are value-judgements, whereas in fact they are merely different kinds of value-judgement: it is no less an evaluation to say that 'X was a period of decline' than to say that 'X was good' or 'X was beautiful'. The difference is rather that the first statement does not entail approval or the same degree of commitment by the person making it as the other statements do. The latter therefore offer a greater range of variation. But since many of the most far-reaching events of the past have been the outcome of acts per-formed in the name of moral imperatives, the historian can no more eschew moral issues than any other aspect of human agency. He does not, however, have to be morally committed as an histor-ian, whatever his sympathies as an individual. In writing of the rights and wrongs of the Crimean War a historian is no more a moralist than a general. He is concerned with events which occurred in a context: what he cannot find there he cannot put there, just as he cannot ignore what he finds. It is in that sense that he cannot impose the standards of the present upon the past: as an Anglican or democrat it is as irrelevant historically to condemn the thirteenth century for being Catholic or feudal as to dismiss Aristotle for not knowing Newtonian physics. From that point of view the issue of moral judgements is an irrelevance. That does not mean on the other hand that the historian must succumb to relativism. Unless he has a conception of what he is studying, he could hardly begin to write history. For that, he must have some order of priorities which enables him to place events and measure their significance. That involves some wider view of mankind and history. It is here that the historian's *Weltanschauung* (which is inseparable from his temperament and sympathies) enters into his study, not by introducing mere preconception, but in providing the spectacles through which he looks at the world. Ultimately his outlook must be founded upon his notion of what man is, what he takes to be right and wrong, progress and regress, and so on. According to how these are conceived, as we men-tioned previously, history will be written: in that sense the historian's model of man and his values combine to provide his model of history. To that extent it will also influence his approach to history. Marxist historians tend to concentrate on economic and social history from the standpoint of the exploited classes. The classic form of liberal history on the other hand was institutional and political. Today the stress has moved nearer to the Marxist emphasis, a direct reflection of the preoccupations of contemporary society with social and economic change. But beyond the workings of the *Zeitgeist* – which can be exaggerated – there is the logic of the subject which in its development points to new problems and new fields, usually as the result of individual pioneering and the influence of a powerful personality. In these ways the historian's initial point of departure, like his standpoint and emphases, lies outside history, as he himself must stand outside the events with which he is concerned. Nevertheless, his history, in order to be accepted as history, must be mediated by those events. He must therefore treat them by the criteria and methods which are appropriate, above all through recognizing the norms of the epoch to which they belong, whether they concern thirteenth-century estate management or scholastic philosophy.

Accordingly, the concept of an epoch will be governed by how its events are conceived. For those who considered the Tudor sovereigns as despots, the period covered by their reigns may be characterized as Tudor Despotism; similarly terms like the Age of Enlightened Despots or the Dark Ages take their definition from what are regarded as their dominant traits. But, again in contrast to the natural sciences, the same periods of time may also be evaluated by different or conflicting criteria which can coexist without invalidating each other. Thus for other historians Tudor Despotism may cede to Tudor Constitutionalism, in which the rise of parliament is seen as the main element; others may reject the very notion that seventeenth- and eighteenth-century kings were significantly more enlightened or despotic than their predecessors or successors, and so dismiss the title as inappropriate to the period; others again may invoke quite other criteria which lead to notions like the Reformation or the Scientific Revolution, and so set their temporal boundaries at variance with those of other epochs, one cutting across the other.

All these are common occurrences in the writing and study of history: they owe as much to the framing of new terms of reference as to new evidence. The main changes in history, as in other branches of knowledge, come through the constant interaction between hypothesis and data; a new model like that of say the Scientific Revolution itself transforms the way in which the evidence is treated. But that does not thereby exclude what previously held; it merely superimposes upon the pre-existing model of the age in which it falls a new additional pattern which may be reconcilable with what is already there, or may only, because of radically different criteria, be related temporally as coexisting for a certain time. The unequal coexistence of diverse phenomena is one of the characteristics of history as the study of the past; there is no conceivable means of relating causally styles of hairdressing in Mayfair with coalmining at Wigan: although they are contemporaneous, the history of each is structurally independent of the other since knowledge of one does not presuppose knowledge of the other. Yet in sharing the same epoch they will presuppose certain common terms which help to define both: say the state of the economy, the effects of strikes or inflation, or changing attitudes as they concern fashion and coal. It is that community, bringing diverse things into a contemporal relation, which gives periods their *raison d'être*. Before considering how they operate in actual historical situations we must consider finally their status.

From what has been said it will be apparent that periods are used nominalistically, as labels. No historian, at least, regards expressions like Tudor Despotism or Age of Enlightened Despots as corresponding to something real or as seizing some real essence; he treats them more as summaries, a convenient shorthand for bringing together diverse series of events. Paradoxically, it is because historians are so aware of the conventional and factitious nature of their categories in the light of the real diversity to which they refer that they tend to deny them any independent conceptual standing. What they describe as a battle of a revolution or a reign is taken to coincide so completely with the events which it describes that they are identical. In fact it is the reverse that is true: like Tolstoy's description of war in *War and Peace*, the sequences of events which constitute a battle were not the same for its participants as they are for the historian: it is reserved for him to endow them with seeming coherence, subsequently in the light of their outcome. As recorded in history, the Battle of Ulm was a

victory for Napoleon; for those who fought there it was a congeries
of innumerable disconnected incidents, just as those living under
the separate reigns of five Tudor monarchs extending for more than
a century were not aware that they belonged to a Tudor Age which
would be subsequently demarcated from that of the Stuarts. Each
takes on these defined characteristics at the hands of the historian,
often centuries after their occurrence.

They are therefore his constructs imposed upon the evidence;
they do not inhere in it. Battle of Ulm or Tudor Monarchy refer
to everything and nothing in particular which falls under them in
a relation which is neither causal nor ontological: merely one of
conforming to a category, which, however closely it may be derived
from the evidence, is arbitrary in that it does not naturally exist as
such, but is the work of the historian. The characteristics which he
identifies as a battle or a reign are at once ideal and comparative.
They belong to no individual thing as such and they are defined
by reference to what is like and unlike. Tudor Epoch, for example,
is a composite picture of, say, masterful kings and queens, sweep-
ing religious change and persecution, national greatness, a golden
age of music and literature, new forms of agriculture and commerce,
exploration, the Spanish Wars, and so on, all defined not only in
terms of the individuals and events constituting it – Henry VIII,
Elizabeth I, the dissolution of the monasteries, Spenser, Shakespeare, Tallis, the Armada – but in relation to what did or did not
occur, in Lancastrian or Stuart England, previously or subsequently. As such it can never be more than an approximation,
which is never fully present at any time or place; it rather provides
the means for measuring individual events against a norm which,
artificially established, is not inviolable but can be modified or
crossed to produce hybrids, like the English Reformation or the
Reformation Parliament, in an almost unlimited range of variations
which is the clearest evidence of their factitious nature.

That leads us to the final consideration, of how historical
models operate. From what we have said, it can be seen that they
consist of three main elements: the specific set of historical events,
the category or categories to which they belong, and the epoch in
which they occur. It is the last which makes an event historical:
epoch or period at once gives a set of occurrences context and
preserves them from fragmenting into their own constituent

categories. It is therefore not enough for the events and categories to be historical; they need some further unifying term which brings them into a coherent relationship and so provides an historical model. This can be illustrated by our earlier example of the persecution of the Huguenots. Let us take the statement 'In 1690 Louis XIV revoked the Edict of Nantes which had protected the Huguenots from persecution and they were forced to flee the country.' This describes a specific set of historical events. But before it can be either stated or understood as such it must form part of a wider complex which enables us to identify it and evaluate it. For that we must invoke each of these three main elements.

Temporally, the persecution of the Huguenots as a historical event forms the point of departure for treating them as a historical problem. Conceptually it rests upon having identified its categories and the epochal sequences to which they belong. In this case the two main ones are the Huguenots as a religious minority and Louis XIV as a seventeenth-century French king. Each must be set in a context of ever-increasing generality. The Huguenots as Protestant and French belong to sequences which take in both: their nature as a Protestant sect, its relation to Protestantism, the opposition between Protestantism and Catholicism as the source of their conflict, which ultimately goes back to the beginnings of the Reformation era. In its French aspect the persecution of the Huguenots converges with the other sequence of seventeenth-century France, and embraces the kind of king Louis XIV was, the nature of his reign, the nature of France as one of the absolutist monarchies which emerged from the post-medieval age, the bearing which the religious strife between Protestant and Catholic in the sixteenth century wars of religion had upon its development, and the circumstances leading to the persecution of the Huguenots. Neither of these is a causal chain but represents the terms with which the initial statement 'Louis XIV persecuted the Huguenots' is convertible if it is to be intelligible historically: that is to provide a context. In practice no historian formally enunciates such sequences because such knowledge is implicit in the concept of the epoch. As we mentioned earlier the model of the reign of Louis XIV must embrace such notions as that of absolute monarchy, the intolerance of religious minorities, the struggle between Catholic and Protestant, as well as a range of individual characteristics which together define it. However they are evaluated, what gives these sequences unity is nothing intrinsic to them as kinds of events in common but the notion of belonging to a temporal continuum.

A term like Age of Absolutism or Early Modern Age is wide enough to bring together disparate events, which in themselves have no inherent connection, because it is at a far enough remove from the evidence to be denuded of specific content. It can thus embrace, say, the conflict between Protestant and Catholic, the emergence of Absolute monarchies, the growth of Dutch sea power, the decline of Spain, the beginnings of the Scientific Revolution, the colonization of America and the East, the over-throw of the Stuarts, changes in painting and architecture, the decline of the universities, to take examples at random, without having to reconcile their intrinsic and circumstantial differences. It serves to do no more than to establish their temporal coexistence and so to provide a context to their contingent connections, as in the collision between the Huguenots and Louis XIV, without which they would not be historically intelligible.

It is this restriction upon content which enables an epoch to act as a unifying term; it does not seek out the common properties which each of its constituents must share as part of a common nature. Rather it constitutes a dossier of the main case histories making up a particular span of time upon which the historian can draw to make a kind of identikit for his particular historical situation, however widely or narrowly defined. Thus in the perse-cution of the Huguenots, he makes use, as we have seen, of the religious and political developments which render it possible to explain what Louis XIV was doing when he revoked the Edict of Nantes. From his knowledge of the Reformation and Absolute Monarchy, he can relate the persecution of the Huguenots to the context of Louis XIV's reign. In doing so he implicitly assumes that, had there been neither a Reformation nor Absolute Monarchies, the persecution could hardly conceivably have occurred in the way in which it did. Logically that does not commit him to determinism, but on the contrary to a view of the contingency of historical events which, because they could have been different, could have set in train different sequences. It is the need to grasp those which have occurred which makes some unifying category necessary.

The historian's models are thus principally directed to the assimilation of the new: a Reformation, the Huguenots, the reign of Louis XIV, Louis as a young king in 1650 and an old king in 1690. He has to show how one situation or group or individual, regarded initially as worthy of study, was succeeded by another. But the new does not emerge evenly; it can occur at innumerable different levels, in social structure, intellectual life, political change, or sheer chance without necessarily entailing change, or at least fundamental change, elsewhere. The discontinuity of change, both in time and area, is perhaps the greatest barrier between history and other disciplines. It accounts for the reluctance of the historian to generalize and for the seemingly anarchic or at least unsystematic nature of a historical standpoint. In fact this springs from the need to preserve the complexities of a historical situation. Only exceptionally can all its events, beyond a very limited range, such as a battle, a persecution, a *coup d'état*, be synchronized into a real unity. For the most part, in occurrence or in mode of occurrence, change is not uniform: there can be an intellectual revolution, as there was in the thirteenth century, without a corresponding social or political evolution; it can be cumulative, as this one was, extending over nearly a century, or sudden like the events following the assassination of the Archduke Ferdinand at Sarajevo in 1914. There can be large-scale political upheavals which can change the political face of a country, as repeatedly in South America or the Middle East, and yet leave its social structure largely untouched. There can be revolutionary innovations – Gutenberg's press, Einstein's theory of relativity – when an age is supposed to be in decline, while philosophy – Plato's, Aristotle's – and law – Roman – can survive for millenia. The historian's model has therefore to embrace all three of the elements previously adumbrated. Or perhaps, put more strictly, he must make use of three different models: the general epochal model, which must be wide enough to catch everything coming within his own categories, acts as the defining element: it tells him at once what he must expect – persecution, absolutism – and what he cannot expect – tolerance or electricity; in that sense he receives his norms from his view of the epoch. The categories act as the comparative model telling him how the events he is examining do or do not differ from those under which they fall. From the conjunction of

the two he is able to frame his conception of Louis XIV's persecution of the Huguenots. It will therefore depend upon his initial
postulates: how much he feels must be included either epochally
or categorically, or both, which is not immediately given in the
actual sequence of events which constitute the persecution.
According to what these are – whether they extend to say economic
criteria, class structure, Louis's own psychopathology, the French
character – the particular model with its appropriate interpretation
will result. Its plausibility will be in proportion to how appropriate these defining criteria are regarded as being. If they cannot
be related to the evidence, or are shown to be at variance with what
are accepted as the norms of the epoch, they will be disputed by
other historians. Much historical discourse revolves around issues
of interpretation because history is written from an irreducible
number of differing initial presuppositions.

We can say, then, that historical models are essentially norm-
defining. They centre upon establishing the criteria by which
actions, generically constant, can be brought into a context
appropriate to the prevailing practices and assumptions of an age.
However they may vary – an economic revolution demands a
different context from a scientific revolution and both from the
life of an individual who was neither economically nor scientifically
revolutionary – they make use of certain common conceptions
which rest upon the model of a period. These act as signposts which
direct the historian to certain defined areas, so that, however little
use he may have for them as such, they help him to steer a course
which keeps him out of alien waters: to know that there was an
Age of Gothic is at least to know that it was not the Age of Baroque.
In practice these divisions do much more by providing him with a
construct in terms of which he approaches his own problem.
However much he may come to modify it, or even to dispense
with it, initially he is as dependent upon his model as the builder
of a house is upon a scaffolding.

NOTE

1 I have discussed the theoretical grounds in *History and Social Theory*,
  London, Merlin, 1969, Part I.

© *Gordon Leff 1972*

Comment

P. J. CAIN

Since I am basically in agreement with Professor Leff's approach and space is limited, I will confine my remarks to one or two areas mainly centred upon the problem of the historian's initial presuppositions.

1. It would have been helpful if Professor Leff had indicated more deliberately the sort of thinking about history which he is attacking. As it stands, the paper does tend to suggest that those who deny any independent conceptual standing to the names of historical periods or institutions have never argued this formally. It could have been pointed out that there are some versions of the doctrine known as 'methodological individualism', for example, which deny conceptual standing to what are called 'social wholes' like period names on the ground that these wholes should be reducible to a set of descriptive statements which are an exhaustive definition of the wholes and that if they are not so reducible they do not have meaning. Professor Leff, on his side, is arguing that period terms are, in fact, irreducible and to some degree indispensable in the writing on, and thinking about, historical events. To put the matter in terminology different from Professor Leff's,[1] terms like 'Renaissance' function in a similar way to what are called, in logic, proper names in that they are not equivalent in meaning to any complete set of descriptive statements, there being no final agreement as to what would actually constitute an exhaustive list of these statements. Many historians agree that there was such a thing as the Renaissance; but they may, and do, disagree about when it began, when it ended, and what events actually constitute

161

it. What they do agree on is that the Renaissance is a distinct historical period because there is something essentially different about it which distinguishes it from what goes before and what comes after.[2] Keeping in mind what Professor Leff calls 'the unequal co-existence of diverse phenomena' at any particular time it is still the case that the historian is primarily interested in the uniqueness of an age, in 'the assimilation of the new'.

2. Wherein this uniqueness may be said to lie depends upon the historian's presuppositions, to which Professor Leff devotes considerable space but which will bear closer scrutiny in view of their critical role in historical inquiry. Using Collingwood's language,[3] one can say that our fundamental vision of what the world of men is like (which is in some way related to the particularity of their environment at any one time), rests ultimately upon 'constellations of absolute presuppositions'. From the subject's point of view at least, these are neither true nor false in that the truth or falsity of things is judged in the light of them. Collingwood did not believe that these groups of presuppositions need have any internal logical consistency although they do make sense of the world for the holder of them.

To relate this to periodization, we can say that our presuppositions give us our sense of period by shaping the historian's views about what is unique or essential in an age. And although there is a sense in which we can talk of the 'presuppositions of an age' it has to be recognized that there may be vast differences in people's presuppositions at any one time (a cause and a consequence of the 'contemporality of diverse phenomena') and because of this historians' sense of period differs, as Professor Leff indicates.

In periodizing we are examining what we regard as the crucial presuppositions of an age, and this, together with the problem of how and why one set of presuppositions gives way to another in one or more areas of life – how periods succeed one another in fact – are among the most interesting and difficult contemporary historical problems.

Perhaps it should be mentioned here that I think Professor Leff occasionally uses the word 'norm' in a way which suggests that these norms are entirely given. But in so far as norm means 'ideas and assumptions of an age' then our view of the norms of the past will depend on the historian's presuppositions and are therefore subject to dispute.

3. Making a 'social whole' intelligible depends upon the ability to convert it 'into a sufficient number of terms to explain it' (describing it). As Professor Leff says, many of these descriptions will be 'implicit in the concept of the epoch' but the degree to which this is so will vary. For instance, historians who agree on fundamental assumptions can take for granted a great deal in communicating with each other: those who do not may have to spell out in great detail what they think. This is not simply a matter of baldly stating presuppositions. Where initial assumptions differ, historians can only communicate by a more or less wide-ranging survey of the evidence in an attempt to show that their own view point can account for the evidence better than that of others. Again, when the historian is speaking to the uninitiated he may have to explain a great deal which could be assumed if he were addressing a more sophisticated audience.

4. An interesting question arising from this paper would be a comparison between the concepts employed in historical inquiry and in the natural sciences. How similar are they? Kuhn's 'paradigms' or 'disciplinary matrix', for instance, sound very like presuppositions. He periodizes past scientific endeavours, denying the idea of unilinear progress and insisting that past scientific achievements should be evaluated in terms of the particular paradigm which governed thought at that particular time. And he also proposes answers to the question why paradigms change which could be useful to the historian.[4]

NOTES AND REFERENCES

1 His own terminology I sometimes find a little confusing. For example, the word 'category' seems to be used in more than one sense in the course of the paper.
2 STALNAKER, R. 'Events, Periods and Institutions in Historians' Language', *History and Theory*, **8**, 1967.
3 COLLINGWOOD, R. G. *Metaphysics*, Oxford, 1940, esp. chs. IV and V.
4 KUHN, T. S. *The Structure of Scientific Revolutions* (2nd ed.), Chicago, University of Chicago Press, 1970.

Theology as a Discipline
of a Modern University

DONALD MACKINNON

At first sight one might be tempted to say that theological study
has no place at all in a modern university. It is a discipline whose
relevance must necessarily be confined to the professional formation of those who are going to minister in the various churches,
and as such it is arguable that its study should be confined to the
seminary-type institutions in which that training in its specialist
aspects is carried on. The amount of public money available to
subvent fundamental research in universities is strictly limited,
and one can understand the attitude of mind of those who regard
it as little short of scandalous that some part of it should be diverted to the prosecution of a subject so intellectually dubious as
theology.

And it must be clear that to very many theology seems more than
a little intellectually dubious. The present writer is a specialist in
the philosophy of religion, and is quite familiar with the taunt
that his religious commitment necessarily spoils him as a philosopher. Theologians are almost invariably recruited from the
ranks of those who believe; how then can they be expected to
obey the imperative to follow the argument whithersoever it leads
them? A scientific hypothesis must by definition be vulnerable to
empirical refutation; the accepted reconstruction of a sequence of
historical events must be abandoned in the light of fresh indisputable evidence; a conception of philosophical method can be
discarded when its assumptions are shown to disregard the complexities of actual discourse. But is not the theologian (and for the
sake of simplicity I confine myself to Christian theology) fettered
to *credenda* that he is not prepared to query? He will analyse them,

certainly; but where, for instance, Christ's divinity is concerned, can he in the last resort allow that the belief that *Christ is divine* is groundless and should be discarded?

Yet the practice of theology in the modern university to some extent at least is a very different and more complex thing than this model allows. Certainly it represents at least in the ancient universities an inheritance from a past in which its truimphalist pretensions gave it a deservedly bad name. Yet in the same time it had undergone a measure of reformation. Thus in Cambridge it had become a school of historical theology, the disciplined historical study of Christian origins. The apparent academic aloofness of this study got it a bad name among the devout, who are often inpatient of the checks exact scholarship imposes upon their spiritual exuberance. Yet the fact that this attempted identification of theology as an academic discipline with a branch of historical study happened is something of great significance. After all, Christianity is a historical religion. If its truth-claims are to be sustained, they can only be sustained if certain contingent historical propositions are true. If the proposition *Jesus Christ was crucified under Pontius Pilate* is false, as the proposition *Charles I died in his bed* is false, *cadit tota quaestio*. Again, if in fact Jesus was executed on a proved charge of gross immorality, or of incitement to undisciplined violence accompanied by generally corrupt behaviour, etc. however much we may condemn the methods of his punishment, we can hardly be expected to revere Him as Saviour and Lord. What sort of man was He? Did He, in fact, speaking as He did against the background of the tangled politics of His age, manifest a total innocence? Or was He in fact another agitator playing with the fires of Jewish resentment of Roman domination? Or was He a fool who believed that a kind of detachment from harsh political realities was possible? Was He in fact a source of trouble or a focus of corruption? These are historical questions: and if Jesus belongs to history, is a man of flesh and blood, it is a theological duty to ask these questions about Him. If we seek to dodge them by saying that they are unanswerable, then we have to defend the perilous gambit of seeking to cut Christian faith loose from its historical roots, and of substituting a product of the cultic imagination of a primitive community for the concrete flesh and blood of the man of Nazareth.

Those academic theologians, then, who identified Christian theology with the historical study of Christian origins were loyal to the essential nature of their faith. They also bore witness in a most important way to that faith's vulnerability by suggesting that there were aspects of it that merited putting to the test in the rigorous school of detached historical study. But a critic might say: why then should such study form an element in a university curriculum? To that I have no immediate answer except to point out that, for good or ill, Christianity is a formative element in our culture. It has supplied the language, the conceptual system, in whose terms men and women in these islands have posed and sought to answer ultimate questions. Or if they have sought an alternative idiom, an alternative conceptual system, it is as an alternative to the Christian tradition in one or other of its forms that they have sought it. I say in one or other of its forms; for where Christianity as an historical phenomenon is concerned we have to reckon with the fact that its differing traditions have supplied the idioms in which men and women have been able to articulate some of their profoundest differences. Think, for instance, of the seventeenth-century conflict of Anglican and Puritan. But when any variant of this tradition is rejected, a new dialect has to be found, and its novelty is self-consciously asserted *vis-à-vis* that form of Christianity most present to the consciousness of the innovator. So in the case of Bertrand Russell, his early schooling in a strictly Evangelical tradition is reflected in his querying the moral excellence of Jesus, in as much as in the received records of his teaching He proclaimed Hell the ultimate destiny of the recalcitrant transgressor, even of the unbeliever.

It is a commonplace to say that we live in a pluralist society, one in which an established church in the sense in which the Church of England is established seems a curious anachronism, obstinately defended on the ground that it preserves the ordained ministers of that Church from some of the worst vices of clericalism. Yet the multitude of beliefs, attitudes, policies of life between which the individual must choose (unless he can afford the luxury of a complete agnosticism) all in one way or another remind the student of a Christian past strongly encapsulated in the present. Thus, if one studies for instance the subtle, rarefied attitude of the 'Bloomsbury circle', with its deep indebtedness to some of the theses of G. E. Moore's *Principia Ethica*, one quickly notices that it embodies a protest not only against the philistine crudities of Bentham's 'Hedonistic Calculus', but also against certain styles of Christian ethics, especially those which have sought to incorporate into their fabric Kant's doctrine of the supremacy in the universe of value of specifically moral excellence. Again, if one turns to the complex phenomenon of Marxism, whether the Marxism of the Thirties, or the contemporary espousal of the ideas of the young Marx (the word 'alienation' is among the most significant of contemporary catchwords), one has to reckon with a doctrine and a method that, apart altogether from their initial Hegelian inspiration, are at heart a profound criticism of the substance of Christian faith. And if one turns to the formidable figure of Lenin, perhaps the greatest atheist of the twentieth century, òne has to reckon with an atheism whose positive quality as a policy of life to which its professor was absolutely committed, only emerges when one puts it over against a pattern of faith that he pitilessly and uncomprisingly rejected. Again if one seeks to articulate the assumptions of our own gentler liberal humanism, one soon is made aware that it is at once indebted to Christian tradition, and profoundly antagonistic towards it. Always it seeks to avoid tumbling headlong into a thoroughgoing utilitarianism, and to do justice to the complexities and profundities of the moral universe to which the utilitarian tradition, even in its most refined form, fails to measure up. Here it suggests (I will say no more) a continued awareness of the riches of the Christian moral tradition, riches incidently which the Churches have frequently, by their perhaps inevitable tendency to legalism (disguised as a fidelity to 'principles'), tended to obscure. Yet it is an awareness that takes the shape of a most resolute attempt to do justice to the profundities, even the absolutes, of the moral life without investing them with a transcendental religious impact. And to understand what is happening here some knowledge of the Christian tradition is essential. *Of course the kind of study implicit in the previous section of my argument is much wider in scope than a new historico-critical investigation of Christian origins:* the latter is of necessity to some extent a genetic investigation, whereas what I am now suggesting is much more a philosophically critical investigation of a system of belief. Inevitably this investigation will take account of the most fundamental questionings to which the system in question has been submitted, and thus must include the sort of interrogation to which its tenets have been submitted by professors of the other great religions of the world. In the present situation a faculty or department of theology must be a place where Christian belief is tested to destruction, where individual *credenda* are submitted to the most meticulous scrutiny. It must be a setting in which the most searching and pervasive discontents in the received traditions of Christian understanding achieve a new self-consciousness, where indeed anciently professed articles of faith may be shown to be less tolerable of sense than may conventionally appear, but where nothing is taken for granted in respect of the historically observable future of Christian institutions.

The university teacher of theology must therefore be a man at once committed and uncommitted. He must be committed to a grave fundamental seriousness about the problems of Christian belief. Such commitment is indeed a necessary condition of his entering into his professional work; he must care. Yet at the same time he must be prepared to find the outcome of his work totally other than his hopes and anticipations. He is unlikely to find the secure resting-place of a well-founded citadel of belief, an impregnable fortress of conviction strong to resist the interrogation and assaults of a prevailingly hostile intellectual climate. Moreover, the further his work advances, the less secure his position. Certainly he will learn to call nonsense by its name, and acquire an impatience alike with a facile positivism and a spurious ecclesiastically inspired apologetic. He will learn, in a hard school, something of the cost of following the argument whithersoever it leads, something of the price of seeking the truth. Certainly it is possible within the Christian tradition to offer an interpretation in terms of spirituality of this experience; but in so far as the Churches, as institutions, are inevitably preoccupied with the problem of their own survival, they are liable to withhold their approval from the genuinely academic theologian, and distribute their accolade rather on the man who, whether by his apologetic dexterity or his scholarship, best serves their own purpose. The kind of tension between commitment and detachment that an academic theologian must know is reflected in his sense (especially if he is a layman, as one may hope more and more academic theologians in the future will be) of being at once involved in and standing apart from the life of the Churches.

In the university community theological study as here interpreted has obviously close relations with philosophy, history, sociology. Yet it has its own underlying dynamic, in that its practitioners will of necessity be men and women deeply disturbed either by questions of religion in general, or of Christian faith in particular. May I here refer to my own experience? There are many times when I crave the intellectual freedom of the professional philosopher, the uninhibited permission to engage with philosophical problems without the constraining sense of a complex of beliefs whose very claim to validity might fall to the ground by the acceptance as authoritative of certain styles of logical analysis. It is as if religious belief held one prisoner in a kind of fundamental dishonesty, as if it were a compulsion to intellectual cheating of which one was powerless to cure oneself, but which none the less one saw as tainting with a deep pervasive flaw one's essays in supposedly rigorous philosophical analysis. And yet on the other side the memory of the person of Christ continually beckons one's intelligence as well as one's will in a direction that at first sight seems quite different, but after a while is seen to engage that same intellectual integrity for which philosophical activity calls. There is a riddle here that will not let one rest until one has solved it, an opening-up of the frontiers of the unknown that calls out one's energies. To speak in these terms is to do no more than state empirical facts; it may indeed be doing no more than record an obsession. Where university life today is concerned, that obsession must justify its indulgence by its fertility in stimulating work that is of value to those who do not share it, even to those who dismiss it as at bottom pathological. To speak in this way is not to deny the immense significance of faith or belittle the intellectually demanding character of fundamental theological inquiry; it is merely to suggest that such inquiry must be justified, where universities of the present are concerned, by its fruits. The kind of discoveries that the theologian makes are not immediately shareable; therefore they must establish their import, I had almost said in quantifiable form, by the renewed vitality they bring to critical philosophy, to social science, to historical study.

The theologian in the university today must live and work

as a man who has to establish his right to exist. He will be guilty of the deepest sort of failure if he takes himself for granted: and yet he must never, in the effort to declare in practice the human point of his studies, deny the special dynamic and objective of his enterprise. He will have his moments of vision, even as he will also have his frequent periods of underlying distaste for his whole involvement in a subject that remains, in the imagination of many critics, academically disreputable. Yet he will from time to time be reminded that his peculiar activity is of service to the university community, that his self-consciously exposed position equips him for a role that is of genuine, even permanent significance.

It is of course essential for the health of theology as a subject that it should be carried on in the setting of a university, and not in the restricted, specially orientated atmosphere of a denominational seminary. Inevitably in the latter setting there is a concentration of emphasis on the confessional orthodoxy of the denomination whose future ministers are there receiving their professional formation at the expense of serious engagement with the work of those great theologians who, by the depth of their intellectual penetration, frequently undermine the foundations of historically recent denominational allegiances, suggesting that the ultimate Christian reality is something as often obscured as expressed by the historical actualities of the Christian Churches. If the supreme maxim of Protestant ecclesiology is *Ecclesia reformata semper reformanda*, in practice the Churches after the Reformation have preferred to emphasize the past participle at the expense of the gerundive; reformation has seemed a thing accomplished once for all, rather than a permanent imperative making Christian men and women ever restless with their received institutions and traditions.

Again, the involvement of theology as a subject in the total life of a university ensures that its emphases are continually fertilized by ideas flowing from other fields of study. I have mentioned history, philosophy, sociology; I should certainly include the critical study of political institutions, ancient and modern. The theologian is very often a philistine; the temples of Philistia are often easier to dwell in than the shrines of the living God. There is for the professional student of theology something peculiarly significant in continued attention to the claims of a genuine literary culture. It is after all in literature rather than in philosophy that one finds the most searching, the most-profound, treatments of the 'problem of evil'; it is in tragedies such as the *Electra* of Sophocles, the *Lear* of Shakespeare, the *Phèdre* of Racine, that one finds the most remorseless determination not to fudge with the intractable, surd element in human life, but to lay it bare as it is, no false consolation sought, no make-believe refuge found. One can learn from a theologically orientated library study a whole new style of engagement with the Gospel tradition, which lays bare its sharp outlines more effectively that do ecclesiastical tradition, on the one hand, and an overoptimistic reductionist liberalism, on the other.

It is indeed most important to remember that a continually exposed theology is not likely to decline into the intellectually slack system of obscure commonplaces which sometimes sells itself as *avant-garde*. It will be very often tentative, untidy, suggestive rather than systematic, aware constantly of inconsistencies that must be eliminated by more rigorous conceptual reconstruction; but it will never seek escape into a fog where all distinction is obliterated and a supposedly generous intellectual tolerance made to do duty for disciplined effort of thought. However incomplete, for instance, the classical Christology, it had the great advantage of refusing to dodge the problems; rather, by its very unsatisfactoriness, it thrust them upon men's notice. We need most certainly to advance beyond the positions of Nicea and Chalcedon; but we shall do so only if we acknowledge our debt to those Church Councils in refusing to dodge issues, raised inescapably by the *mysterium Christi*, by the recognition that in Christ we have to reckon with that One in whom uniquely the frontiers of the unfathomable are opened up.

The theologian is certainly in the university's debt. The very prestige of the exact experimental and observational sciences continually reminds him of the power of their methods, and the complex involved structure of those of his own discipline. Yet that very complex structure is a reminder that in his discipline (for all the criticisms that may be laid against it) there is the meeting-point of a whole variety of intellectual styles. He has to acknowledge the claims of logical rigour, the authority of empirical fact; yet he has also to remember that, where human life is concerned, there are heights and depths calling for a very different sort of reflection if the experience of these realities is not to be diminished and lost. He must be a rootless man, restless and awkward, ill at ease with himself; towards his fellows, at once receptive and committed. It should not be easy to be a theologian in a modern university; indeed it should never have been easy, and if the status of the subject in the structures of the ancient universities once made it so, we must be thankful that it does so no longer. It may not be palatable continually to be on the defensive; yet if theology lives through interrogation, through questioning and being questioned, we should be thankful that its practitioners have continually to make their case for its acceptance as a discipline.

The whole texture of theological existence is changed, changed with the great deliverance that has come to Christianity with the advent of the post-Constantinian age. Since Constantine's conversion, churchmen have kept company with men of power, and not only learnt to talk *de haut en bas*, but have come to see the fundamental Christian mystery as such a communication. The reality of the divine condescension has been lost. Now it has become something that the theologian proves in the pulses of his own radical insecurity. He is no longer protected by the status accruing to one supposedly a master in the accepted spiritual traditions of his society. He has to learn to speak, and sometimes he finds that silence is the only adequate 'system of projection' at his disposal. But because he has thus in a confused and complicated way, continually to defend himself, he is able to learn far more of the reality of apostleship (as the second Epistle to the Corinthians understands it) than he could hope to know when his discipline was endowed in its practice with a great and manifest dignity. For the reality of apostleship is not proved by a quickly effective ministry of apologetic, but by a long and painful apprenticeship to which the individual knows himself constrained by that which will not let him escape.

To end on such a note may seem strange. But what I am trying to say is that the harder the struggle the theologian must fight to secure both a place for his discipline, and more important, for the worthiness of his discipline to occupy such a place, the better the work we may expect from him, the more authentic its style. It is a good thing, even a very good thing, for theology to have to fight for its existence in the university, even as it is for Christianity a profound deliverance to emerge from a situation in which its chief practitioners were compelled to debase the currency of its strange and searching paradoxes, the better to incorporate its profession in the traditionally accepted way of life of established society.

I may seem here to contradict what I said earlier of the extent to which Christianity provided the men and women of our culture with an idiom or conceptual system in terms of which to articulate their engagement with ultimate questions. But here we have to reckon with a diffused Christianity which has always successfully resisted the efforts of so many of the Churches to convert the Christian ethos into the consciously professed assumptions of a supposedly orderly society. It is that Christianity whose influence (even when it is rejected as inadequate to the bitterness of human life, as by Shakespeare in *Lear*: I follow Dr N. Brooke's interpretation[1]) is there present in the substance of the very deepest treatments of the theme of our human lot in literature past and present: whose inwardness indeed merits a new articulation by this indirect invocation of its depths. It is indeed that Christianity of which we learn though deep engagement with the interrogation of its critics, whether they be Bertrand Russell or V. I. Lenin, John Maynard Keynes or D. H. Lawrence, or whether they be found among men of science, simply but searchingly revolted by the historic obscurantism and pettiness of the ecclesiastical temper, its disregard at once for the claims of reason and of compassion.

The very mockery to which he is sometimes exposed at least preserves the theologian from the kind of elaborate make-believe, encouraged, for instance, by the authorities of the Established Church at the time of the Coronation of Elizabeth II, when it was suggested that its whole elaborate and archaic ritual was a kind of representation of the coming of God's Kingdom, that its long ceremonial embodied a veritable *parousia*. At least the theologian knows illusion when he sees it, quickly shocked indeed by the deliberate trivialization of an infinitely complex reality, glad that his own situation is geared without pretence to a world in which (I hope I do not speak irreverently), if he has somewhere to lay his head, he does not know whether his successor will share his fortune. It is for him to let his worth be proved, and his honesty is in a measure preserved by the fact that he cannot hope to fix the judges. So the university keeps the theologian to his job, and in so doing, maybe *malgré tout*, serves well the cause of its own intellectual health.

REFERENCE

1 BROOKE, NICHOLAS. *King Lear*, London, Arnold, 1963.

Comment

G. R. DUNSTAN

Professor MacKinnon writes as the Apostle Paul wrote in the Epistle to the Romans, searching a self painfully sensitive to conflicting claims, obedient to that posterior centre of unity from which both claims derive and in which both subsist, yet torn by them in the self to a depth which honesty can contemplate but not assuage. On Paul the claims were of two communities, the Old Israel and the new – both, as he was bound to say, from God and both one in God, but seemingly irreconcilable in Paul's own person. So he struggled to be free from that from which he could not be free, which was Judaeism, in order to live with that to which he was newly bound, the Christian Church; and *perhaps* it was Paul's own very striving with the problem of division in himself which, with tragic inadvertence, assured the perpetuation of that division between Jew and Christian throughout subsequent time. For Professor MacKinnon the claims are of two professions, the one to the Christian faith, brought to him (whether he likes the fact or not) through the historic Christian Church, and formulated in the dogmatic statements and attendant literature of Christian theology; the other to academic philosophy, brought to him through the tradition of the open pursuit of truth in the university. Both professions, he would allow, meet where they originate, in truth itself; yet him they divide. And over the years an indebted and admiring reader of Professor MacKinnon is made to wonder whether his struggles too to reconcile his two professions may not also, with tragic inadvertence and inevitability, widen the schism outside himself and leave for others an inheritance of sharper division.

175

Professor MacKinnon is sensitive to the suspicion, in an academic community, that the substance and method of his own
discipline, the philosophy of religion, are intellectually dubious.
He lives with the risk that the historical foundations of the Christian faith are assailable on historical grounds, and with the impu-
tation that, because *credenda*, faith-statements, lie at the centre of
his commitment, he is inhibited from pursuing the truth wherever
it might lead, as – the argument runs – his academic colleagues are
not. The reader of his paper may fairly ask, does he exaggerate this
isolation? Is he projecting upon his Senior Combination Room a
preoccupation which is evidently of critical importance to himself?

Next, the historical analysis of the origins of Christianity and of
the theological tradition of which Christianity is the fount, pursued in a 'school of historical theology', is justified as a proper
university discipline on the ground that Christianity and the
theological tradition have been a formative element in our culture,
both in what they have entrenched and in the reactions they have
occasioned; it is as important to study what Lord Russell, the
Hegelians, and the Marxists reject, as to study those Christian
institutions whose occasional manifestations of 'triumphalism'
Professor MacKinnon so much deplores. Yet again, it must be
asked, is he forcing two entities out of one? The Christian faith
and its rejection are not two entities; rejection is one of the Christian *credenda*, essential to the theological understanding of Christ
himself, essential to the understanding and formulation of the
Christian faith in the perennial intellectual debate, essential to the
Christian *askesis* or formation of Christian character. The university would be, on this showing, one of the many proper embodi-
ments of this engagement to be expected in a world which has, in
its history, taken Christianity seriously. This, I think, Professor
MacKinnon would allow; but he would not allow anything 'to be
taken for granted in respect of the historically observable future of
Christian institutions'. But is this limitation essential to his
discipline? or does he, again, exaggerate, setting himself a standard
which few if any other disciplines would share? Does the academic
student of law, for instance, or of education or public administration take nothing for granted about future institutional embodi-
ment, or does he not rather presuppose some *organa vocis* in which
the concepts of his study will find expression?

It is in the second part of his paper, when he is dealing less with the inheritance of the past (and is therefore only occasionally provoked into shooting at ecclesiastical clay pigeons) and more with the present engagement, that Professor MacKinnon by clarity of vision penetrates to something like a solution to his own problem. In a notable passage he writes of his craving for the intellectual freedom of the professional philosopher, and then of the constraint upon him, upon intelligence and will, of the person of Christ. But in facing this riddle he *is* the perennial Christian philosopher. Aquinas and the rest wrestled no less with the truth that they saw in Christ and the truth to which their logic led them. But is this necessity confined only to religious philosophers, or to philosophers of religion? It would not occur readily to a natural scientist to use the word *credenda* for the complex of axioms or presuppositions upon which his edifice of assurance rests and from the acceptance of which his further researches become possible. He lives under the shadow of possibility that his axioms might be overthrown, as those of earlier generations have been – and some day they may be; but it would be absurd to suppose that he could work without axioms; or that he would not passionately defend them against some trivializer who suggested that he ought to be 'free' of them. The claim on intelligence and will of which Professor MacKinnon writes cannot, of its very nature, be empirically validated, for it *may* be an illusion; neither can its beckoning be but more than partially – even minimally – obeyed. Yet he cannot deny its presence or its power. These facts are among the inescapable *data* of his science as a philosopher; they are authenticated as part of the genuine religious experience throughout the literature of his subject, both in the sacred 'scriptures' and in the theological tradition.

The exploration of this experience is certainly a multidisciplined task, and its deep entrenchment in what we may call the humanity of man points to its relevance to other disciplines centred on man. It is not easy to find, therefore, any objective reason for Professor MacKinnon's sense of professional inferiority in the university, for his occasional fears that his subject is 'academically disreputable', to be defended and ever fought for. We may agree entirely with his belief that the study of theology is advantageously pursued within the cross-fertilization of university

life without sharing his adverse judgement upon its pursuit in a
seminary: he rightly attests the value of the classical, Chalce-
donian, Christology, for its refusal to dodge the problems, and he
may well conclude, would he but reflect again upon both history
and present experience, that an obstinate fidelity to the *truths*
enshrined in these old formulae (incomplete in formulation as they
must necessarily be) and the detachment to reflect further upon
them, are far from incompatible with cloistered scholarship, and
may indeed be characteristic of it. Similarly, we may share with
him an awareness of the dangers attending a complacent resting on
'establishment' by men whose very profession binds them to keep
mind and conscience sensitive to truth, to just complaint, to proper
and inherent drives towards change, to the most demanding
because inarticulate call for compassion – a danger present to the
law, medicine, the universities, the civil administration, as well as
the Church. We hold ourselves free, nevertheless, to reserve the
language of 'debasing the currency of its strange and searching
paradoxes' and the like for recognized betrayals of integrity, and
to find some other language to describe genuine involvement –
including a necessary cultural and symbolic expression – with the
total life of society as a duty inherent in the profession itself, an
involvement which often requires the practitioner to make the
best of several legitimate conflicting claims, and denies him the
luxury of 'acting on principle' if by that is meant obeying the
clear dictates of only one. To insist on this is to claim that there is
a basic unity, and the possibility of resolution, where some of
Professor MacKinnon's language would seem to heighten diversity
and discord.

© *G. R. Dunstan 1972*

Models for Grammars

JAMES PETER THORNE

In his book *The Structure of Scientific Revolutions* Kuhn has argued that the traditional view of the history of science, that sciences develop through the gradual accumulation of data and the gradual extension of theories to cover the data, is quite false. Kuhn points out that in nearly every case what, in retrospect, appeared to be new and crucial data, far from being new were available long before an accepted theory was rejected, and only came to be seen as crucial in the context of the theory that took its place. As the title of his book suggests, Kuhn's view of the history of science is that all significant developments are, in a quite literal sense, revolutionary, and that just as the concept of the state changes in political revolutions, so, in the case of scientific revolutions, the concept of the science – what scientists are prepared to accept as facts – changes; so that in an important sense it is no longer about what it used to be about.

The recent history of linguistics seems to afford striking confirmation of Kuhn's thesis. The publication of Chomsky's book *Syntactic Structures* in 1957 brought about a revolution in linguistics of exactly the kind Kuhn describes. For about fifty years before this date ideas about the way in which language should be studied were for the most part formed in response to positivistic – more especially behaviouristic – pressures. True, other, more tangible, forces can also be seen to have been at work; notably the fact that in America, where as an academic discipline linguistics had originally been closely associated with anthropology, linguists were faced with the immense practical problem of the existence of a vast number of American Indian languages, most of

179

which had never been seriously studied, and many of which were in imminent danger of dying out. Under these circumstances it is hardly surprising that a linguist's education should mainly be devoted to training as a fieldworker, and that his main task should be seen as that of assembling a corpus of sentences of various languages so that at least some data concerning them would be available. Before the days of efficient tape-recorders this meant that the linguist was faced, in the field, with the problem of working out an adequate transcription for the utterances he elicited from his informants. This is one reason why, in what came to be called 'structural linguistics', it was the study of the sound structure of languages ('phonemic analysis') that commanded most attention – so much so that the study of their syntactic and semantic structures was largely neglected. But behaviourist influences were another, and more powerful, reason. No matter how strictly one formulates the criteria for what is to count as observable, the sounds of a language will be counted as observable. The acceptance of behaviourist dogmas encouraged linguists in the belief that it was only those aspects of language structure that are, in a very narrow sense, observable which could provide data for a 'scientific' linguistics. To those who are not behaviourists what appears to be a totally unrealistic picture of the relationship between linguists and language came to be accepted. Strenuous (one might even say 'superhuman') efforts were made to try to overcome the effects of the fact that the linguist knew that what he was studying was a language and that, in the nature of things, he already had a native speaker's intuitive knowledge of at least one language. (The structuralists always lay great emphasis on what their successors would regard as being superficial differences between languages.) The linguist was urged to follow out as far as possible 'mechanical' procedures in analysing his data in order to ensure that the divisions he imposed upon them were only in response to the recognition of empirical clues. These procedures came to be looked upon as more important than the results they produced; the question of what set of criteria the taxonomies thus formed were to be evaluated by being left strictly in abeyance. The following quotation from Leonard Bloomfield's *Language*, for over thirty years a basic textbook in structural linguistics, provides a clear summary of these views and of the theories – which Bloomfield calls 'materialist'[1] – which lay behind them.

The danger here lies in mentalistic views of psychology, which may tempt the observer to appeal to purely spiritual standards instead of reporting the facts. To say, for instance, that combinations of words which are 'felt to be' compounds have only a single high stress (e.g. *blackbird* as opposed to *black bird*), is to tell exactly nothing, since we have no way of determining what the speaker may 'feel': the observer's task was to tell us, by some tangible criterion, or, if he found none, by a list, which combinations of words are pronounced with a single high stress. The worker who accepts the materialistic hypothesis in psychology is under no such temptation; it may be stated as a principle that in all sciences like linguistics, which observe some specific type of human activity, the worker must proceed exactly as if he held the materialistic view. This practical effectiveness is one of the strongest considerations in favour of scientific materialism.

One reason for calling *Syntactic Structures* 'revolutionary' is that its orientation is explicitly mentalistic. That is the main reason why structuralists could not, and do not, understand it, and why there can be no genuine discussion between them and the proponents of Chomsky's ideas. In Kuhn's telling phrase, they 'talk through' rather than talk to each other. What Bloomfield dismisses under the disparaging label of 'spiritual' Chomsky sees as being the most important evidence available to the linguist. This is because he regards the primary goal of linguistics not as that of setting up taxonomies which could be constructed by someone who does not know the language he is working with, but as that of constructing models of what the native speaker of the language intuitively knows about its structure. Chomsky, as it were, looks at language not from the outside but from the inside. The importance of his work – not only for linguistics but for the social sciences in general – lies in the fact that he has demonstrated that the investigation of this intuitive knowledge can be conducted in a quite rigorous and objective way.[2]

What, according to Chomsky, are the kind of facts that the

native speaker knows about the structure of his language? Consider the sentence

The boy kicked the ball.

Among the information which must be available to anyone who understands the utterance that the sentence represents is the following. It is a well-formed ('grammatical') English sentence in a sense that *Ball the kicked boy the* is not. *The, boy,* and *kicked* are all separate elements or units, in a sense that in this sentence *all* and *kick* are not. *The* and *boy* go together to form a unit in a sense which *boy* and *kicked* do not. *Boy* and *ball* are the same kind of units in a sense that *ball* and *kicked,* or *kicked* and *the,* or *the* and *ball* are not.

Regarding this information there are three points to be made. The first – which cannot have failed to occur to the reader already – is that these facts are of precisely the kind that traditional grammarians have been concerned with for at least the last three thousand years, and for dealing with which they have, during this time, developed an extremely useful technical vocabulary which includes such terms as *sentence, word, noun, verb, noun phrase, subject, object,* etc. Adopting a useful device from traditional grammar we can represent structural information about the sentence *The boy kicked the ball* in a very natural way by means of a tree-diagram, thus:

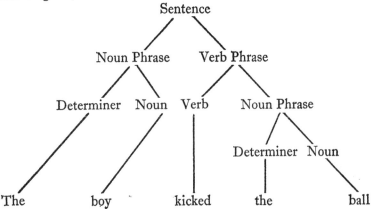

(Like all the analyses given in this paper this one has been considerably simplified in order to facilitate the exposition. Some of the deficiences of this particular analysis are discussed below.) In

view of the way in which it seems most people are taught grammar at school, it is perhaps necessary to emphasize that the information which is conveyed by the use of technical grammatical vocabulary is not of an esoteric nature. Quite the opposite. When I say that in the case of the sentences we are discussing *the* is a word and *boy* is a word and that together they form a noun phrase, I am using technical terms to convey information about the sentences possessed by anyone who understands English. Indeed they would not be said to understand English unless they possessed this information; which, of course, is not to say that they have to understand the technical vocabulary. Obviously people understand English who have never even heard of words like 'noun' or 'verb' or even, conceivably, the word 'word'. But they could not be said to know English unless they had available to them information about the structure of English sentences that is conveyed through the use of these terms. Notice, moreover, that given a knowledge of English and a familiarity with the terminology, with regard to the kind of facts we have been discussing it is virtually inconceivable that there should be any disagreement. If you were to deny that in the case of the sentence under consideration *boy* was a noun, I should be as surprised as I would be if, being present now in the room in which I am sitting, you were to deny that the piece of paper upon which I am writing is rectangular in shape and white in colour. That facts of this kind are obvious does not make them any the less important but it does, perhaps, make them less interesting. It is a result of their being – in a sense which will be made clearer as we go on – facts about the superficial structure of language. One of the important consequences of Chomsky's approach to linguistics is that it makes it possible for us to uncover facts about language structure that are not obvious and that are not immediately available, even to the native speaker of the language.

The second point is that the kind of structural information we have been discussing is what would be traditionally described as 'syntactic'. There is not room here for anything more than a passing reference to the current controversy about whether it is possible to draw a distinction between syntactic and semantic structure.[3] The decision has profound implications for linguistic theory. Here we need notice only that proponents of both points of view, when they talk about the structure of a sentence (other than its phonological structure), are essentially concerned with its meaning.

The third point about the information contained in the tree-diagram is that none of it relates directly to what can be observed. For example, there is nothing in the pronunciation of *boy* and *ball* that tells one that they are both nouns, or even that they are both words (listening carefully to a tape-recording of a conversation should be enough to convince most people that, contrary to what is popularly believed, speakers do not always make short pauses before and after words, though, of course, these are the places, rather than in the middle of words, where they are most likely to make pauses). The point that nothing of what we know about the syntactic or semantic structure of an utterance relates directly to what we can observe about it is so obvious that it is easy not to notice it. But it explains why this kind of information lies beyond the reach of structuralist analytical techniques.

The kind of information contained in a model of what the native speaker (or one who has acquired a native speaker's knowledge) knows about the structure of his language, will, therefore be of the same kind, and expressed in the same terminology, as that found in traditional grammars (with the important difference that in traditional grammars the information tends to be restricted to what we have termed information about the superficial structure of the language). What above all distinguishes grammars as Chomsky conceives of them from traditional grammars – and this relates to the former being explicitly models of the native speaker's knowledge of the structure of his language – is that they are constructed in such a way as to meet certain formal constraints. Of these, three are particularly important.

The first relates to the fact that probably everyday we hear a sentence we have never heard before, but immediately we hear it – assuming it is a well-formed sentence in a language we know – we know its structure (understand what it means). It would not be regarded as odd if we were to say to someone that we had just heard a new word, but it would certainly be regarded as odd if we were to say that we had just heard a new sentence. A moment's consideration shows that there is no upper bound to the number of sentences in any natural language. To say that I know English, therefore, is to say that I know an unlimited (not just a very large) number of sentences, though for obvious reasons I will only actually hear or utter a finite number of them. If a grammar is to qualify as a model of my knowledge of English, one of the conditions it must meet, therefore, is that it should supply information about an unbounded set of sentences.

The second formal condition that a grammar must meet relates to the fact that this information is in some sense 'inside' us. It follows from the fact that we are finite beings that at the same time as covering an unbounded set of cases a grammar must be finite. At first sight this might appear a paradox but consideration of the following, more familiar, case will show that it is not. Suppose you write down numbers on a blackboard. No matter what number you write down I can immediately write down a larger number simply by adding one to your number. We might, therefore, want to say that I know infinitely many numbers. But clearly I have not acquired this knowledge as a result of learning them. My ability to produce an infinite set of numbers is, in this case, the result of my having mastered a simple set of rules for generating numbers; and clearly this set of rules is finite. Similarly, a grammar must take the form of a finite set of rules for generating an unbounded set of sentences. Systems of this kind are studied in recursive function theory. One of Chomsky's most important contributions to linguistics has been to show that it is in this part of mathematics – more particularly, the branch called 'restricted infinite automata theory' – that the foundations of the subject are to be sought.[4] The concept of a grammatical rule is, of course, as old as the study of grammar itself. Looking at the problem from another point of view we see that what a grammar of this kind reflects is the fact that, although there is no upper bound to the number of well-formed sentences in a language, a sentence qualifies for membership of this set only as a result of its being constructed in accordance with the (finite) rules of the language. For example, it is a rule of English that a noun phrase may be formed by a determiner (like *the*) followed by a noun (like *boy*). This information can be expressed in a rule of the kind

$$N(\text{oun}) \ P(\text{hrase}) \longrightarrow D(\text{eterminer}) + N(\text{oun})$$

where the symbol $\longrightarrow$ is to be interpreted as 'is to be rewritten or expanded as'. If we now add rules of the kind

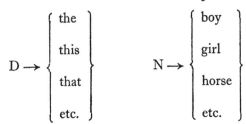

(where the brackets indicate that one, but only one, of the items they contain is to be chosen to expand the symbol on the left-hand side of the equation) we have a set of rules for constructing certain types of English noun phrases. Moreover, these rules will generate only well-formed English noun phrases. They will not generate phrases like *boy the* or *the this*. When we look at the set of rules that have been involved in the construction of a particular noun phrase we find that they constitute an analysis of it.

The third formal condition that a grammar must meet relates the fact that it is intended to be a model of what the native speaker intuitively knows about the structure of his language. Obviously the construction of such a model can be undertaken only by somebody who is a native speaker or by somebody who has acquired a native speaker's knowledge of the language. But this means that he faces very special problems regarding the completeness of the model he builds. It is always possible that his belief that he has provided in the grammar a complete, objective statement of the structure of a particular sentence is an illusion resulting from his having a complete intuitive knowledge of its structure. Probably the only way of overcoming this difficulty is to ensure that the rules of the grammar are 'effectively computable'. That is to say, they must be set up in such a way that the generation of sentences, together with their analyses, is the result of the rules of the grammar being followed out in a purely automatic manner.

Probably nothing else in Chomsky's work has caused more misunderstanding than his claim that grammars must be effectively computable (perhaps because many people subconsciously feel antipathetic to this way of talking about the capacities of human beings). It is particularly important to understand that, although the grammar has to be set up in such a way that it will automatically generate sentences and their analyses, this does not mean that it is intended to be a model, or part of a model, of the way in which we actually produce sentences. To repeat, a grammar is a model of what we know about the structure of a language. It is not intended to be a model of how we apply this knowledge in producing or understanding sentences. Obviously the latter is a legitimate study (and obviously any model we might produce of this activity would have to incorporate a grammar) but it is not what we are concerned with when we construct a grammar. The only reason for setting a grammar up in the form of a finite set of effectively computable rules is in order to meet demands of completeness and objectivity; the failure to attempt to meet such demands rendering the whole enterprise trivial.

If we accept the idea that a grammar must consist of a finite set of effectively computable rules then there are certain classes of grammatical models that we can immediately reject.

Of these the most interesting are those called 'phrase-structure' grammars.[5] A phrase-structure grammar has rules of the following kind:

$$S \rightarrow NP + VP + \langle Adverb \rangle$$

$$NP \rightarrow \begin{cases} D + N \\ Pronoun \end{cases}$$

$$V \rightarrow \begin{cases} Vintransitive \\ Vtransitive + NP \end{cases} + \langle Adverb \rangle$$

$$D \rightarrow \begin{cases} the \\ that \\ etc. \end{cases}$$

$$N \rightarrow \begin{cases} boy \\ girl\ ball\ book \\ etc. \end{cases}$$

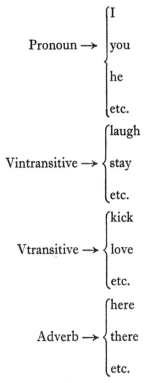

Pronoun → { I, you, he, etc. }

Vintransitive → { laugh, stay, etc. }

Vtransitive → { kick, love, etc. }

Adverb → { here, there, etc. }

Where $<\ >$ indicates that it is optional whether the items contained therein form part of the expansion of the symbol on the left-hand side of the arrow.

A grammar of this kind is capable of generating sentences together with analyses of the tree-diagram type attached to them. But it is important to notice that the rules themselves do not generate tree-diagrams directly. The immediate output of the set of rules above would be structures like the following

```
S
NP + VP
D  + N  + VP
the + N  + VP
the + boy + VP
the + boy + V      + NP
the + boy + kicked + NP
```

the + boy + kicked + D + N
the + boy + kicked + the + N
the + boy + kicked + the + ball

A structure of this kind is called a 'derivation'. Given a derivation it is a straightforward matter to produce a tree-diagram from it through the purely automatic process of cancelling out each occurrence of any symbol except the first, and then drawing lines linking it with the symbol or symbols which now lie directly beneath it. Thus *NP* will be linked to *D + N*, *D* to *the*, and *N* to *boy* etc.

The rules in a phrase-structure grammar can only be partially ordered. Although with regard to the set of rules given above the rule that introduces the symbol *V* cannot, of course, apply before the rule that introduces the symbol *VP* there is, for example, no reason for our insisting that the rules which expand *VP* should apply before those that expand *NP*. This means that for any given set of rules and any given sentence a number of derivations will be produced. For example, an alternative derivation for the sentence *The boy kicked the ball* is one starting

S
NP + VP
NP + V + NP

The reader can easily produce several more for himself, all of them cancelling out to the same tree-diagram. However, it is important to understand that they cancel out to the same tree-diagram only because the grammar meets certain conditions. For example, it contains no rules which rewrite more than one symbol at a time. That is, there are no rules of the kind

NP + VP → D + N + V + NP

If there were such rules then a derivation would be produced of the following kind

S
NP + VP
D + N + V + NP

Remembering that it is part of the process for generating sentences, and, therefore, must be implemented in a fully automatic way, it is obvious that, given such a derivation, there is nothing to direct the algorithm to produce a tree-diagram of the desired form

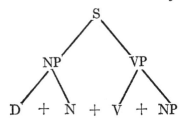

as opposed say to

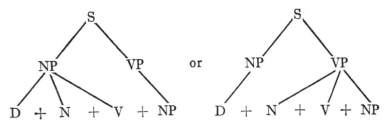

This is not the only restriction that has to be imposed upon the kind of rules that a phrase-structure grammar can contain if it is to meet the condition that for any given set of rules and any given sentence all the possible derivations are to be equivalent in the sense of reducing to the same tree-diagram. They must also comply with the restriction that in the case of no symbol that is introduced shall there be a rule that has the effect of removing it. But consider the imperative sentence

Stay here.

and the analysis

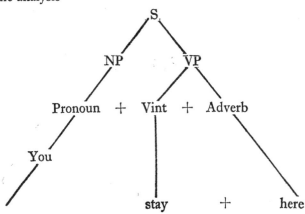

Notice first, that this analysis could only be attached to the sentence *Stay here* by a grammar containing the rule You → ø (where ø is to be interpreted as a blank, that is to say, the rule has the effect of deleting the symbol *you*). Notice, second, that what this analysis claims is that although the word *you* cannot be observed to be part of the sentence *Stay here*, in the sense that one does not hear it when the sentence is uttered or read it when the sentence is written down, it nevertheless forms part of its structure. In fact, it claims that it is the subject. This accords exactly with what traditional grammarians said about the meaning of sentences of this kind – as they put it, in sentences like this the subject is 'understood'. Evidence that the subject understood in this sentence is the word *you*, comes from the fact that *You stay here* is an exact paraphrase of *Stay here*, whereas *John, stay here, Gentlemen, stay here, Cat Stevens, stay here*, or any other noun phrase you care to suggest is not. But this fact cannot be represented in a phrase-structure grammar because the analysis which adequately represents it, given above, has to come from a derivation like

$$
\begin{array}{l}
\text{S} \\
\text{NP } + \text{VP} \\
\text{Pronoun } + \text{VP} \\
\quad \text{You } + \text{Vint } + \text{Adverb} \\
\quad \text{You } + \text{stay } + \text{Adverb} \\
\quad \text{You } + \text{stay } + \text{here} \\
\quad\quad \text{stay } + \text{here}
\end{array}
$$

and there is nothing in such a derivation to indicate whether what has happened is that *you* has been deleted or whether, for example, *you* has been rewritten as *stay*, *stay* has been rewritten as *here* and *here* has been deleted.

The inability to assign correct analyses to even one type of sentence is a sufficient reason for rejecting a grammar, but it is easy enough to find examples of other kinds of sentences whose structure cannot be adequately represented by a grammar with rules of this form. Consider the sentence

I put the book back.

In this case too a phrase-structure grammar cannot assign a correct analysis. Perhaps the best it can do is the following

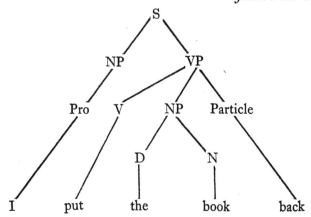

This analysis brings out the fact that the verb *put*, the noun phrase *the book*, and the particle *back*, all go together to make up the verb phrase, but it fails to bring out the fact that anyone who knows English will feel that within the verb phrase *put* and *back* go together to form a unit; irrespective of the fact that they do not occur next to each other in this sentence, as they do, however, in the sentence

I put back the book.

The analysis of which is:

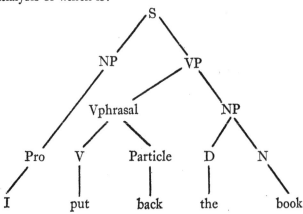

(Assuming now that we add to the set of phrase-structure rules above, a rule

VP → V phrasal + NP

as an alternative expansion of *VP*, and where *V particle* represents the class of verbs including those like *put, look, turn,* etc. which together with particles form phrasal verbs like *put back, look up, turn on,* etc.). Moreover, careful consideration of this analysis leads one to the realization that, as far as the most important structural facts are concerned, it is also the correct analysis of the sentence, *I put the book back.* Just as the correct analysis of *You stay here* is also the correct analysis of *Stay here.* This, of course, relates to the fact that both pairs of sentences are exact paraphrases of each other. It therefore seems that what is needed to capture this insight is a grammar which would assign, what it is natural to call, the same 'underlying' or 'deep-structure' analyses to each of these pairs of sentences, but which would in each case generate two different sentences; the sentences *Stay here* and *I put the book back* being generated as the result of the application of rules playing no part in the generation of the sentences *You stay here* and *I put back the book,* these rules having no effect on the basic meaning structure of the sentence, but merely, as it were, that of distorting and obscuring the enduring underlying pattern, in the one case by deleting an element in the underlying structure, in the other by permuting elements in it. But we have already shown that a phrase-structure grammar cannot contain rules for deleting symbols, and it is also easy to show that phrase-structure rules which have the effect of permuting symbols also, inevitably, have the effect of producing absurd analyses. For example, the only way we can get the grammar given above to assign the analysis

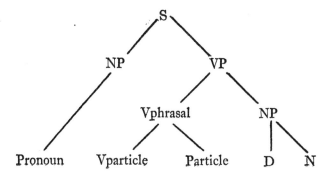

to the sentence *I put the book back* is by accepting in the grammar
rules like

$$\text{Particle} \rightarrow \text{NP}$$

$$\text{NP} \quad \rightarrow \text{Particle}$$

which are clearly absurd.

In Syntactic Structures Chomsky lays the foundations for the
study of a class of grammars which are able to assign analyses to
sentences via rules which delete and (in a non-absurd way) permute symbols and are thus able adequately to represent the structure of sentences of the kind we have been discussing. These are
called transformational grammars and the rules which delete and
permute symbols are called transformational rules. The name
transformational grammar is perhaps misleading since it gives the
impression that a grammar of this kind contains only transformational rules. In fact, a transformational grammar is a grammar that
contains both transformational and phrase-structure rules; transformational rules being rules which operate upon the output of
phrase-structure rules. That is, unlike phrase-structure rules, they
are not rules for rewriting one symbol as another (or others) but
rules for rewriting one tree-diagram as another. It is important to
bear this in mind because the way transformational rules are
written down tends to obscure this fact. It is impossible in a brief
non-technical exposition of this kind to provide any account of the
formal nature of transformational rules. But it is less important to
understand their formal nature than to understand the way in
which they enable us to represent the kind of facts about sentences
that we have just been discussing. Chomsky claims that the complete analysis of every sentence consists of two parts, the first
called the 'deep-structure analysis' (the term from now on being
used as a technical term) which is a tree-diagram generated by
phrase-structure rules and which, essentially, represents the
meaning of the sentence, the second – the 'surface structure
analysis', again a tree-diagram, but this time one generated by
much more complicated transformational rules from a deep-
structure tree, and relating much more closely to the observable
utterance, being in fact, the input to the phonological component
of the grammar which interprets it in phonological terms.

Thus in the case of the sentence

I put the book back.

the complete analysis consists of the deep-structure tree

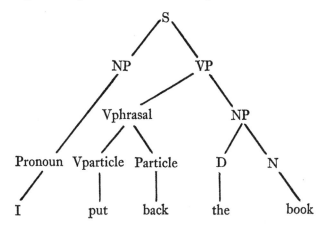

together with a surface-structure tree

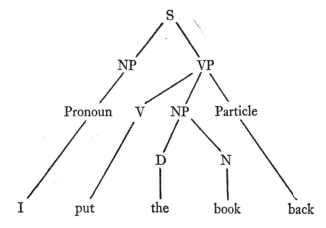

generated by the transformational rule

X + Vparticle + Particle + NP + Y → X + Vparticle
+ NP + Particle + Y

which is to be read as follows; for any tree-diagram reducing to
the structural description that occurs on the left-hand side of the

equation where *Vparticle, Particle,* and *NP* stand for any particle verb, particle, or noun phrase and *X* and *Y* stand for any, and any number, of grammatical symbols (so that as well as the generation of sentences like *I put the book back,* the rule will also cover that of sentences like *The old man hung his coat up on a nail*), another tree-diagram, the structural description of which occurs on the right-hand side of the equation, can be constructed and will be a correct surface-structure representation of it. The grammar containing both phrase-structure and transformational rules can, then, deal in a very natural way with sentences like *I put back the book* and *I put the book back,* which have the same meaning but a different appearance, by assigning them the same deep structure but different surface structures. It deals equally well with what one might regard as the converse case, that is, with sentences like *I hate boring students.* The fact that this sentence has two different meanings (or rather that there are two sentences here) is not reflected in the surface. One may intend either of the two possible interpretations while pronouncing it in exactly the same way. A transformational grammar will reflect this by containing transformational rules which will operate upon the two different deep structures to produce identical surface-structure representations.

Transformational grammarians claim that in the case of all sentences a complete analysis consists of distinct deep- and surface-structure analyses or, to put it another way, that transformational rules are involved in the generation of all sentences. We have shown that this is so in the case of sentences like *Stay here* and *I put the book back,* but up to now we have talked about the structure of sentences like *You stay here* and *I put back the book* as if correct analyses could be assigned to them by phrase-structure rules alone. This is only because we have deliberately ignored the fact that the analyses that have been assigned to these sentences in the course of the discussion are incomplete.

Consider again the sentence

The boy kicked the ball.

The phrase-structure rules given above would assign to this sentence the analysis

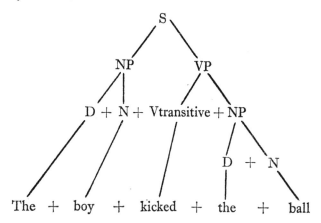

When we look at this analysis a little more carefully we see that it fails to represent all the structural information associated with the sentence. Anyone who knows English knows that *kicked* is further analysable into two elements (morphemes) the verb *kick* and the past-tense marker *-ed*. At first sight there seems to be no problem in emending the grammar to cover this by adding rules of the kind

$$\text{Vtransitive} \rightarrow \text{M(ain)V} \cap \left\{ \begin{array}{l} \text{Present tense} \\ \text{Past tense} \end{array} \right\} + \text{NP}$$

where $\cap$ indicates a morpheme juncture. The analysis produced by this new set of rules would be

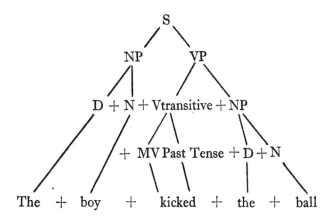

Now take the sentence *The boy has kicked the ball*, and notice that we cannot analyse *kicked* here in the way we analysed it in the previous sentence, taking *-ed* as a past-tense marker. In fact, *The boy has kicked the ball* is a present-tense sentence, as shown by the well-formedness of the sentence *The boy has kicked the ball now*, as opposed to, *The boy has kicked the ball yesterday*. (Cf. *The boy kicked the ball yesterday* and *The boy kicked the ball now*.) But tense does not constitute the only difference between the two sentences. In *The boy has kicked the ball* the verb is also marked for perfective aspect (which, roughly speaking, indicates completeness of action) this being associated with two elements, the so-called auxiliary verb *have* and the past participle ending on the main verb – which also happens in this case to have the phonological form *-ed*. What then tells us that the sentence is present tense? Clearly in this case it is the ending on the auxiliary verb (cf. the past-tense sentence *The boy had kicked the ball*). To summarize: in the sentences *The boy kicked the ball* the verb phrase is past tense and in the sentence *The boy has kicked the ball* it is present tense. In the latter case it is also marked for perfective aspect, which is realized by a complex discontinuous element comprising both the auxiliary verb *have* and the *-ed* ending on the main verb. When, so to speak, the position at the end of the main verb is occupied by the participle, the tense marker gets added to the auxiliary verb. Exactly the same thing happens in sentences where the verb phrase is marked for continuous aspect; that is those containing the discontinuous element (*be – – Present participle*, the phonological representation of forms produced by adding tense markers to the auxiliary verb, *be⌢Present tense* and *be⌢Past tense*, being *is* and *was*, as in *The boy is kicking the ball* and *The boy was kicking the ball*.

Now look at the sentence

The boy has been kicking the ball.

Here the verb phrase has both perfective and continuous aspect. When both occur the elements associated with perfective aspect come before those associated with continuous aspect, so that it is the present participle ending that is attached to the main verb, the past participle now being added to the auxiliary verb *be*, where its phonological realization is *-en*, and the tense marker being added to *have*. It is an interesting, and perhaps rather surprising, fact that these clear, if rather cumbersome, informal descriptions of the structure of the verb phrase cannot be adequately translated into phrase-structure rules. This is not to say that a phrase-structure grammar could not generate these verb phrases and their correct analyses. It can, but only as a result of having a different rule for each kind of verb phrase. One would need one rule

$$V \rightarrow MV \frown Tense$$

for sentences like

> The boy kicks the ball.

Another rule

$$V \rightarrow have \frown Tense + MV \frown Past\ participle$$

for sentences like

> The boy has kicked the ball.

Another

$$V \rightarrow be \frown Tense + MV \frown Present\ participle$$

for

> The boy is kicking the ball.

and yet another

$$V \rightarrow have \frown Tense + be \frown Past\ participle$$
$$+ MV \frown Present\ participle$$

for

> The boy has been kicking the ball.

But this is to miss the generalization contained in the informal descriptions given above; the fact that there is a persistent pattern underlying all four verb phrases. In a transformational grammar this can be expressed in just two rules which will generate all well-formed verb phrases. One phrase-structure rule

$$V \rightarrow Tense + \langle have \frown Past\ participle \rangle$$
$$+ \langle be \frown Present\ participle \rangle + MV$$

and one transformational rule

$$X + \begin{Bmatrix} Tense \\ Past \\ participle \\ Present \\ participle \end{Bmatrix} + \begin{Bmatrix} have \\ be \\ MV \end{Bmatrix} + Y \rightarrow X + \begin{Bmatrix} have \\ be \\ MV \end{Bmatrix} \frown \begin{Bmatrix} Tense \\ Past \\ participle \\ Present \\ participle \end{Bmatrix} + Y$$

This states that whenever an underlying tree-diagram contains one of the elements in the first pair of brackets followed immediately by one of the elements in the second, a new tree is to be produced in which the order of the elements is reversed and the sign connecting them changed from a word boundary to a morpheme boundary. This rule will apply once to a tree whose structural description is

$$X + \text{Tense} + \text{MV} + Y$$

to produce a tree with the structural description

$$X + \text{MV} \frown \text{Tense} + Y$$

as in the case of the sentence

The boy kicked the ball.

It will apply twice in cases where the structural description is

$$X + \text{Tense} + \text{have} + \text{Past Participle} + \text{MV} + Y$$

or $\quad X + \text{Tense} + \text{be} + \text{Present participle} + \text{MV} + Y$

as in the case of the sentence

The boy has kicked the ball.

and   The boy was kicking the ball.

and three times when the structural description is

$$X + \text{Tense} + \text{have} + \text{Past participle} + \text{be}$$
$$+ \text{Present participle} + \text{MV}$$

as in the case of the sentence

The boy has been kicking the ball.

The reason for preferring this analysis is not merely that it requires fewer rules – though this, of course, is an attractive feature – but, as we have already indicated, that it states a fact about the structure of English verb phrases that the phrase-structure analysis fails to capture. The latter implies that each type of verb phrase is constructed in a different way, the former makes the less obvious but, once it is pointed out, much more plausible suggestion, that they are all formed in essentially the same way. If this analysis is accepted, since every well-formed English sentence contains at least one verb phrase, then transformational rules will play a part in the generation of every English sentence.

But the transformational analysis of the verb phrase has a further advantage. Consider the sentences

John did not arrive.

and

John has not arrived.

The positive versions of these negative sentences are

John arrived.

and

John has arrived.

The question we are concerned with is why it is, in the case of sentences which are marked for aspect, the positive differs from the negative sentence only through the presence of the negative particle *not*, whereas in the case of the sentences which are not marked for aspect, in addition to the particle *not* there is also present the verb *do* which, moreover, takes the tense ending instead of the main verb. If we accept the transformational analysis of the verb phrase it turns out that we can provide a very natural explanation for these facts. Let us assume that a grammar which could generate both positive and negative sentences will have as its first rule

$$S \rightarrow <Neg> + NP + VP$$

Then the underlying structure for

John has not arrived

will be a tree-diagram with the structural description

$$X + Neg + NP + Tense + have$$
$$+ \text{ Past participle} + MV + Y$$

Clearly in this case the transformational rule which puts the negative particle into its surface-structure position has to move it to a position between *have* and *Past Participle*, to produce a tree with the structural description

$$X + NP + Tense + have + Neg$$
$$+ \text{ Past participle} + MV + Y$$

The rule forming the surface realization of the verb phrase will now operate upon this structure to generate the sentence

John has not arrived.

Now let us consider the underlying structure of

John did not arrive.

Assuming that this is

$$X + Neg + NP + Tense + MV + Y$$

then the effect of rule that moves the negative particle is to place
it between the elements *Tense* and *MV*. (Thus there are really
two rules which move *Neg*. The first moves it to a position immediately after *Tense*, the second moves it to a position immediately after *have* or *be* if the effect of the first rule has been to
place the *Neg* in a position immediately in front of these elements.)
In this case only the first rule is applicable, producing a tree-
diagram with the description

$$X + NP + Tense + Neg + MV + Y$$

But notice that in this case the rule for the verb phrase cannot
apply. This states that elements like *Tense* and *MV* reverse their
position only if one immediately precedes the other, and in this
case they are separated by *Neg*. But this now suggests why this
sentence contains the verb *do*; its role being that of a carrier to
which the separated tense element can be attached. All we need is a
transformational rule which introduces *do* into tree-diagrams with
the structural description

$$X + NP + Tense + Neg + MV + Y$$

giving

$$X + NP + Tense + do + Neg + MV + Y$$

and emend the verb phrase rule by adding *do* to the list comprising
have, *be*, and *MV*, and the desired surface structure will be
generated. Notice that in allowing transformational rules to introduce elements like *do* we are in no way impugning the claim
that transformational rules do not affect the meaning of the
sentence. The verb *do* in this sentence is clearly a meaningless
element; as we have suggested, its role in the sentence is merely
to provide a verbal element for the tense marker to be attached to.
A phrase-structure grammar could generate these sentences but
it would fail to assign analyses which provide the kind of explanation of the structure that is implicit in the transformational analysis.[6]

This analysis of the verb phrase (which is essentially that proposed by Chomsky in *Syntactic Structures*) is a good example of a non-obvious hypothesis about language structure. The reason for accepting this hypothesis is not just that it provides a satisfactory account of the verb phrase itself, but that it also turns out to be the basis of an equally satisfactory account of certain kinds of negative sentences. A grammar is a theory of the structure of a language, and in constructing a grammar a linguist is subject to the same constraints and liberties as someone constructing a theory in, say, physics or biology. Among these is the right to feel that he is on the right track when, as in this case, by making only a small increase in the complexity of his theory he is able greatly to extend the data that it covers.

At this point it is perhaps necessary to enter a *caveat*. The nature of transformational rules is still not properly understood. One thing that is certain, however, is that in their present form they are too powerful.[7] Some less general formulation needs to be found which will limit the types of transformational rules. At the moment any type of deletion and any type of permutation is permitted. This means that for any postulated deep structure transformational rules exist which will relate it to the desired surface structure. For this reason the claim that is sometimes made that transformational theories have shown that the deep structure of all natural languages is the same must, for the time being at least, be regarded as being without foundation.

This is not to say that the hypothesis that all languages have the same deep structure is not a reasonable one. Indeed one might almost say that the whole of transformational linguistics is directed towards substantiating it. English, Arabic, Chocktaw, and Chinese are quite different phenomena, but we have a deep-seated intuition that in spite of their observable differences each of them is a language. Transformational grammarians are committed to the attempt to discover the basis for this intuition; to discover those formal characteristics which all languages possess and which make them languages.

The hypothesis that all languages have the same deep structure is connected with another hypothesis, which is that language is innate. Like the first hypothesis this has been put forward in many different versions so that it can either be a very strong or a very weak hypothesis. At the moment there seems to be little point in trying to arbitrate between them. But there is, perhaps, some point in trying to explain why Chomsky should seek to revive the rationalist hypothesis as far as language is concerned.[8] If there is one lesson to be learned from Chomsky's work it is that the structure of language is far more complex than it is generally recognized to be and that many of the structural characteristics of sentences relate to what can be observed only in a very indirect way. It is hardly surprising, therefore, that anyone who has made a serious study of it should find it difficult to accept theories which postulate no special predisposition in the child for mastering language structure and which put at his disposal only procedures of the kind described in behaviourist learning theories, and that he should be attracted to the idea that the child is in some way, 'pre-programmed' for this specific purpose.

NOTES

1 Bloomfield (1935), p. 38. Esper (1968) gives an interesting account of the history of these ideas and their influence on linguistics.
2 See Chomsky and Halle (1968).
3 See Chomsky (1969) and Lakoff (in press).
4 See the articles by Chomsky and Miller in Luce, Bush & Galanter (1963) and (1965).
5 For a fuller account of phrase-structure grammars see Postal (1964) and Lyons (1970).
6 For a full account of the grammar of negative sentences see Klima 'Negation in English' in Fodor and Katz (1964).
7 See Peters and Ritchie (1969).
8 See Chomsky (1959), (1965), and (1968).

BIBLIOGRAPHY

BLOOMFIELD, L. *Language*, London, Allen and Unwin, 1935.
CHOMSKY, N. *Syntactic Structures*, The Hague, Mouton, 1957.
CHOMSKY, N. 'Review of Skinner "Verbal Behaviour" ', *Language*, **35**, 26–58, 1959. Reprinted Fodor & Katz, 1964.
CHOMSKY, N. *Aspects of the Theory of Syntax*, Cambridge, Mass., MIT Press, 1965.
CHOMSKY, N. *Language and Mind*, New York, Harcourt, Brace & World, 1968.
CHOMSKY, N. *Deep Structure, Surface Structure and Semantic Interpretation*, MIT (Mimeo), 1969.

CHOMSKY, N. & HALLE, M. *The Sound Pattern of English*, New York, Harper & Row, 1968.

ESPER, E. *Mentalism and Objectivism in Linguistics*, New York, Elsevier, 1968.

FODOR, J. & KATZ, J. (eds). *The Structure of Language: Readings in the Philosophy of Language*, Englewood Cliffs, N. J., Prentice-Hall, 1964.

KUHN, T. *The Structure of Scientific Revolutions*, Chicago, University of Chicago Press, 1962.

LAKOFF, G. (in press). 'On Generative Semantics', in Jakobovits & Steinberg (eds), *Semantics*, London, Cambridge University Press.

LUCE, R., BUSH, R. & GALANTER, E. (eds). *Handbook of Mathematical Psychology*, Vol. II, New York, Wiley, 1963.

LUCE, R., BUSH, R. & GALANTER, E. (eds). *Readings in Mathematical Psychology*, Vol. II, New York, Wiley, 1965.

LYONS, J. *Chomsky*, London, Fontana/Collins, 1970.

PETERS, P. & RITCHIE, R. 'A Note on the Universal Base Hypothesis', *Journal of Linguistics*, **5**, 150–2, 1969.

POSTAL, P. *Constituent Structure: A Study of Contemporary Models of Syntactic Description*, The Hague, Mouton, 1964.

Comment

R. B. LEES

Elaborating somewhat on Thorne's instructive introduction, we may summarize the central notion thus: Chomsky's programme proposes to gain insight into some features of the mind by studying certain aspects of linguistic intuitions. It assumes that a normal, expert user of a natural language L has memorized its vocabulary but has come to know its SENTENCES by having mastered a set G of compositional RULES which determine exactly the relation between pronunciations and meanings in L. Accordingly, the paramount task of linguistics is to formulate for each language L_i such a set G_i of principles, its GRAMMAR, under certain plausible constraints. For example (1) each G_i must be an instantiation of a general form which characterizes human languages, i.e. Language; (2) each L_i contains a countably infinite set of (fully) grammatical sentences S_j^i; (3) each S_j^i has a specifiable internal organization of parts, the choice and arrangement of which determine the meaning and pronunciation of S_j^i; (4) the grammar G_i can plausibly be imputed to the knowledge of every native user of L_i and can form an essential part of the mental equipment he requires to understand an arbitrary sentence of L_i; etc. Any of these constraints may have to be relaxed or strengthened more or less as research progresses. The phenomena studied, the linguistic intuitions of users of L_i, must obviously be considered in a more or less idealized form, presumably the less so as more knowledge is gained. Thus, (1) speakers who differ somewhat in their judgements will be accorded slightly different G-s, even if they are said to speak the same language; (2) every S_j^i is judgeable by each user of L_i as grammatical and as containing its fixed con-

206

stituents; (3) certain S_j are judged to be exact paraphrases of one another, though perhaps different in style; (4) each user is presumed to be master of more than one variant of L_i; etc.

The current favourite candidate for the form of G is one or another variant of a so-called TRANSFORMATIONAL GENERATIVE grammar, i.e. one which relates sound and meaning in part by means of rules capable of transforming constituent trees by ellipsis or attachment of sub-trees. There are many degrees of freedom in the choice of elements in such a model – in fact, too many, as Thorne remarks. For example, in Chomsky's so-called classical model, each S_j is assigned to a deep-structure tree of constituents the terminal nodes of which are morphemes, each of which in turn has a particular semantic, syntactic, and phonological characterization; the tree is transformed in a certain way to a surface-structure tree, and these two trees are interpreted semantically and phonetically, respectively. Thus, one must choose in G_i (1) the rules which generate recursively all the deep structures (rules which, because they must be recursive, cannot in general be ordered); (2) the lexicon of morphemes, each with its semantic syntactic, and phonological descriptions, say in terms of binary features; (3) the grammatical transformation rules; (4) the rules of semantic and phonetic interpretation; etc. Naturally, there are no algorithms to determine whether a given linguistic distinction is correctly formulated as a difference in (1) choice of base elements, (2) arrangements of these on a tree, (3) choice of semantic or syntactic features characterizing one or more morphemes, (4) transformational derivation, (5) semantic interpretation, (6) the position of one or more rules prior to, within, or subsequent to a CYCLE of ordered transformational rules, etc., or any combination of these.

For any given generally accepted choice there is usually much plausible evidence. For example, to Thorne's support for describing imperative sentences in English as derivatives from an abstract underlying (deep) structure with a subject *you*, itself subsequently deleted in the transformational derivation, we may add the stronger argument that there is no other plausible way to explain the heavy restriction in such imperative sentences on subsequent reflexive pronouns to only the forms *yourself* and *your own*. Or again, for his example of why one must assume that certain verbs contain a particle, as *up* in *Max looked the information up*, there would otherwise by no reasonable explanation for the absence of nominals such as **Max's looking of the information up* . . . (parallel to, say, *Max's sending of the information to Japan* . . .).

There are, of course, many difficult open questions in current research. For example, no one has developed a satisfactory account of how a person understands an UNgrammatical utterance, though we might well expect that as insight is gained into how we understand grammatical sentences some reasonable view will emerge. Further, we do not now know how to construe the language of infants, nor how infants acquire their abilities. We do not now know whether and, if so, how language evolved. No one has yet provided a satisfactory way to describe our knowledge of idioms; we do not know how correctly to describe derivative morphology and other partially productive constructions. We are not sure what a 'natural phonetic description' would be like, nor how correctly to describe sentence intonation.

Much current controversy centres on the choice between two alternative views on the position of semantic rules in a grammar. Chomsky's classical model has them as interpretative, projecting from the meanings of the morphemes and the syntactic form of the deep structure of a sentence to its meanings. A sizeable group of his older students and some others would assume rather that the grammar as a whole interprets phonetically in underlying semantic representation, itself perhaps specified by some semantic base-rules, and that there is no uniformly definable syntactic base for sentences. Chomsky conjectures that at our present level of understanding neither model is strongly enough constrained for the two to be distinguished empirically, i.e. that they are notational variants.[1] Many would view the former model to be supported by an (empirical) finding that there is a universal syntactic base, in Chomsky's sense, languages differing among themselves only in morphemes, some transformational rules, and phonology.

Peters and Ritchie reached the result cited by Thorne after investigating the empirical significance of the universal-base hypothesis; they show, in effect, that ANY BASE can be made universal and thus that the choice of base cannot be made on empirical grounds. In fact, as has been feared for some time, transformational rules, as now conceived on good evidence, are so powerful that a transformational grammar is equivalent to a universal Turing machine, i.e. can compute ANY partial recursive function. Therefore, until stronger constraints can plausibly be imposed on these concepts, there is no hope of distinguishing empirically between two alternative transformational models for language.[2]

Recently some radically different proposals have been mooted. As we noted, a grammar must, of course, serve within a larger account of HOW a language-user puts to USE the knowledge the grammar represents. Bever and others have suggested that linguistic intuitions are not correctly captured by a transformational grammar but that rather they must be represented in terms of the 'perceptual strategies' which a person uses to decode a sentence as parts of it are received and processed successively.[3] Perhaps these psycholinguists would not go quite that far, for the evidence is strong in favour of the claim that a person does have the kind of independent syntactic knowledge a transformational description implies. Thus, we may expect the truth to fall somewhere in between.

Thus we see that the central issue in linguistics today is wide open, namely, what is the form of a person's knowledge of his language.

NOTES AND REFERENCES

1 See, for example, CHOMSKY, N. A., 'Deep Structure, Surface Structure and Semantic Interpretation', in Jakobovits and Steinberg, *Semantics*, Cambridge University Press (forthcoming).

2 Nor is this state of affairs altered by the addition of new freedoms, even if linguistically motivated, such as, for example, so-called 'global derivational constraints', as proposed by Lakoff, Postal, and others; see LAKOFF, G., 'Global rules', *Language*, **46**, 627–39, 1970.

3 See, for example, BEVER, T. G., *A Survey of Some Recent Work in Psycholinguistics*, IBM Research Center, Yorktown Heights, N.Y., 1968.

© *R. B. Lees 1972*

Pure Mathematics: moons not hers?

JOHN PYM

My aim is first to show you the kind of thing mathematics is. This I shall try to do by means of an example, and as it is necessarily quite simple, in the second section I shall attempt to describe a more significant result. In the third section, I discuss some questions more philosophical in nature.

I. THE ORDINARY MATHEMATICIAN'S VIEW OF HIS SUBJECT

The book which has most influenced the contemporary mathematician's view of his subject began to be written in 1939, and chapters of it are still appearing. *Éléments de mathématique* is written by a group of Frenchmen under the pseudonym N. Bourbaki,[1] and the rules for membership of the group, though informal, seem to be very strict. It could be said that Bourbaki had illusions about what he was going to do. The only picture in the book occurs at the beginning; it is presented entirely without comment; and it is a photograph of a marble showing Hercules cleaning out the Augean stables. To be fair, many people would see some truth in this picture.

What concerns us here is Bourbaki's view of mathematics. (I am not suggesting that he was the first to take this standpoint – it can be found in the works of Euclid.) Fortunately, the first sentence of the introduction to his work is very much to the point: 'Depuis les Grecs, qui dit "Mathématique" dit "démonstration".' Mathematics is about proving things, but anyone who recalls school geometry will remember that it has a very special idea of proof. To tell you what I mean by mathematics, I must tell you what I mean by proof.

At this point I could launch into a philosophical discussion of the nature of proof, but this might only tangle you up in my prejudices. I shall allow myself the luxury of giving my opinion later. I hope to convey an impression of what a proof is by actually showing you one. Of course, several would be better, and you should try to bear in mind what you remember of school geometry. Mainly because the subject is intuitively accessible, I have chosen a geometrical example.

Geometry is about points and lines. It is impossible to say exactly what these words mean for reasons which should become clear later, but so that the proof makes sense, I will try to give a provisional description. Roughly, a *point* is just a mark of position; it has no size in the sense of length or area. The word *line* is to be interpreted as meaning 'straight line with infinite extent in both directions'. Thus a line never ends. Lines have no width, and if two different lines meet, where they cross is a point. I shall call two lines *parallel* if they are identical or else do not meet.

We now come to the proof. It is usual (and helpful) to precede it by a statement of what is to be proved:

THEOREM. There is a one-to-one correspondence between the points of a line and the points of any other line which intersects it.

One-to-one correspondence means just what it says: we can make the points of the lines correspond in pairs in such a way that every point of the first corresponds to exactly one of the second and vice versa. (This may be understood as saying that the two lines have the same number of points.) To illustrate the concept, I give an example which has nothing to do with the theorem. Take two

Figure 1

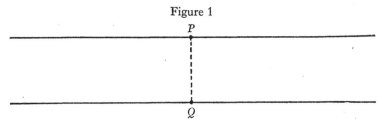

horizontal lines, and let two points correspond if and only if one is vertically above the other (e.g. the points *P* and *Q* in *Figure 1*).

The proof consists of the numbered statements which follow. The explanatory remarks and the picture (*Figure 2*) have nothing to do with it (except for the important fact that they help in understanding).

Figure 2 ·

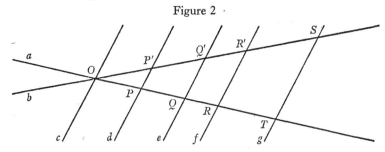

(i) Let the lines a, b intersect in the point O.

(ii) There is a line c through O distinct from both a and b.

This provides a setting for the rest of the proof. We next construct the correspondence.

(iii) Let P be any point on a.

(iv) There is a line d through P parallel to c.

(v) The line d is not parallel to b.

(vi) The line d meets b in a point which we shall denote by P'.

(vii) We let P' correspond to P.

As P was any point on a, we have seen how we can assign to each point of a a point of b. Two things must now be shown. First, that to different points of a, different points of b are assigned, and, secondly, that each point of b is assigned to some point of a. We consider the first of these.

(viii) Let Q, R be two distinct points of a.

(ix) The line e through Q parallel to c meets b in Q'.

(x) The line f through R parallel to c meets b in R'.

(xi) The lines e, f are parallel.

(xii) The lines e, f are not identical.

(xiii) The lines e, f do not meet.

(xiv) The point Q' is distinct from R'.

And now the second.

(xv) Let S be a point of b.

(xvi) Let g be the line through S parallel to c.

(xvii) The line *g* is not parallel to *a*.

(xviii) The line *g* meets *a* in a point *T*.

(xix) The line through *T* parallel to *c* is *g*.

(xx) The line *g* meets *b* in *S*.

(xxi) Thus *S* is *T'*.

The proof is now complete.

The point of a proof is that it should be absolutely incontrovertible. There should no longer be any question of doubting the truth of the theorem. Every statement in the proof should be a necessary logical consequence of those which precede it.

In fact, one has only to look at statement (ii) to see that this ideal has not been attained: and indeed it cannot be attained. There must be some statements in a proof which are unsupported. However I can offer you four statements on which this proof can be made to rest.

(A) Given any two distinct points, there is exactly one line on which they both lie.

(B) On any one line lie at least three distinct points.

(C) Any point lies on at least three distinct lines.

(D) Let any line *l* and any point *P* not on *l* be given. Then there is exactly one line *m* on which *P* lies which has the property that no point lies on both *l* and *m*.

(The last statement looks simpler if we introduce a definition. Call *l* and *m* parallel if either *l* = *m* or no point lies on both *l* and *m*. Then (D) is equivalent to: given any line *l* and any point *P*, there is exactly one line on which *P* lies which is parallel to *l*.)

We can now say what a proof does. If the truth of statements (A)–(D) is admitted, then as a matter of logical necessity the truth of the theorem must be admitted. What is more, the proof does not really make sense until it is given a context by writing down these statements, for if a different set of statements was chosen in place of (A)–(D) then the statements (i)–(xxi) might not be a proof at all.

A mathematical theory is determined by giving a collection of statements which are called *axioms* which are to play the role of (A)–(D) in the theory. Every theorem in the theory must ultimately derive from these axioms. I shall call the theory which (A)–(D) determine an *affine geometry*.

It now looks as if every mathematical theory must begin by facing the problem of justifying its axioms. But mathematics is more subtle than this: it avoids the problem by denying its axioms any real content. Let us see how this works.

Most of the words in our axioms are simple ones from ordinary English, but there are three ideas which require clarification: point, line, lies on. The mathematician says that it does not matter at all what 'points' and 'lines' are understood to be, or what the relation 'lies on' is taken to be; but if, under any interpretation, the axioms (A)–(D) are true, then under the same interpretation the theorem must be true. Indeed, if you look at (i)–(xxi) you will find that all you need to know is that 'point', 'line', and 'lies on' satisfy (A)–(D) and not what these terms actually mean.

To convince you that I mean what I say, let me give a ridiculous example. Suppose we have a village in which each boy addresses certain of the adult males as 'uncle', and suppose an anthropologist observes the following facts.

(a) Given any two different boys, there is exactly one adult they both call uncle.

(b) Any adult is called uncle by at least three different boys.

(c) Any boy calls at least three different adults uncle.

(d) Let any adult l and any boy P who does not call l uncle be given. Then there is exactly one adult m who is called uncle by P and is such that no boy calls both l and m uncle.

Then, whatever the anthropologist may conclude, the mathematician will say, 'What an interesting example of an affine geometry'. And he will also be able to say that his theorem, under the correct interpretation, is true, that is that if two uncles have a common nephew, they have the same number of nephews (which the anthropologist, who has been busy checking (d), has probably failed to notice).

Next we consider an example of an affine geometry which looks just as trivial but has important features about it. As 'points' we take the nine letters A B C D E F G H I. As 'lines' we take the twelve triples (ABC) (DEF) (GHI) (ADG) (BEH) (CFI) (CEG) (AFH) (BDI) (AEI) (CDH) (BFG). A 'point' 'lies on' a 'line' if the letter appears in the triple. (I have tried to illustrate this geometry in *Figure 3*. To find a 'line' on this diagram you take the letters

ʄFigure 3

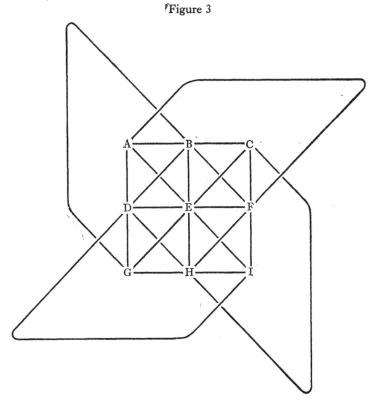

on the lines drawn, but you are not allowed to turn a corner, except where is it rounded off.) It is easy to check that the axioms are satisfied; observe for example, that the only triple containing F 'parallel' to (BDI) is (AFH). Observe also that the theorem is true, for every triple contains three letters.

Let us again take stock of the situation. When I do affine geometry, I deduce everything from axioms (A)–(D). Since these axioms are satisfied by ordinary Euclidean geometry (in the right interpretation), I am assured that everything I prove will be true for Euclidean geometry. But now I also see that my axioms are satisfied by my collection of nine letters, so anything I prove must be true of this as well. When I do affine geometry, I am simultaneously talking about Euclidean geometry and about my collection of nine letters – and about who knows what else besides.

It is in this sense that we are to understand Bertrand Russell's remark: 'Mathematics is the subject in which we never know what we are talking about.'[2]

I shall call an example of a theory, that is something for which the axioms of a theory are satisfied, a *realization* of the theory. (The technical term is 'model', but this word carries a very different sense in the vocabulary of this collection of essays.)

The study of the realizations of theories has lead to some of the deepest results of modern mathematics. I shall give a simple example of the kind of result which can be proved, and provide a more significant one in the next section. Consider this statement:

(E) Every line has at least four points.

Can this be proved in affine geometry? If it can, then the statement must be true for every realization, but it is obviously false for the realization on the nine letters. Thus, (E) cannot be proved. Can (E) be proved to be false? In that case, it would be false for every realization, but (E) is obviously true for ordinary Euclidean geometry. Thus, (E) cannot be proved false in affine geometry. A statement which can neither be proved in a theory, nor proved false in a theory, is called *undecidable* in that theory. (Of course, it may be provable in other theories, for (E) is true in Euclidean geometry.)

I have slipped in a second example of a proof here, for I have proved that (E) is undecidable in the theory of affine geometry. Admittedly, I gave the proof very informally, and you might justifiably be puzzled as to what theory this proof is in, or what axioms I am referring it to. I shall say a little about this later.

I would like to draw your attention to one feature of the result. It is obviously qualitative and not quantitative. It tells us something about the limitations of the statements (A)–(D). Almost certainly, more of modern mathematics is qualitative than quantitative in nature.

Let me sum up what I have said so far. Mathematics consists of proofs, which are strict logical arguments based on clearly stated axioms. A system of axioms may be applicable to more than one situation – indeed, axioms do not define situations, but they describe unknown relationships between unknown quantities. Finally, I pointed out that there may be statements which are undecidable with respect to a particular theory.

II. A GLIMPSE OF MATHEMATICAL LOGIC

The subject of mathematical logic has for the layman – and I count myself one of these – an air of mystery and fascination. Here, if anywhere, we should find certainty. Indeed, to study logic, the sure foundation of reason, by using mathematics, where reason has reached its purest form, might yield insights into the foundations of truth itself. I hope to show that this dream is too wild, but I also hope that some of the mystery will remain.

Another reason for the popularity of logic is that here mathematics comes nearest to suffering the fate of many of the social sciences. Its technical terms often seem to make sense in ordinary language, and its results are therefore open to interpretation in ways which are misleading. I shall try to present one of the important theorems of the subject as it might appear at first glance, and give a more sophisticated view later. I shall not be able to state the theorem precisely in this essay, but I hope the impression I leave you with will not be altogether false.

In 1931, a paper appeared which was shattering in its impact.[3] Its author, K. Gödel, would on this count alone rank as one of the very great mathematicians. Comparable discoveries might be the theory of relativity in physics or the role of DNA in biology. Suddenly it was seen that an end mathematicians had been confidently working towards since the turn of the century was unattainable.

In its simplest terms, the question is about arithmetic. *Arithmetic* is just the study of the numbers, 1, 2, 3, 4, and so on. What mathematicians would like to have done is to write down a collection of axioms on which this study could be based. What Gödel's theorem appears to say is (in part) this:

> If any finite number of true statements of arithmetic are considered as axioms, there can be found another statement which is undecidable in the theory they define.

('Undecidable' is used in the sense of the last section.) Notice that the theorem does not provide something which might be called an 'absolutely undecidable' statement; the one you find will depend on the axioms you choose. But notice that it does say that a finite number of axioms cannot tell you everything about arithmetic (Gödel's theorem also says that some infinite systems of axioms are not sufficient) and in this lies its importance.

I want to digress for a moment to indicate how this kind of theorem is sometimes applied outside of mathematics. A statement which is true of a simple system like the whole numbers ought *a fortiori* to be true of more complicated systems like the universe or a man. We ourselves are finite beings. We have lived for only a finite time, have met only a finite number of statements, known only a finite number of things. Because we can at any time know only a finite number of true statements about a man, for example, Gödel's theorem suggests that there will be statements about this man whose truth or falsity we cannot decide at that time; and as there are only a finite number of men alive, even if they pooled their knowledge, undecidable statements would still remain. Here we have a lever to prise out determinism, and slip in free will. This argument is, of course very rough, but there is no point in refining it, for I am going to strike at its root.[4]

Let us return again to arithmetic. The existence of undecidable statements for a theory implies that we do not know what we are talking about in the sense discussed above: we can find different realizations of the theory. But in arithmetic (in spite of our having met only a finite number of statements in our lives) we do know what we are talking about – it is the numbers 1, 2, 3, and so on. It is obvious to me that I know what these numbers are, and I hope it is obvious to you, for I do not know what arguments I could use to support my claim. Notice that I am not saying that I know all facts about the whole numbers (for example, I do not know what the millionth prime number is) but I am saying that I can recognize a whole number when I see one, and that you can too. Gödel's theorem seems to deny this.

What is wrong? When a mathematician is going to treat a subject he begins by writing down a system of axioms. I have taken Gödel's theorem out of its context, but to understand it properly, I must provide one. Now the objects under discussion are 'statements of arithmetic' and the relation between them is 'proof'. I am not in a position to write down the axioms usually used, but what I shall try to do is to explain what sort of arithmetical statement they correspond to.

First, you are allowed to use the symbols 1, 2, 3, and so on. You can use symbols n, m, p, q (and any others) as variables which may take any whole number as a value. You can use the symbols = (equals), + (plus), × (times), < (less than). You can use the words 'and', 'or', 'not', 'there is . . . with the property' and 'for every'. (In fact all the other usual arithmetical operations – e.g. subtraction and division – can be defined in terms of these.) Finally, every statement must contain only a finite number of these symbols. Thus, examples of allowable statements are:

$5 \times 7 = 7 \times 5$
There is n with the property $n + n = 1$
For every n, $n < n + 1$

(The middle statement is allowable but false; the other two are true.) In particular, observe that each statement can contain only a finite number of the symbols 1, 2, 3, and so on.

A more precise statement of Gödel's theorem can now be given:

If a finite number of true statements of the above kind are taken as axioms, there can be found another statement of the same kind which is undecidable in the theory they define.

The most important restriction here is the one concerning finiteness, and this may not appear very severe. But it does get us out of our difficulty, for the statement which tells us that we know that we are talking about is something like this:

either $n = 1$ or $n = 2$ or $n = 3$ or . . .

which has an infinite number of symbols in it.[5]

The first version of Gödel's theorem I offered was, strictly speaking, false. There are statements which I think we must be prepared to recognize as true and which implicitly contain an infinite number of symbols, for example, 'The whole numbers are 1, 2, 3, and so on'. If these are allowed, then finite axiom systems for the whole of arithmetic can be found.

Various kinds of finiteness are of crucial importance in mathematics. However, I doubt whether most of the sentences we ordinarily use share the kind of finiteness Gödel's theorem requires. If analogues of results in logic are held to be true in other situations, then the reasons urged in their support should be examined closely, for the analogy is likely to be a very bad one indeed.

III. SOME PHILOSOPHICAL QUESTIONS

I began by saying that the most important characteristic of mathematics is proof, and so I ought to try to say what I think 'proof' means. Let me begin with a side-issue.

In mathematical logic, things are proved about proofs. This looks like a second-order activity: what are we to think of it? It seems to me that if we are to say anything about proof, we should be allowed to use the best arguments available to do it, and of course, for the mathematician, this means using proofs. I see nothing wrong with this: after all, we use language to discuss words.

Is a proof just a good argument? This is not how I imagine it. A proof has to be absolutely conclusive, it has to be irrefutable. If a proof establishes the truth of something you would rather not believe it is no good marshalling evidence to support your point of view; you must find a mistake, and then the 'proof' is seen never to have been a proof after all. On the other hand, if you ask what criteria I use in judging whether I am looking at a proof or not, I have to confess that I 'just know'. This knowledge seems to have been acquired by the ordinary processes of learning: I read examples, I tried writing proofs of my own, I had mistakes corrected by my teachers. I was not given a definition of proof.

Those who do mathematical logic of course must know something precise about what they mean by proof, just as they have to know what they mean by statement. Formally, what they do is to write down certain relationships between statements which are to be called proofs, but informally we can say that these correspond to the application of a few rules. Although ordinary mathematicians would certainly agree that an argument using only these rules was a proof, it seems on the face of it unlikely that everything we would ever wish to call a proof should fall under these rules. I am afraid I do not know enough about the subject to give a definite answer here.

I have claimed that I 'just know' what a proof is. It is reasonable to ask whether other mathematicians agree with my conception. On the whole they do (after all, I learned it from them), but there is a small group, the intuitionists, who do not. The most essential feature of the intuitionist position is that it is constructivist. To see what this means, suppose I am given a particular equation and I want to prove that it has a solution. The intuitionist says that to do this I must show how a solution can actually be found; the ordinary mathematician has another alternative: he can prove that the proposition 'this equation has no solution' is false.

Of course, a proof written by an intuitionist is perfectly acceptable to an ordinary mathematician. Moreover, both kinds of mathematician require a proof to have the virtues I listed above. The difference is that the intuitionist doubts whether one of the logical rules (the law of the excluded middle, which says roughly that if a statement is false its negation is true) has the required aura of certainty about it. The quarrel is perhaps not about what the nature of proof is but about which arguments partake of this nature.

I do not want to overstate the importance of this controversy. Intuitionists form a very small minority of mathematicians, and the ordinary mathematician is happy to admit the work they do as part of mathematics. I have mentioned it only because it is almost the only controversy in the subject.

My view of proof, then is inconsistent. To be a proof an argument must be absolutely conclusive, but I recognize proofs simply by knowing that they are.

I now turn to another kind of question. I have said that mathematics is formally the study of axiom systems. Is a mathematician prepared to consider any collection of statements as axioms, and how does he decide what to do?

There is one logical restriction on the axioms which may be employed. What the mathematician most wishes to avoid is making a mistake, and unless he takes some care he might build a mistake into his axioms. For example, if he wishes to write down axioms with which he can do some arithmetic, he will naturally want his axioms to enable him to prove that $2 + 2 = 4$ and that 3 and 4 are not equal, but if he is very careless he may also be able to prove $2 + 2 = 3$. If the axioms do encapsulate a mistake, they are called inconsistent; otherwise they are consistent.

It now looks as if a mathematician must begin a theory by proving that his axioms are consistent, and indeed he would like to do this. However it is a consequence (not an immediate one –

it requires a lot of significant mathematics) of the theorem of Gödel discussed above that this is impossible to do for most theories. The word 'impossible' here is an expression of faith rather than of fact; what is proved is that certain methods of proving consistency cannot work, and faith enters because it is hard to see how any other methods could be regarded as satisfactory. This failure to prove consistency is one of the reasons why intuitionists have abandoned ordinary mathematics, for their system avoids this problem.

There are two directions in which the mathematician tries to do something to meet the demand for consistency. One is to prove that a new theory is consistent provided some other known theory is (to give a rough example which would not be used for this purpose in practice, since a two-dimensional plane can be placed within three-dimensional space, if three-dimensional geometry is consistent then so must two-dimensional geometry be). The other is to find a realization of the theory, for then if a contradiction was possible in the theory, it would also have to be present in the realization (thus, if from axioms true for arithmetic it could be proved that $2 = 3$, then 2 really would have to equal 3, and therefore it is impossible to obtain the contradiction $2 = 3$ from axioms true for arithmetic). This method sometimes gives a real proof of consistency, but the trouble is that most realizations of mathematical theories are themselves rather abstract. I do not want to pursue the subject further here.

The role which realizations play in a theory is much more significant than I have suggested so far. When a mathematician decides what theory to study, or what to try to do in it, he usually has one or more realizations in mind. It is because he wishes to know things about the realizations that he has chosen his particular set of axioms, and the questions he wants to answer about the realizations determine what he does. (Again I am allowing realizations to be abstract, even so far as to say at this point that one mathematical theory may be a realization of another.) In realizations the mathematician finds both the inspiration and the justification of his work. And it is here that he gives his main answer to the intuitionist: in the most real of realizations, the sciences, his theories seem to yield good results.

Mathematics is not a tale told by a few (clever) idiots signifying nothing. It aims at understanding, sometimes an understanding of the real world, sometimes of an abstract one. It is not a game played by choosing a (consistent) set of axioms and making any move allowed by the laws of logic. It is done with an end in view. Sometimes it is said that as every theorem of a theory can be deduced from its axioms, then the whole theory is already present in the axioms. This contains an obvious truth; but the same truth is here: the vocabulary of Latin and the rules of its grammar already contain the Aeneid. It requires understanding to construct a mathematical theory. The mathematician is asked not whether he followed the rules – that is taken for granted – but what he won.

Finally, I want to raise a question which is more immediately relevant to the interests of the Subject–Object Relations Group, namely the relationship between a theory and the world it is attempting to describe. I want to suggest Euclidean geometry as being a theory which it might well be worth discussing in this context. First, because it is a theory everybody learned something about in school. Second, because it is undoubtedly useful (the Egyptians built pyramids with it, Newton used it to find the consequences of his theory of gravitation). Third, because the question of the truth of the theory will not intrude, for as a description of the world the theory is false (on one level because the surface of our world is curved but on a deeper level because of the general theory of relativity). I do not want to suggest that every theory is false, or that every theory fits the world as well as geometry does, but I do think that the relationship between geometry and reality might be simpler to consider than that between quantum theory or psychoanalytic theory and reality.

Indeed, in the case of geometry, I doubt whether any problem exists. What I mean is that I do not see how any explanation could do other than obscure a picture which is already clear.

I want to conclude with my favourite quotation from Wittgenstein[6] and I shall try to make it relevant. Wittgenstein is discussing the word 'Moses' and he points out how difficult it is to give it a definite meaning. For example, it might mean 'the man who as a child was taken out of the Nile by Pharaoh's daughter' or 'the man who led the Israelites through the wilderness' and it makes sense to ask if these men were the same. To draw my analogy, I would like to suggest that some formal aspects of the word 'Moses' are quite precise, for example, its spelling and the fact that it is a noun. In a similar way, geometry is formally exact, but in its application may be approximate. Wittgenstein writes: 'Soll man sagen, ich gebrauche ein Wort, dessen Bedeutung ich nicht kenne, rede also Unsinn? – Sage, was du willst, solange dich das nicht verhindert, zu sehen, wie es sich verhalt. (Und wenn du das siehst, wirst du Manches nicht sagen.)' In Anscombe's translation: 'Should it be said that I am using a word whose meaning I don't know, and so am talking nonsense? – Say what you choose, so long as it does not prevent you from seeing the facts. (And when you see them there is a good deal that you will not say.)'

NOTES AND REFERENCES

1 BOURBAKI, N. *Éléments de mathématique*, Paris, Hermann, 1939.
2 RUSSELL, B. *Mysticism and Logic*, London, Allen & Unwin, 1918, ch. 5.
3 GÖDEL, K. 'Uber formal unentscheidbare Sätze der Principia Mathematica und verwandter Systeme', *Monatsh. Math. Phys.*, 1931, **38**, 173–98.
4 A full version of the argument can be found in *The Freedom of the Will* by LUCAS, J. R. (Oxford, 1970). Lucas discusses various objections to the use of Gödel's theorem in this context, but I hope that the reader will find his dismissal (on page 125) of the one given in this essay a little too brief.
5 Mathematicians will find this statement woefully inadequate. To discover what is intended, they can turn, for example, to page 286 of *Models and Ultraproducts* by BELL, T. R. and SLOMSON, A. B. (North Holland, 1969).
6 WITTGENSTEIN, L. *Philosophische Untersuchungen*, I, 79. English translation by ANSCOMBE, G. E. M. *Philosophical Investigations*, Oxford, Blackwell, 1953.

Comment

VIVIAN HUTSON

It is very clear from reading the collection of essays in this volume that the term 'model' has a number of almost completely different meanings. The term itself, at least as applied in any of the senses here, seems fairly recent. However, the idea of a model is very important in the development of modern thought, in particular in mathematics, logic, and philosophy, and, perhaps because of its fundamental character, it has been difficult to make the idea precise. In fact it seems sure that lack of a clear definition held up the development of mathematics and science for close on two thousand years – from the time of Aristotle until perhaps the seventeenth century. This statement needs justification and I shall try to provide this later. But, granting for the moment that it is true, should not some agreed and reasonable definition be reached for 'model'?

Of course the answer is yes. As a mathematician I would like to say 'And mathematicians can provide a clear and useful definition.' However, immediately a difficulty appears. For the term model is used in mathematics in two quite distinct senses. In the interesting article by Dr Pym the use of the term by the pure mathematician is illustrated (in fact he uses 'realization' there as a substitute for the normal mathematical term 'model' to avoid any possibility of confusion with the less precise definitions currently in vogue), and a precise definition may be supplied without too much difficulty. But 'model' to an applied mathematician or physicist means something quite different.

To simplify matters let us suppose that we can rid our minds of the doubts raised in them by the last section of Dr Pym's article

225

about the nature of proof in mathematics, and let us agree that mathematics is a structure obtained by rigorous deduction from a consistent set of axioms. It will be convenient here to use the term 'mathematical system' to mean a particular set of axioms together with the deductions that may be made from it. Consider now some physical system. This might be sets of lines drawn with a ruler on a sheet of paper or it might be the nucleus of an atom. The aim of the physicist is to obtain a model for the system. The model is a *mathematical* system which represents the physical system as well as possible. There are good and bad models. How good the model is will be judged on the basis of how well it predicts the behaviour of the physical system.

Let us now consider the consequences referred to above of not having a reasonably clear definition of model. The trouble started, perhaps paradoxically, in one of the most productive periods of mathematical and logical innovation, the period from Pythagoras to Euclid. At this time the main preoccupation of mathematicians was the system defined by geometrical figures in the plane. Euclid produced what the physicist would now call a model for the system, that is a set of axioms – the five postulates, together with logical deductions from these axioms; the mathematical system is of course now known as Euclidean geometry. This was a giant stride forward in mathematics and justifiably received great attention from logicians and mathematicians. Unfortunately at the very basis of this great discovery a fundamental fallacy became encapsulated. The fallacy was the belief that the axioms were in some sense universally true. To be a little more precise it was believed that they could be classified as self-evident and could in some way be established on physical grounds. The model was thus completely identified with the physical system. Of course we now know that the question of the universal truth of a set of axioms does not arise – merely the consistency of the set. Any non-Euclidean geometry, such as the geometry used in the general theory of relativity, is just as 'true' as Euclidean geometry. Euclidean geometry merely predicts the properties of lines in a plane more accurately, and so is a better model for this particular physical system.

Had there been a continuing period of productive thought in Greece it is possible or even likely that the role of the axioms would have been clarified. However that may be, the fallacy persisted for nearly two thousand years and almost completely arrested the development of mathematics. For it was nearly impossible for the mathematician to construct a new and interesting theory, faced as he was with the task of establishing in some absolute sense the 'truth' of this theory. On the other hand the progress of the physical sciences was also held up; first, through lack of satisfactory mathematical techniques, and, second, because it seemed necessary that physical systems should behave according to simple mathematical laws (for example, it was at one time thought that the orbits of the planets must be circles).

The clarification of these difficulties did not really begin until about the seventeenth century, and was not completed until the nineteenth century.

Freed of this confusion the concept of a model as defined above has been of immense importance in science and in particular has led to great progress in the field of physics. The concept seems somehow fundamental to our thinking and this definition might with profit be more widely adopted. It is not of course necessary for the system to be modelled by a mathematical system, merely that another presumably simpler system be constructed which in some sense reproduces or approximates the original system. It may be that in the social sciences this concept is already used and will lead to progress as dramatic as that which has sprung from it in physics.

© *Vivian Hutson 1972*

Order, Consciousness, and Meaning: the broader theme

Part II Introduction

Part II incorporates a number of papers of a more general and cross-disciplinary nature and falls roughly into three overlapping sections. The first focuses on what was termed by Professor Bohm 'the implicate order' of the world we encounter. The similarities and differences on the one hand between nature, social phenomena, and human thought, and on the other hand between the various groups of disciplines specializing in different fields of knowledge also belong here. The second section approaches what was referred to by Shanin as 'models of the second type' ('submerged . . . at the back of our mind') – the deep predispositions of the human mind which influence cognition. The social programming of human beings, the dialectical character of such processes, the influence of communication, and the fact that we live in 'second-hand worlds' will also fit here. The third section comes to stress the human, social, and ethical context of scholarship and its perspectives. The crucial issues of the philosophy and sociology of knowledge are here again treated not by specialized philosophers and sociologists of knowledge; a critical discussion of the social sciences by one of the most eminent social scientists of our generation is followed by a scientist's discussion of knowledge versus meaning in contemporary science.

It may be fitting to stress here once more the relative character of the book's division into parts. For example, the paper by MacKinnon could fit into the last section of Part II, the paper by Ramon is relevant to those by Bauman and Brittan and so on. The overlapping character of the issues in different parts and papers does indeed truly represent the essential unity of scholarship and the relative character of its division which this publication accepts as a credo.

Beyond Atomism and Holism– The concept of the holon[1]

ARTHUR KOESTLER

> *Hierarchical organization on the one hand, and the*
> *characteristics of open systems on the other, are*
> *fundamental principles of living nature.*
>
> L. von Bertalanffy

When one talks about hierarchic organization as a fundamental principle of life, one often encounters a strong emotional resistance. For one thing, hierarchy is an ugly word, loaded with ecclesiastic and military associations, and conveys to some people a wrong impression of a rigid or authoritarian structure. Apart from this, the term is often wrongly used to refer simply to order of rank on a linear scale or ladder (e.g. Clark Hull's 'habit-family hierarchies'). But that is not at all what the term is meant to signify. Its correct symbol is not a rigid ladder but a living tree – a multilevelled, stratified, outbranching pattern of organization, a system branching into subsystems; a structure encapsulating substructures; a process activating subprocesses and so on. As Paul Weiss said at the Alpbach Symposium: 'The phenomenon of hierarchic structure is a real one, presented to us by the biological object, and not the fiction of a speculative mind.' It is at the same time a conceptual tool, a way of thinking, an alternative to the linear chaining of events torn from their multidimensionally stratified contexts.

All complex structures and processes of a relatively stable character display hierarchic organization, and this applies regardless of whether we are considering inanimate systems, living organisms,

233

social organizations, or patterns of behaviour. The linguist who thinks primarily in terms of Chomsky's hierarchic model experiences a *déja vu* reaction – towards the physiologist's intra-cellular hierarchy; and this may equally apply to Bruner's presentation of the hierarchic structure of voluntary action. In this essential respect – and in some others that I shall mention – these processes in widely different fields are indeed isomorphic. The hierarchic tree-diagram may equally serve to represent the branching-out of the evolution of species – the tree of life and its projection in taxonomy; it serves to represent the stepwise differentiation of tissues in embryonic development; it may serve as a structural diagram of the parts-within-parts architecture of organisms or galaxies, or as a functional schema for the analysis of instinctive behaviour by the ethologist (Tinbergen, 1951; Thorpe, 1956); or of the phrase-generating machinery by the psycholinguist. It may represent the locomotor hierarchy of limbs, joints, individual muscles, and so down to fibres, fibrils, and filaments (Herrick, 1961; Weiss, 1950, etc.); or, in reverse direction, the filtering and processing of the sensory input in its ascent from periphery to centre. It could also be regarded as a model for the subject-index of the Library of Congress, and for the organization of knowledge in our memory-stores; lastly, as an organizational chart for government administrations, military and business organizations; and so on.

This almost universal applicability of the hierarchic model may arouse the suspicion that it is logically empty; and this may be a further factor in the resistance against it. It usually takes the form of what one may call the 'so what' reaction: all this is old hat, it is self-evident – followed by the *non sequitur* 'and anyway, where is your evidence?' Well, hierarchy may be old hat, but I would suggest that, if you handle it with some affection, it can produce quite a few lively rabbits – which can even be tested in the laboratory.

EVOLUTION AND HIERARCHIC ORDER

One of my favourite examples to illustrate the merits of hierarchic order is an amusing parable invented by Herbert Simon. The parable concerns two watchmakers, Hora and Tempus. Both make watches consisting of a thousand parts each. Hora assembles his watches bit by bit; so when he pauses or drops a watch before it is finished, it falls to pieces and he has to start from scratch. Tempus, on the other hand, puts together subassemblies of ten parts each; ten of these subassemblies he makes into a larger sub-assembly of a hundred units; and ten of these make the whole watch. If there is a disturbance, Tempus has to repeat at worst nine assembling operations, and at best none at all. If you have a ratio of one disturbance in a hundred operations, then Hora will take four thousand times longer to assemble a watch – instead of one day, he will take eleven years. And if, for mechanical bits, we substitute amino acids, protein molecules, organelles, and so on, the ratio between the time-scales becomes astronomical.

This is one basic advantage of employing the hierarchic method. The second is, of course, the incomparably greater stability and resilience to shock of the Tempus type of watch and its amenability to repair and improvement. Simon concludes: 'Complex systems will evolve from simple systems much more rapidly if there are stable intermediate forms than if there are not. The resulting complex forms in the former case will be hierarchic. We have only to turn the argument round to explain the observed predominance of hierarchies among the complex systems Nature presents to us. Among possible complex forms, hierarchies are the ones that have the time to evolve.' If there is life on other planets, we may safely assume that, whatever its form, it must be hierarchically organized.

Motor manufacturers discovered long ago that it does not pay to design a new model from scratch by starting on the level of elementary components; they make use of already existing sub-assemblies – engines, brakes, etc. – each of which has developed from long previous experience, and then proceed by relatively small modifications of some of these. Evolution follows the same strategy. Once it has taken out a patent it sticks to it tenaciously. The patented structure, organ, or device acquires a kind of autonomous existence as a subassembly. The same make of organelles functions in the cells of mice and men; the same make of contractile protein serves the streaming motion of amoeba and the finger muscles of the piano-player; the same homologous design is maintained in the vertebrate forelimb of man, dog, bird, and whale. Geoffroy de St Hilaire's *loi du balancement*, and d'Arcy

Thompson's transformation of a baboon's skull into a human skull by harmonious deformations of a Cartesian coordinate lattice, further illustrate the hierarchic constraints imposed on evolutionary design.

AUTONOMOUS HOLONS

The evolutionary stability of these subassemblies – organelles, organs, organ-systems – is reflected by their remarkable degree of *autonomy* or self-government. Each of them – a piece of tissue or a whole heart – is capable of functioning *in vitro* as a quasi-independent whole, even though isolated from the organism or transplanted into another organism. Each is a subwhole which, towards its subordinated parts, behaves as a self-contained whole, and towards its superior controls as a dependent part. This relativity of the terms 'part' and 'whole' when applied to any of its subassemblies is a further general characteristic of hierarchies.

It is again the very obviousness of this feature which tends to make us overlook its implications. A part, as we generally use the word, means something fragmentary and incomplete, which by itself would have no legitimate existence. On the other hand, there is a tendency among holists to use the word 'whole' or 'gestalt' as something complete in itself which needs no further explanation. But wholes and parts in this absolute sense do not exist anywhere, either in the domain of living organisms or of social organizations. What we find are intermediary structures on a series of levels in ascending order of complexity, each of which has two faces looking in opposite directions: the face turned towards the lower levels is that of an autonomous whole, the one turned upward that of a dependent part. I have elsewhere (1967) proposed the word 'holon' for these Janus-faced subassemblies – from the Greek *holos* = whole, with the suffix *on* (neutr*on*, prot*on*) suggesting a particle or part. The concept of the holon is meant to supply the missing link between atomism and holism; and to supplant the dualistic way of thinking in terms of 'parts' and 'wholes', which is so deeply engrained in our mental habits, by a multilevelled stratified approach.

FIXED RULES AND FLEXIBLE STRATEGIES

The term holon may be applied to any stable subwhole in an organismic, cognitive, or social hierarchy which displays rule-governed behaviour and/or structural gestalt constancy. Thus biological holons are self-regulating 'open systems' (von Bertalanffy, 1952) governed by a set of fixed rules which account for the holon's coherence, stability, and its specific pattern of structure and function. This set of rules we may call the *canon of the holon*.[2] The canon determines the fixed, invariant aspect of the open system in its steady state (*Fliessgleichgewicht* – dynamic equilibrium); it defines its pattern and structure. In other types of hierarchies, the canon represents the codes of conduct of social holons (family, tribe, nation, etc.); it incorporates the 'rules of the game' of instinctive rituals or acquired skills (behavioural holons); the rules of enunciation, grammar, and syntax in the language hierarchy; Piaget's schemes in cognitive hierarchies, and so on. The canon represents the constraints imposed on any rule-governed process or behaviour. But these constraints do not exhaust the system's degrees of freedom; they leave room for more or less flexible strategies, guided by the contingencies in the holon's local environment.

It is essential at this point to make a sharp categorical distinction between the fixed, invariant canon of the system and its flexible (plastic, variable) strategies. A few examples will illustrate the validity of this distinction. In *ontogeny*, the apex of the hierarchy is the zygote, and the holons at successive levels represent successive stages in the development of tissues. Each step in differentiation and specialization imposes further constraints on the genetic potential of the tissue, but at each step it retains sufficient developmental flexibility to follow this or that evolutionary pathway, within the range of its competence, guided by the contingencies of the cell's environment – Waddington's (1957) 'strategy of the genes'. Turning from embryonic development to the *instinctive activities* of the mature animal, we find that spiders spin webs, birds build nests according to invariant species-specific canons, but again using flexible strategies, guided by the lie of the land; the spider may suspend its web from three, four, or more points of attachment, but the result will always be a regular polygon. In *acquired skills* like chess, the rules of the game define the permissible moves, but the strategic choice of the actual move depends on the environment – the distribution of the chessmen on the board. In *symbolic operations*, the holons are rule-governed cognitive structures variously called 'frames of reference', 'universes of discourse', 'algorithms', etc., each with its specific 'grammar' or canon; and the strategies increase in complexity on higher levels of each hierarchy. It seems that life in all its manifestations, from morphogenesis to symbolic thought, is governed by rules of the game which lend it order and stability but also allow for flexibility; and that these rules, whether innate or acquired, are represented in coded form on various levels of the hierarchy, from the genetic code to the structures in the nervous system responsible for symbolic thought.

TRIGGERS AND SCANNERS

Let me discuss briefly some specific characteristics of what one might loosely call *output hierarchies*, regardless of whether the output is a baby, or a sentence spoken in English. However much their products differ, all output hierarchies seem to have a classic mode of operation, based on the trigger–releaser principle, where an implicit coded signal which may be relatively simple, releases complex, pre-set mechanisms. Let me again run through a few examples. In *phylogeny*, Waddington (1957) and others have convincingly shown that a single favourable gene-mutation can act as a trigger to release a kind of chain-reaction which affects a whole organ in a harmonious way. In *ontogeny*, the prick of a fine platinum needle on the unfertilized egg of a frog or sheep triggers off parthenogenesis. The genes act as chemical triggers, catalysing reactions. The implicit four-letter alphabet of the DNA chain is spelled out into the explicit, twenty-letter alphabet of amino acids; the inducers or evocators, including Spemann's 'general organizer', again turn out to be relatively simple chemicals which need not even be species-specific to activate the genetic potentials of the tissue. In *instinct behaviour*, we have releasers of a very simple kind – the red belly of the stickleback, the spot under the herring-gull's beak, which trigger off the appropriate behaviour (Tinbergen, 1951). In the performance of *acquired skills* you have the same process of stepwise filling in of details of implicit commands issued from the apex of the hierarchy, such as 'strike a match and light this cigarette' or 'sign your name', or 'use your phrase-generating Chomsky machine' – to transform an unverbalized image into innervations of the vocal chords.

The point to emphasize is that this spelling-out process from intent to execution, cannot be described in terms of simple response images transferred from classical mechanics, only as a series of discrete steps from one Open Sesame, activated by a combination lock, to the next. The activated holon, whether it is a government department or a living kidney, has its own canon which determines the pattern of its activity. Thus the signal from higher quarters does not have to specify what the holon is expected to do; the signal merely has to trigger the holon into action by a coded message. Once thrown into action, the holon will spell out the implicit command in explicit form by activating its subunits in the appropriate strategic order, guided by feedbacks and feed-forwards from its environment. Generally speaking, *the holon is a system of relations which is represented on the next higher level as a unit, that is, a relatum.*

If we turn now to the *input hierarchies* of perception, the operations proceed, of course, in the reverse direction, from the peripheral twigs of the tree towards its apex; and instead of trigger–releasers we have the opposite type of mechanism, a series of filters, scanners, or classifiers through which the input traffic must pass in its ascent from periphery to cortex. First you have lateral inhibition, habituation, and presumably some efferent control of receptors. On the higher levels are the mechanisms responsible for the visual and acoustic constancy phenomena, the scanning and filtering devices which account for the recognition of patterns in space and time, and enable us to abstract universals and discard particulars. The colloquial complaint 'I have a memory like a sieve' may be derived from an intuitive grasp of these filtering devices that operate first all along the input channels, then along the storage channels.

How do we pick out a single instrument in a symphony? The whole medley of sounds arriving at the ear-drum is scrambled into a linear pressure-wave with a single variable. To reconstruct the timbre of an instrument, to identify harmonies and melodies, to appreciate phrasing, style, and mood, we have to abstract patterns in time as we abstract visual patterns in space. But how does the nervous system do it? If one looks at an LP record with a magnifying glass, one is tempted to ask the naïve question why the nervous system does not produce engrams by this simple method of coding, instead of being so damned complicated. The answer is, of course, that a linear engram of this kind would be completely useless for the purpose of analysing, matching, and recognizing input patterns. The chain is a hopeless model; we cannot do without a tree.

In motor hierarchies, an implicit intention or generalized command is particularized, spelled out, step by step, in its descent to the periphery. In perceptual hierarchies, we have the opposite process. The peripheral input is more and more de-particularized, stripped of irrelevancies during its ascent to the centre. *The output hierarchy concretizes, the input hierarchy abstracts.* The former operates by means of triggering devices, the latter by means of filtering or scanning devices. When I intend to write the letter R, a trigger activates a functional holon, an automatic pattern of muscle contractions, which produces the letter R in my own particular handwriting. When I read, a scanning device in my visual cortex identifies the letter R regardless of the particular hand that wrote it. Triggers release complex outputs by means of a simple coded signal. Scanners function the opposite way: they convert complex inputs into a simple coded signal.

INTERLOCKING HIERARCHIES AND FEEDBACK CONTROL

I have used the term 'interlocking' or 'interlacing' hierarchies. Of course hierarchies do not operate in a vacuum. This truism about the interdependence of processes in an organism is probably the main cause of confusion which obscured from view its hierarchic structure. It is as if the sight of the foliage of the entwined branches in a forest made us forget that the branches originate in separate trees.

The most obvious example of interlocking hierarchies is the sensorimotor system. The sensory hierarchy processes information and transmits it in a steady upward flow, some of which reaches the conscious ego at the apex; the ego makes decisions which are spelled out by the downward stream of impulses in the motor hierarchy. But the apex is not the only point of contact between the two systems; they are connected by entwining networks on various levels. The network on the lowest level consists of reflexes like the patellary. They are shortcuts between the ascending and descending flow, like loops connecting opposite traffic streams on a motor highway. On the next higher level are the networks of sensorimotor skills and habits such as touch-typing or driving a car, which do not require the attention of the highest centres – unless some disturbance throws them out of gear. But let a little dog amble across the icy road in front of the driver, and he will have to make a 'top-level' decision whether to slam down the brake, risking the safety of his passengers, or run over the dog. It is at this level when the pros and cons are precariously balanced, that the subjective experience of free choice and moral responsibility arises.

But the ordinary routines of existence do not require such moral decisions, and not even much conscious attention. They operate by means of feedback loops, and loops-within-loops, which form the multilevelled networks linking the input and output hierarchies. So long as all goes well and no dog crosses the road, the strategy of riding a bicycle or driving a car can be left to the automatic pilot in the nervous system – the cybernetic helmsman. But one must beware of using the principle of feedback control as a magic formula. The concept of feedback without the concept of hierarchic order is like the grin without the cat. All skilled routines follow a pre-set pattern according to certain rules of the game. These are fixed, but permit constant adjustments to variable environmental conditions. *Feedback can only operate within the limits set by the rules* – by the canon of the skill. The part which feedback plays is to report back on every step in the progress of the operation, whether it is overshooting or falling short of the mark, how to keep it on an even keel, when to intensify the pace and when to stop. But it cannot alter the intrinsic pattern of the skill. To quote Paul Weiss (1951) at the Hixon Symposium: 'The structure of the input does not produce the structure of the output, but merely modifies intrinsic nervous activities, which have a structural organization of their own.' One of the vital differences between the simple stimulus–response model and ours is that, according to the former, the environment determines behaviour, whereas according to the latter, feedback from the environment merely guides or corrects or stabilizes pre-existing patterns of behaviour.

Moreover, the cross-traffic between the sensory and motor hierarchies works both ways. The input guides the output and keeps it on an even keel; but motor activity in its turn guides perception. The eye must scan; its motions, large and small – drift, flicker, tremor – are indispensable to vision; an image stabilized on the retina disintegrates into darkness (Hebb, 1958). Similarly with audition: if you try to recall a tune, what do you do? You hum it. Stimuli and responses have been swallowed up by feedback loops within loops, along which impulses run in circles like kittens chasing their tails.

A HIERARCHY OF ENVIRONMENTS

Let us carry this inquiry into the meaning of current terminology a step further, and ask just what that convenient word 'environment' is meant to signify. When I am driving my car, the environment in contact with my right foot is the accelerator pedal, its elastic resistance to pressure provides a tactile feedback which helps to keep the speed of the car steady. The same applies to the 'feel' of the wheel under my hands. But my eyes encompass a much larger environment than my feet and hands; they determine the overall strategy of driving. The hierarchically organized creature that I am is in fact functioning in a hierarchy of environments guided by a hierarchy of feedbacks.

One advantage of this operational interpretation is that the hierarchy of environments can be extended indefinitely. When the chess-player stares at the board in front of him, trying to visualize various situations three moves ahead, he is guided by feedbacks from imagined environments. Most of our thinking, planning, and creating operates in such imaginary environments. But – to quote Bartlett (1958) – all our perceptions are inferential constructs, coloured by imagination, and so the difference is merely one of degrees. The hierarchy is open-ended at the top.

REGULATION CHANNELS

When the centipede was asked in which order he moved his hundred legs, he became paralysed and starved to death because he had never thought of it before and had left his legs to look after themselves. When an intent is formed at the apex of the hierarchy, such as signing a letter, it does not activate individual motor units, but triggers off patterns of impulses which activate subpatterns and so on. But this can only be done one step at a time: the higher centres do not normally have dealings with lowly ones, and vice versa. Brigadiers do not concentrate their attention on individual soldiers – if they did, the whole operation would go haywire. Commands must be transmitted through 'regulation channels'.

This statement looks trivial, but ignoring it carries heavy penalties of a theoretical or practical order. The stimulus–response theorist's vague reference to 'intervening variables' is a face-saving manœuvre to sweep all the essential problems of complex human behaviour, including language, under the laboratory carpet.

MECHANIZATION AND FREEDOM

A skilled activity, such as writing a letter, branches into subskills which, on successively lower levels of the hierarchy, become increasingly mechanized, stereotyped, and predictable. The choice of subjects to be discussed in a letter is vast; the next step, phrasing, still offers a great number of alternatives, but is more restricted by the rules of grammar, the limits of one's vocabulary, etc.; the rules of spelling are fixed, with no leeway for flexible strategies, and, lastly, the muscle contractions which depress the typewriter keys are entirely automatized. Thus a *subskill or behavioural holon on the (n) level of the hierarchy has more degrees of freedom* (a larger variety of alternative strategic choices permitted by the canon) *than a holon on the (n − 1) level.*

However, all skills tend with increasing mastery and practice to become automatized routines. While acquiring a skill we must concentrate on every detail of what we are doing; then learning begins to condense into habit as steam condenses into drops; with increasing practice we read, write, type, drive 'automatically' or 'mechanically'. Thus we are all the time transforming 'mental' into 'mechanical' activities. In unexpected contingencies, however, the process can be reversed. Driving along a familiar road is an automatized routine; but when that little dog crosses the road, a strategic choice has to be made which is beyond the competence of automatized routine, for which the automatic pilot in my nervous system has not been programmed, and the decision must be referred to higher quarters. The *shift of control* of an ongoing activity from one level to a higher level of the hierarchy – from 'mechanical' to 'mindful' behaviour – seems to be of the essence of conscious decision-making and of the subjective experience of free will.[3]

The tendency towards the progressive mechanization of skills has its positive side: it conforms to the principle of parsimony. If I could not hit the keys of the typewriter 'automatically' I could not attend to meaning. On the negative side, mechanization, like rigor mortis, affects first the extremities – the lower subordinate branches of the hierarchy, but it also tends to spread upward. If a skill is practised in the same unvarying conditions, following the same unvarying course, it tends to degenerate into stereotyped routine and its degrees of freedom freeze up. Monotony accelerates enslavement to habit; and if mechanization spreads to the apex of the hierarchy, the result is the rigid pedant, Bergson's *homme automate*. As von Bertalanffy wrote, 'organisms *are not* machines, but they can to certain extent *become* machines, congeal into machines' (1952).

Vice versa, a variable environment demands flexible behaviour and reverses the trend towards mechanization. However, the challenge of the environment may exceed a critical limit where it can no longer be met by customary routines, however flexible – because the traditional 'rules of the game' are no longer adequate to cope with the situation. Then a crisis arises. The outcome is either a breakdown of behaviour – or alternatively the emergence of new forms of behaviour, of original solutions. They have been observed throughout the animal kingdom, from insects onward, through rats to chimpanzees, and point to the existence of unsuspected potentials in the living organism, which are inhibited or dormant in the normal routines of existence, and only make their appearance in exceptional circumstances. They foreshadow the phenomena of human creativity which – as discussed elsewhere (1964 and 1967) – must remain incomprehensible to the stimulus–response theorist, but appear in a new light when approached from the hierarchic point of view.

SELF-ASSERTION AND INTEGRATION

The holons which constitute an organismic or social hierarchy are Janus-faced entities: facing upward, towards the apex, they function as dependent parts of a larger whole facing downward. Organelles, cells, muscles, neurons, organs, all have their intrinsic rhythm and pattern, often manifested spontaneously without external stimulation, in that they tend to persist in and assert their characteristic pattern of activity. This *self-assertive tendency* is a fundamental and universal characteristic of holons, manifested on every level of every type of hierarchy: in the regulative properties of the morphogenetic field, defying transplantation and experimental mutilation; in the stubbornness of instinct rituals, acquired habits, tribal traditions, and social customs; and even in a person's signature, which he can modify but not sufficiently to fool the expert. Without this self-assertive tendency of their parts, organisms and societies would lose their articulation and stability.

The opposite aspect of the holon is its *integrative tendency* to function as an integral part of an existing or evolving larger whole. Its manifestations are equally ubiquitous, from the 'docility' of the embryonic tissues, through the symbiosis of organelles in the cell, to the various forms of cohesive bonds, from flock to insect state and human tribe.

We thus arrive at a polarity between the self-assertive and the integrative tendency of holons on every level. This polarity is of fundamental importance to our concept. It is in fact implied in the model of a multilevelled hierarchy, because the stability of the hierarchy depends on the equilibration of the two opposite tendencies of its holons. Empirically the postulated polarity can be traced in all phenomena of life; in its theoretical aspect it is not derived from any metaphysical dualism, but may rather be regarded as an application of Newton's third law of motion (action and reaction) to hierarchic systems. We may even extend the polarity into inanimate nature: wherever there is a relatively stable dynamic system, from atoms to galaxies, stability is maintained by the equilibration of opposite forces, one of which may be centrifugal or separative or inertial, and the other a centripetal or attractive or cohesive force, which keep the parts in their place in the larger whole, and hold it together.

Under conditions of stress, part of an organism may become overstimulated and tend to escape the restraining control of the whole (cf. Child, 1924). This can lead to pathological changes of an irreversible nature, such as malignant growths with untrammelled proliferation of tissues that have escaped from genetic restraint. There is a whole gamut of mental disorders in which some subordinate part of the mental hierarchy exerts its tyrannical rule over the whole, from the insiduous domination of 'repressed' complexes to the major psychoses, in which large chunks of the personality seem to have 'split off' and lead a quasi-independent existence. Aberrations of the human mind are frequently due to the obsessional pursuit of some part-truth, treated as if it were the whole truth – of a holon masquerading as a whole.

If we turn from organismic to *social hierarchies*, we again find that under normal conditions the holons (clans, tribes, nations, social classes, professional groups) live in a kind of dynamic equilibrium with their natural and social environment. However, under conditions of stress, when tensions exceed a critical limit, some social holon may get overexcited and tend to assert itself to the detriment of the whole, just like an overexcited organ. It should be noted that the canon which defines the identity and lends coherence to social holons (its laws, language, traditions, rules of conduct, systems of belief) represents not merely negative constraints imposed on its actions but also positive precepts, maxims, and moral imperatives.

The single individual constitutes the apex of the organismic hierarchy, and at the same time the lowest unit of the social hierarchy. Looking inward, he sees himself as a self-contained, unique whole; looking outward, as a dependent part. No man is an island, he is a holon. His *self-assertive* tendency is the dynamic manifestation of his unique wholeness as an individual; his *integrative* tendency expresses his dependence on the larger whole to which he belongs, his partness. Under normal conditions, the two opposite tendencies are more or less evenly balanced. Under conditions of stress, the equilibrium is upset, manifested in emotional behaviour. The emotions derived from the self-assertive tendencies are of the well-known aggressive, defensive, hunger, rage, and fear type, including the possessive component of sex. The emotions derived from the integrative tendency have been largely neglected by contemporary psychology; one may call them the self-transcending or participatory type of emotions. They arise out of the human holon's need to be an integral part of some larger whole – which may be a social group, a personal bond, a belief-system, nature, or the *anima mundi*. The psychological processes through which this category of emotions operates are variously referred to as projection, identification, empathy, hypnotic rapport, devotion, love. It is one of the ironies of the human condition that both its glory and its predicament seem to derive not from the self-assertive but from the integrative potentials of the species. The glories of art and science, and the holocausts of history caused by misguided devotion, are both nurtured by the self-transcending emotions.

These scant remarks on a complex subject, which cannot be pursued here, are merely meant to indicate the wider implications of the hierarchic approach. To conclude, even this fragmentary outline ought to make it clear that in the model presented there is no place for such a thing as an aggressive or destructive instinct in organisms; nor does it admit the reification of the sexual instinct as the *only* integrative force in human or animal society. Freud's Eros and Thanatos are relative late-comers on the stage of evolution: a host of creatures that multiply by fission or budding are ignorant of both. In the present view, Eros is an offspring of the Integrative, destructive Thanatos of the Self-Assertive, tendency, and Janus the symbol of the polarity of these two irreducible properties of living matter – that *coincidentia oppositorum* which von Bertalanffy is so fond of quoting, and which is inherent in the open-ended hierarchies of life.

NOTES

1 The discussion is based on a paper delivered to the Alpbach Symposium, 5–9 June 1968; see Koestler and Smithies (1969).

2 Cf. the 'organizing relations' or 'laws of organization' of earlier
writers on hierarchic organization (for example Lloyd Morgan,
Woodger (1929), Needham (1941)), and the 'system-conditions'
in general systems theory.
3 These considerations may have bearing on the mind–body problem
discussed elsewhere (Koestler, 1967).

REFERENCES

BARTLETT, F. C. *Thinking*, London, Allen & Unwin, 1958.
VON BERTALANFFY, L. *Problems of Life*, London, Watts; New York,
Harper, 1952.
CHILD, C. M. *Physiological Foundations of Behaviour*, New York, Hafner,
1924.
GALANTER, E. See Miller, G. A., 1906.
HEBB, D. O. *A Textbook of Psychology*, Philadelphia, Saunders, 1958.
HERRICK, C. J. *The Evolution of Human Nature*, N.Y., Harper, 1961.
JENKINS, J. See Koestler, A., 1965.
KOESTLER, A. *The Act of Creation*, London, Hutchinson, 1964.
KOESTLER, A. and JENKINS, J., 'Inversion Effects in the Tachisto-
scopic Perception of Number Sequences', *Psychon. Sci.* **3**, 1965.
KOESTLER, A. *The Ghost in the Machine*, London, Hutchinson, 1967.
KOESTLER, A. and SMITHIES, J. R., eds. *Beyond Reductionism*, London,
Hutchinson, 1969.
MACLEAN, P. 'Psychosomatic Disease and the "Visceral Brain"',
Psychosom. Med. **11**, 338–53, 1949.
MILLER, G. A., GALANTER, E., and PRIBRAM, K. H. *Plans and the
Structure of Behavior*, New York, Holt, 1960.
NEEDHAM, J. *Time, the Refreshing River*, London, Allen & Unwin, 1941.
PENFIELD, W. and ROBERTS, L. *Speech and Brain Mechanisms*,
Princeton, Princeton University Press, 1959.
PRIBRAM, K. H. See MILLER, F. A., 1960.
ROBERTS, L. See PENFIELD, W., 1959.
SIMON, H. J. 'The Architecture of Complexity', *Proc. Amer. Philos.
Soc.* **106** (6), 1962.
THORPE, W. H. *Learning and Instinct in Animals*, London, Methuen;
Cambridge, Mass.; Harvard University Press, 1956.
TINBERGEN, N. *The Study of Instinct*, Oxford, Clarendon Press, 1951.
WADDINGTON, C. H. *The Strategy of the Genes*, London, Allen & Unwin,
1957.
WEISS, P., ed. *Genetic Neurology*, Chicago, 1950.
WEISS, P., in *Hixon Symposium*, ed. Jeffress, L. A. New York, Hafner
1951.
WOODGER, J. H. *Biological Principles*, London, Kegan Paul, 1929.

Indication of a
New Order in Physics

D. BOHM

I. INTRODUCTION

Revolutionary changes in physics have always involved the perception of new order and attention to the development of new ways of using language that are appropriate to the communication of such order.

In this article, we shall start with a discussion of certain features of the history of the development of physics that can help to give some insight into what is meant by perception and communication of a new order. We shall then go on to present our suggestions regarding the new order that is indicated by the consideration of the theory of relativity and quantum theory.

Now, in ancient times, there was only a vague qualitative notion of order in nature. With the development of mathematics, notably arithmetic and geometry, the possibility arose for defining forms and ratios more precisely, so that, for example, one could describe the detailed orbits of planets, etc. However, such detailed mathematical descriptions of the motions of the planets and other heavenly bodies implied certain general notions of order. Thus, the ancient Greeks thought that the Earth was at the centre of the universe, and that surrounding the Earth were spheres, which approached the ideal perfection of celestial matter, as one got further and further away from the Earth. The perfection of celestial matter was supposed to be revealed in circular orbits, which were regarded as the most perfect of all geometrical figures, while the imperfection of earthly matter was thought to be shown in its very complicated and apparently arbitrary movements.

Thus, the universe was both perceived and discussed in terms of a certain overall order; i.e. the order of degrees of perfection, which corresponded to the order of distance from the centre of the Earth.

Physics as a whole was understood in terms of notions of order closely related to those described above. Thus Aristotle compared the universe to a living organism, in which each part had its proper place and function, so that all worked together to make a single whole. Within this whole, an object could move only if there was a force acting in it. Force was thus thought of as a *cause* of motion. So the order of movement was determined by the order of causes, which in turn depended on the place and function of each part in the whole.

The general way of perceiving and communicating order in physics was, of course, not at all in contradiction with common experience (in which, for example, movement is possible as a rule only when there is a force which overcomes friction). To be sure, when more detailed observations were made on the planets, it was found that their orbits are not actually perfect circles. But this fact was accommodated within the prevailing notions of order by considering the orbits of planets as a superposition of *epicycles*, i.e. circles within circles. Thus, one sees an example of the remarkable capacity for *adaptation* within a given notion of order, adaptation that enables one to go on perceiving and talking in terms of essentially fixed notions of this kind, in spite of factual evidence that might at first sight seem to necessitate a thorough-going change in such notions. With the aid of such adaptations, men could for thousands of years look at the night sky and see epicycles there, almost independently of the detailed content of their observations.

It seems clear, then, that a basic notion of order, such as was expressed in terms of epicycles, could never be decisively con-tradicted, because it could always be adjusted to fit the observed facts. But eventually a new spirit arose in scientific research, which led to the questioning of the *relevance* of the old order, notably by Copernicus, Kepler, and Galileo. What emerged from such questioning was in essence the proposal that the difference between earthly and celestial matter is not actually very significant. Rather, it was suggested that a key difference is between the motion of matter in empty space and its motion in a viscous medium. The basic laws of physics should then refer to the motion of matter in empty space, rather than to its motion in a viscous medium. Thus, Aristotle was right to say that matter as commonly experienced moved only under the action of a force, but he was wrong in supposing that this common experience was relevant to the fundamental laws of physics. From this it followed that the key difference between celestial and earthly matter was not in its degree of perfection but rather in that celestial matter generally moves without friction in a vacuum, whereas terrestrial matter moves with friction in a viscous medium.

Evidently, such notions were not generally compatible with the idea that the universe is to be regarded as a single living organism. Rather, in a fundamental description, the universe now had to be regarded as analysable into separately existing parts or objects (e.g. planets, atoms), each moving in a void or vacuum. These parts could work together in interaction more or less as do the parts of a machine but could not grow, develop, and function in response to ends determined by an 'organism as a whole'. The basic order for description of movement of the parts of this 'machine' was taken to be that of successive positions of each constituent object at successive moments of time. Thus a new order became relevant, and a new usage of language had to be developed for the description of this new order.

In the development of new ways of using language, the Cartesian coordinates played a key part. Indeed, the very word 'coordinate' implies a function of *ordering*. This ordering is achieved with the aid of a grid. Thus, in two dimension, the grid is constituted of two perpendicular sets of uniformly spaced lines. Each set of lines is

Figure 1

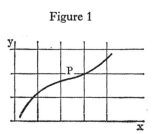

evidently an order (similar to the order of the integers). A given curve is then determined by a *coordination* between the x-order and the y-order.

Coordinates are evidently not to be regarded as natural objects. Rather, they are merely convenient forms of description set up by us. As such, they have a great deal of arbitrariness or conventionality (e.g. in orientation, scale, orthogonality, etc. of coordinate frames). Despite this kind of arbitrariness, however, it is possible, as is now well known, to have a non-arbitrary general law expressed in terms of coordinates. This is possible if the law takes the form of a relationship that remains *invariant* under changes in the arbitrary features of the descriptive order.

To use coordinates is in effect to order our attention in a way that is appropriate to the mechanical view of the universe, and thus similarly to order our perception and our thinking. It is clear, for example, that though Aristotle very probably would have understood the meaning of coordinates, he would have found them of little or no significance for his aim of understanding the universe as an organism. But once men were ready to conceive of the universe as a machine, they would naturally tend to take the order of coordinates as a universally relevant one, valid for all basic descriptions in physics.

Within this new Cartesian order of perception and thinking, which had grown up after the Renaissance, Newton was able to discover a very general law. It may be stated thus: 'As with the order of movement in the fall of an apple, so with that of the moon, and so with *all*.' This was a new perception of law, i.e. universal harmony in the order of nature, as described in detail through the use of coordinates. Such perception is a flash of very penetrating insight, which is basically *poetic*. Indeed, the root of the word 'poetry' is the Greek *poieīn*, meaning 'to make' or 'to create'. Thus, in its most original aspects, science takes on a quality of poetic communication of creative perception of new order.

A somewhat more 'prosaic' way of putting Newton's insight is to write: A : B : : C : D. That is to say, 'As the successive positions, A, B of the apple are related, so are the successive positions, C, D of the moon.' This constitutes a generalized notion of what may be called *ratio*. Here we take ratio in its broadest meaning (e.g in its original Latin root) which includes all of *reason*, which includes not only numerical ratio or proportion $\left(\dfrac{A}{B} = \dfrac{C}{D}\right)$, but also general qualitative similarity.

Rational law is not restricted to an expression of *causality*. Evidently reason, in the sense that is meant here, goes far beyond causality, which latter is a special case of reason. Indeed, the basic form of causality is: 'I do a certain action X and cause something to happen.' A causal law then takes the form: 'As with such causal actions of mine, so with certain processes that can be observed in nature.' Thus, a causal law provides a certain *limited kind* of reason. But more generally, a *rational* explanation takes the form: 'as things are related in a certain idea or concept, so they are related in fact'.

It is clear from the preceding discussion that in finding a new structure of reason or rationality, it is crucial *first* to discern relevant differences. To try to find a rational connection between irrelevant differences leads to arbitrariness, confusion, and general unfruitfulness (e.g. as with epicycles). So we have to be ready to drop our assumptions as to what are the relevant differences, though this has often seemed to be very difficult to do, because we tend to give such high psychological value to familiar ideas.

II. WHAT IS ORDER?

Thus far, the term order has been used in a number of contexts that are more or less known to everyone, so that its meaning can be seen fairly clearly from its usage. But the notion of order is evidently relevant in much broader contexts. Thus we do not restrict order to some regular arrangement of objects or forms in lines or in rows (e.g. as with grids). Rather we can consider much more general orders, such as the *order of growth of a living being, the order of evolution of living species, the order of society, the order of a musical composition, the order of painting, the order which constitutes the meaning of a communication*, etc. If we wish to inquire into such broader contexts, the notions of order to which we have referred earlier in this article will evidently no longer be adequate. We are therefore led to the general question: 'What is order?'

The notion of order is so vast and immense in its implications, however, that it cannot be defined in words. Indeed, the best we can do with order is to try to 'point to it' tacitly and by implication in as wide as possible a range of contexts in which this notion is relevant. We all know order implicitly, and such 'pointing' can perhaps communicate a general and overall meaning of order, without the need for a precise verbal definition.

To begin to understand order in such a general sense, we may first recall that in the development of classical physics, the perception of a new order was seen to involve the discrimination of new relevant differences (positions of objects at successive moments of time) along with new similarities that are to be found in the differences (similarity of 'ratios' in these differences). It is being suggested here that this is the seed or nucleus of a very general way of perceiving order, i.e. *to give attention to similar differences and different similarities*.

Let us illustrate these notions in terms of a geometric curve. To simplify the example we shall approximate the curve by a series of straight line segments of equal length. We begin with a straight line. As shown in *Figure 2*, the segments in a straight line all have

Figure 2

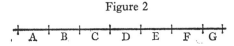

the same direction so that their only difference is in position. The difference between segment A and segment B is thus a space displacement which is similar to the difference between B and C, and so on. We may therefore write

$$A1:B::B:C::C:D::D:E$$

This expression of 'ratio' or 'reason' may be said to define a curve of *first class*; i.e. a curve having only one independent difference. Next we consider a circle, as illustrated in *Figure 3*. Here,

Figure 3

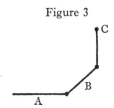

the difference between A and B is in direction, as well as in position. Thus, we have a curve with two independent differences – which is therefore one of *second class*. But we still have a single 'ratio' in the differences, $A: B:: B: C$.

Now we come to a helix. Here the angle between lines can turn in a third dimension. Thus we have a curve of *third class*. But it, too, is determined by a single ratio, $A: B:: B: C$.

Thus far we have considered various *kinds* of similarities in the differences, to obtain curves of first, second, third, classes, etc. However, in each curve, the similarity (or ratio) between successive steps remains invariant. But now we can call attention to curves in which *this similarity is different* as we go along the curve. In this way, we are led to consider not only *similar differences* but also *different similarities of the differences*.

We can illustrate this notion by means of a curve, which is a chain of straight lines in different directions (see *Figure 4*).

Figure 4

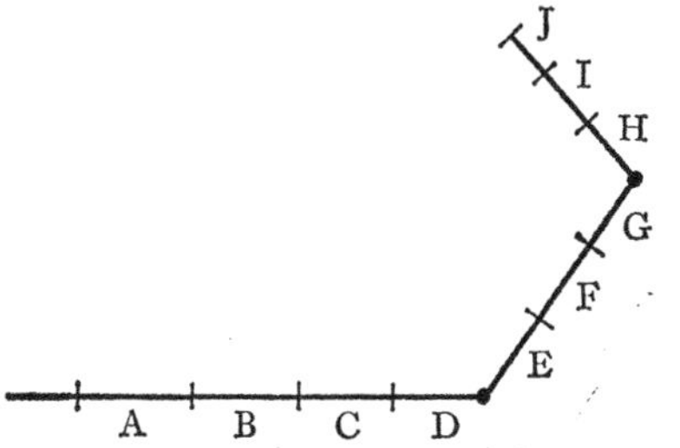

On the first line (ABCD) we can write
$$S_1$$
$$A: B:: B: C$$
The symbol S_1 stands for 'the first kind of similarity' – i.e. in direction along the line (ABCD). Then we write for the lines (EFG) and (HIJ)
$$S_2 \qquad\qquad S_3$$
$$E: F:: F: G \quad \text{and} \quad H: I:: I: J$$
where S_2 stands for 'the similarity of the second kind' and S_3 for 'the similarity of the third kind'.

We can now consider the differences of successive similarities $(S_1, S_2, S_3, \ldots)$ as a *second degree of difference*. From this, we can develop a *second degree of similarity in these differences*. $S_1: S_2:: S_2: S_3$.

By thus introducing what is in effect the beginning of a hierarchy of similarities and differences, we can go on to curves of arbitrarily high degrees of order. As the degrees become indefinitely high, we are able to describe what have commonly been called 'random' curves – such as those encountered in Brownian motion. This kind of curve is not determined by any finite number of steps. Nevertheless it would not be appropriate to call it 'disordered', i.e. *having no order whatsoever*. Rather, it has a certain kind of order, which is of an indefinitely high degree.

In this way, we are led to make an important change in the general language of description. We no longer use the term 'disorder' but instead we distinguish between different degrees of order (so that, for example, there is an unbroken gradation of curves, beginning with those of first degree, and going on step by step to those that have generally been called 'random').

It is important to add here that order is not to be identified with *predictability*. Predictability is a property of a special kind of order such that a few steps determine the whole order (i.e. as in curves of low degree). But there can be complex and subtle orders which are not in essence related to predictability (e.g. a good painting is highly ordered, and yet this order does not permit one part to be predicted from another).

III. ON THE DEVELOPMENT OF NEW NOTIONS OF ORDER
       IN RELATIVITY AND QUANTUM THEORY

As has been pointed out earlier, classical physics implies a certain basic change in key notions of order, relative to those prevailing in ancient times. This change is most centrally characterized by the introduction of Cartesian coordinates, to describe the movements of particles with in principle unlimited precision. As indicated in Section I, this mode of description goes together with the analysis of everything into small quasi-rigid bodies (or their idealization as extensionless particles) which are considered as working together in interaction, as if in a machine.

The first real break in such classical notions of order and structure came with the theory of relativity, which dropped the idea of absolute simultaneity. Instead, the order of time (and space) was taken to be, in certain ways, relative to a frame of coordinates, appropriate to the speed of movement of a particular observer (or equivalently, that of his observing instruments). This new order implied that the complete analysis of the world into distinct and separate quasi-rigid bodies could no longer be carried out.[1] Rather, one had to start with the concept of a universal and continuous field, which pervades the whole of space. 'Particles' were taken to be structures in this field, which had central regions of high intensity, but which extended with lower intensity beyond these regions over all space and merged with the structures of all other 'particles' (including those that constitute our observing instruments). Thus, the new order involved in relativity theory implied *unbroken wholeness* in the constitution of the world, rather than *division into separately existent parts in interaction.*

Quantum theory involved yet further changes in our notions of order, which are very far-reaching and deep in their implications. Indeed, it was seen that the indeterminancy principle (which is a key aspect of this theory) constitutes a limitation on the applicability of classical notions of a well-defined order of movement of matter, as specified by particle orbits referred to coordinate frames. This limitation is in essence an outcome of the introduction of the *quantum of action,* from which the inference is drawn that 'particles' can 'jump' from one discrete orbit to another, without passing through a continuous series of intermediate orbits. Such a discrete notion of movement implies that the world is to be thought of as more like an unbroken network of indivisible links than like an interacting system of separately existing objects.

IV. ON THE NEED FOR A NEW ORDER IN PHYSICAL
CONCEPTS

Although the new notions of order and structure involved in the quantum theory were very different in detail from those brought in by relativity theory, they were nevertheless deeply similar, in that they signified unbroken wholeness of all existence, rather than analysis into interacting parts. Nevertheless, in spite of this deep similarity, it has not proved to be possible to unite relativity and quantum theory in a consistent way. Moreover, each of these theories, when considered by itself, still has serious internal problems that have not yet been solved satisfactorily. Indeed, although considerable technical progress has been made in the ability to find mathematical formulae that fit new experimental data, it cannot be said that there is, at present, a coherent body of theoretical understanding that would, as it were, be at the core of our knowledge of physics. Rather, in this regard, the current situation can best be described as one of 'crisis', which has indeed persisted with no essential change over the past forty years or more.[2]

A more careful examination of this crisis suggests that the time may well be ripe for the perception of a new order, within which these problems will not arise. Such an order would be as different from that of current physics as that of the latter is from the order of classical physics, and as the order of classical physics is from that of the physics of ancient times. In other words, what may be required is to regard current physical theories as clues or indications pointing towards a different sort of physical theory, rather than as solid and well-established frameworks, within which we are to continue to elaborate ever more detailed structures of theory, in response to the continual development of new experimental facts.

V. ON THE PERCEPTION OF NEW ORDERS IN PHYSICS

One may now ask why physicists are generally so slow to consider new notions of order, even when there is considerable evidence indicating the need to do so. Of course, the tendency to regard certain familiar notions of order as if these were permanent and unchangeable is by no means a new one. Indeed, it can be seen that over its entire historical development the task of physics has, on the whole, been taken to be to *accommodate* new observational evidence by means of adaptations within accepted notions of order, rather than to inquire into the possibility of developing new notions of order. This kind of adaptation began (as pointed out in Section I) with the Ptolemaic epicycles, which continued to be used from ancient times until the advent of the work of Copernicus, Kepler, Galileo, and Newton. As soon as the basic notions of order in classical physics had been fairly clearly expressed, it was then supposed that further work in physics would consist of adaptation within this order to accommodate new facts. This continued until the appearance of relativity and the quantum theory. It can accurately be said that since then the main line of work in physics has been adaptation within the general orders underlying these theories, to accommodate the facts to which these in turn have led.

It is thus clear that accommodation within already existing frameworks of order has generally been considered to be the main activity to be emphasized in physics, and that the perception of new orders has been regarded as something that happens only occasionally, perhaps in revolutionary periods, during which what is thought of as the normal process of accommodation has broken down.[3]

It is pertinent to this subject to consider Piaget's[4] description of all intelligent perception in terms of two complementary movements, *accommodation* and *assimilation*. From the roots *modus* meaning 'measure' and 'con' meaning 'together' one sees that to accommodate means 'to establish a common measure'. Examples of accommodation are fitting, cutting to a pattern, adapting, imitating, conforming to rules, etc. On the other hand, 'to assimilate' is 'to digest' or to make into a comprehensive and inseparable whole (which includes oneself). And thus, to assimilate means 'to understand'.

It is clear that, in intelligent perception, primary emphasis has in general to be given to assimilation, while accommodation tends to play a relatively secondary role, in the sense that its main significance is as an aid to assimilation.

Of course, we are able in certain sorts of contexts just to accommodate something that we observe, within known orders of thought, and in this very act it will be adequately assimilated. However, it is necessary in more general contexts to give serious attention to the possibility that the old orders of thought may cease to be relevant, so that they can no longer coherently be adapted to fit the new fact. As has been brought out earlier, one may then have to see the irrelevance of old differences, and the relevance of new differences, and thus one may open the way to the perception of new orders, new measures, and new structures.

Clearly, such perception can appropriately take place at almost any time, and does not have to be restricted to unusual and revolutionary periods, in which one finds that the older orders can no longer be conveniently adapted to the facts. Rather, one may be continually ready to drop old notions of order in various contexts, which may be broad or narrow, and to perceive new notions that may be relevant in such contexts. Thus, understanding the fact by assimilating it into new orders can become what could perhaps be called the normal way of doing scientific research.

To work in this way is evidently to give primary emphasis to something similar to *artistic perception*. Such perception begins by observing the whole fact in its full individuality, and then by degrees articulates the order that is proper to the assimilation of this fact. It does not begin with abstract preconceptions as to what the order has to be, which are then adapted to the order that is observed.

What then is the proper role of accommodation of facts within known theoretical orders and structures? Here, it is important to note that facts are not to be considered as if they were independently existent objects, that we might find or pick up in the laboratory. Rather, as the Latin root of the word, *factum*, indicates, the fact is 'what has been made' (e.g. as in 'manufacture'). Thus, in a certain sense, we 'make' the fact. That is to say, we give it order, form, and structure, with the aid of our theoretical concepts. For example, starting with the notions of order prevailing in certain times, men 'made' the fact about planetary orbits by describing and measuring epicycles. In terms of classical physics, the fact was 'made' in the order of planetary orbits, expressed quantitatively through positions and times. In general relativity, the fact was 'made' in the order of Riemannian geometry, quantitatively expressed in terms of concepts such as 'curvature of space'. And in the quantum theory, the fact was made in the order of energy levels, quantum numbers, symmetry groups, etc., along with appropriate quantitative measures (e.g. scattering cross sections, charges, and masses of particles).

It is clear, then, that changes of order in the theory ultimately lead to new ways of doing experiments and to new kinds of instruments, which in turn lead to the 'making' of correspondingly ordered and measured facts of new kinds. In this development, the experimental fact serves in the first instance as a test for theoretical notions. Thus, as has been pointed out earlier, the general form of theoretical explanation is that of a generalized kind of ratio or reason. 'As A is to B in our structure of thinking, so it is in fact': This ratio or reason constitutes a kind of 'common measure' or 'accommodation' between theory and fact.

As long as such a common measure prevails, then of course the theory need not be changed. If the common measure is found not to be realized, then the first step is to see whether it can be re-established by means of adjustments within the theory without a change in its underlying order. If, after reasonable efforts, a proper accommodation of this kind is not achieved, then what is needed is a fresh perception of *the whole fact*. This now includes not only the results of experiments, but also the *failure of certain lines of theory to fit the experimental results, in a 'common measure'*. Then, as has been indicated earlier, one has to be very sensitively aware of all the relevant differences which underlie the main orders in the old theory, to see whether there is room for a change of overall order. It is being emphasized here that this kind of perception should properly be interwoven continually with the activities aimed at accommodation, and should not have to be delayed for so long that the whole situation becomes confused and chaotic, apparently requiring the revolutionary destruction of the old order to clear it up.

This implies, for example, that there is no need to go on indefinitely with theories, such as relativity and quantum theory, which have led to insoluble problems and to persistent incoherence in efforts to bring them together. Rather, conceptual and theoretical 'experimentation' with new orders, in terms of which such problems would not arise, can usefully be carried out at any time.

In such 'experimentation', it is necessary to proceed slowly and patiently. Thus it will not be appropriate to try immediately to apply new notions of order to current problems that have arisen in the detailed consideration of specialized aspects of the presently available set of experimental facts. Instead, what is called for is very broadly to assimilate *the whole* of the fact of physics into the proposed new notion of order. After this fact has generally been 'digested', we can begin to glimpse new ways in which such notions of order can be tested and extended in various directions.

A premature demand for 'relating the theory to empirical fact' is indeed equivalent to forcing the theory to fit itself into existing frameworks of order, in terms of which this fact is given expression and general structure. To do this is, in effect, to prevent any new order from being *seriously* considered. That is to say, it is important that one does not try *always* to force a theory to fit the kinds of facts that may be appropriate in currently accepted general orders of description. Rather, we have also to be ready where necessary to consider changes in what is meant by fact, changes which may be required for assimilation of such fact into new theoretical notions of order.

VI. UNDIVIDED WHOLENESS OF THEORETICAL NOTIONS OF ORDER AND OF MODES OF INSTRUMENTATION – THE LENS AND THE HOLOGRAM

In the above discussion, fact and theory are seen to be different aspects of one whole, in which analysis into separate but interacting parts is not relevant. This is true quite generally for every phase of the development of science, but it is especially significant to emphasize the inseparability of fact and theory in the context of current developments in physics. For here we have seen that the *content* of physics (notably relativity and quantum theory) is such as to imply undivided wholeness in the structure and constitution of the universe. But now we see, in addition, that there is in our *manner of working* in physics a similar undivided wholeness of fact and theoretical modes of understanding.

Such undivided wholeness in the factual content of physics and in its modes of theoretical understanding implies the need to consider a *new order of fact*; i.e. the fact about the way in which modes of theoretical understanding and of observation and instrumentation are related to each other. Until now, we have more or less just taken such relationship for granted, without giving serious attention to the manner in which it arises, very probably because of the belief that the study of the subject belongs to 'the history of science' rather than to 'science proper'. However, it is now being suggested that the consideration of this relationship is essential for an adequate understanding of science itself.

An example of the very close relationship between instrumentation and theory can be seen by considering the *lens*, which was indeed one of the key features behind the development of modern scientific thought. The essential feature of a lens is, as indicated in *Figure 5*, that it forms an *image* in which a given point, P, in the object corresponds (in a high degree of approximation) to a point, Q, in the image:

Figure 5

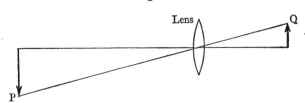

By thus bringing the correspondence of specified features of object and image into such sharp relief, the lens greatly strengthened man's awareness of the various parts of the object, and of the relationships between these parts. In this way it furthered the tendency to think in terms of analysis and synthesis. Moreover, it made possible an enormous extension of this classical order of analysis and synthesis to objects that were too far away, too big, too small, or too rapidly moving to be thus ordered by means of unordered vision. As a result, scientists were encouraged to extrapolate their ideas, and to think that such an approach would be relevant and valid, no matter how far one went, in all possible conditions, contexts, and degrees of approximation.

But as has already been seen, relativity and quantum theory imply undivided wholeness, in which analysis into distinct and well-defined parts is no longer relevant. Is there an instrument that can help give a certain immediate perceptual insight into what can be meant by undivided wholeness, as the lens did for what is to be meant by analysis of a system into parts? It is being suggested here that one can obtain such insight by considering a new instrument, called a *hologram*. (The name is derived from the Greek words *holos*, meaning 'whole' and *gramma* from *graphein* meaning 'something written'. Thus, the hologram is an instrument that, as it were writes the whole.)

As shown in *Figure 6*, coherent light from a laser is passed

Figure 6

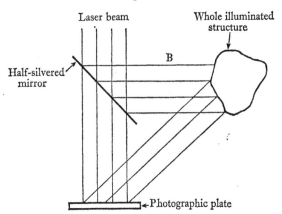

Laser beam   Whole illuminated
                                  structure

B

Half-silvered
mirror

←Photographic plate

through a half-silvered mirror. Part of the beam goes on directly to a photographic plate, while another part is reflected so that it illuminates a certain whole structure. The light reflected from this whole structure also reaches the plate, where it interferes with that arriving there by a direct path. The resulting interference pattern which is recorded on the plate, is not only very complex but also usually so fine that it is not even visible to the naked eye. Yet, it is somehow relevant to the whole illuminated structure, though only in a highly implicit way.

This relevance of the interference pattern to the whole illuminated structure is revealed when the photographic plate is illuminated with laser light. As shown in *Figure 7*, a wave front is then created, which is very similar in form to that coming off the original illuminated structure. By placing the eye in this wave, one in effect sees the whole of the original structure, in three dimensions, and from a range of possible points of view (as if one

Figure 7

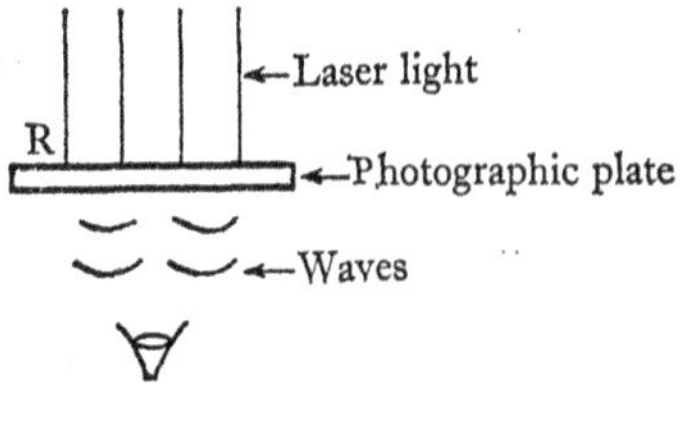

R

←Laser light

←Photographic plate

←Waves

were looking at it through a window). If we then illuminate only a small region, R, of the plate, we *still see the whole structure*, but in somewhat less sharply defined detail and from a decreased range of possible points of view (as if we were looking through a smaller window).

It is clear then that there is no one-to-one correspondence between parts of an 'illuminated object' and parts of an 'image of this object on the plate'. Rather, the interference pattern in each region, R, of the plate is relevant to the whole structure, and each region of the structure is relevant to the whole of the interference pattern on the plate.

Because of the wave properties of light, even a lens cannot produce an exact one-to-one correspondence. A lens can therefore be regarded as a limiting case of a hologram.

We can, however, go further and say that in their overall ways of indicating the meaning of observations, typical experiments as currently done in physics (especially in the 'quantum' context) are more like the general case of a hologram than like the special case of a lens. For example, consider a scattering experiment. As shown in *Figure 8*, what can be observed in the detector is generally relevant to the whole target, or at least to an area large enough to contain a great many atoms.

Figure 8

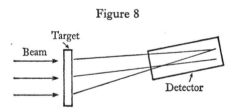

So we may say that in current research in physics, an instrument tends to be relevant to a whole structure, in a way rather similar to what happens with a hologram. To be sure, there are certain differences. For example, in current experiments with electron beams, or with X-rays, these latter are seldom coherent over appreciable distances. If, however, it should ever prove to be possible to develop something like an electron laser or an X-ray laser, then experiments will directly reveal 'atomic' and 'nuclear' structures, without the need for complex chains of inference of the sort now generally required, as the hologram does for ordinary large-scale structures.

VII. IMPLICATE AND EXPLICATE ORDER

What is being suggested here is that the consideration of the difference between lens and hologram can play a significant part in the perception of a new order that is relevant for physical law. As Galileo noted the distinction between a viscous medium and a vacuum, and saw that physical law should refer primarily to the order of motion of an object in a vacuum, so we might now note the distinction between a lens and a hologram, and consider the possibility that physical law should refer primarily to an order of undivided wholeness of the content of a description similar to that indicated by the hologram rather than to an order of analysis of such content into separate parts indicated by a lens.

But then, when Aristotle's ideas on movement were dropped, Galileo and those who followed him had to consider the question of how the new order of motion was to be described in adequate detail. The answer came in the form of Cartesian coordinates extended to the language of the calculus (differential equations, etc.). But this kind of description is of course appropriate only in a context in which analysis into distinct and autonomous parts is relevant, and will therefore in turn have to be dropped. What then will be the new kind of description appropriate to the present context?

As happened with Cartesian coordinates and the calculus, such a question cannot be answered immediately in terms of definite prescriptions as to what to do. Rather, one has to observe the new situation very broadly and tentatively, and to 'feel out' what may be the relevant new features. From this there will arise a discernment of the new order, which will articulate and unfold in a natural way (and not as a result of efforts to make it fit well-defined and preconceived notions as to what this order should be able to achieve).

We can begin such an inquiry by noting that in some subtle sense, which does not appear in ordinary vision, the interference pattern in the whole plate can distinguish different orders and measures in the whole illuminated structure. For example, the illuminated structure may contain all sorts of shapes and sizes of geometric forms (indicated in *Figure 9a*), as well as topological relationships, such as inside and outside (indicated in *Figure 9b*), and intersection and separation (indicated in *Figure 9c*). All of these lead to different interference patterns and it is this difference that is somehow to be described in detail.

Figure 9a   Figure 9b   Figure 9c

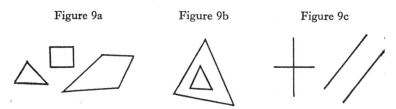

The differences indicated above are, however, not only in the plate. Indeed, the latter is of secondary significance, in the sense that its main function is to make a relatively permanent 'written record' of the interference pattern of the light that is present in each region of space. More generally, however, in each such region the movement of the light implicitly contains a vast range of distinctions of order and measure, appropriate to a whole illuminated structure. Indeed, in principle, this structure extends over the whole universe and over the whole past, with implications for the whole future. Consider, for example, how, on looking at the night sky, we are able to discern structures covering immense stretches of space and time, which are in some sense contained in the movements of light in the tiny space encompassed by the eye (and also how instruments, such as optical and radio telescopes, can discern more and more of this totality, contained in each region of space).

There is the germ of a new notion of order here. This order is not to be understood solely in terms of a regular arrangement of *objects* (e.g. in rows) or as a regular arrangement of *events* (e.g. in a series). Rather, a *total order* is contained, in some *implicit* sense, in each region of space and time.

Now, the word 'implicit' is related to the verb 'to implicate'. This means 'to fold inwards' (as multiplication means 'folding many times'). So we are led to consider the notion that each such region contains a total structure 'folded up', in a way that is, in some sense, similar to that in which a concept contains implications 'within' it.

It will be useful to illustrate what is meant here with the aid of some further examples of implicate order. Thus, in a television broadcast, the visual image is translated into a time order, which is 'carried' by the radio wave. Points that are near each other in the visual image are not necessarily 'near' in the order of the radio signal. Thus, the radio wave carries the visual image in a 'folded up' or implicate order. The function of the receiver is then to 'unfold' this order, and thus to *explicate* it, in the form of a new visual image.

A more striking example of implicate order can be demonstrated in the laboratory, with a transparent container full of a very viscous fluid, such as treacle, and equipped with a mechanical rotator that can 'stir' the fluid very slowly but very thoroughly. If an insoluble droplet of dye is placed in the fluid, and the stirring device is set in motion, the ink drop is gradually transformed into a thread that extends over the whole fluid. The latter now appears to be distributed more or less at 'random' so that it is seen as some shade of grey. But if the mechanical stirring device is now turned in the opposite direction, the transformation is reversed, and the droplet of dye suddenly appears, reconstituted.

When the dye was distributed in what appeared to be a random way, it nevertheless had *some kind* of order which is different, for example, from that arising from another droplet, originally placed in a different position. But this order is *folded up* or *implicated* in the 'grey mass' that is visible in the fluid. Indeed, one could thus 'fold up' a whole picture. Different pictures would look indistinguishable and yet have different implicate orders, which differences would be revealed when they were explicated, as the stirring device was turned in a reverse direction.

What happens here is evidently similar in certain crucial ways to what happens with the hologram. To be sure there are differences. Thus, in a fine enough analysis, one could see that the *parts* of the ink droplet remain in a one-to-one correspondence, as they are stirred up and the fluid moves continuously. On the other hand, in the functioning of the hologram, there is no such one-to-one correspondence. So in the hologram (as also in experiments in a 'quantum' context), there is no way ultimately to reduce the implicate order to a finer and more complex type of explicate order.

All this calls attention to the relevance of a new distinction between implicate and explicate order. Generally speaking, the laws of physics have thus far referred mainly to the explicate order. Indeed, it may be said that the principle function of Cartesian coordinates is just to give a clear and precise description of explicate order. But now we are proposing that in the formulation of the laws of physics, primary relevance is to be given to the implicate order, while the explicate order is to have a secondary kind of significance (e.g. as happened with Aristotle's notions of movement, after the development of classical physics). Thus, it may be expected that a description in terms of Cartesian coordinates can no longer be given a primary emphasis, and that a new kind of description will indeed have to be developed for discussing the laws of physics.

VIII. THE HOLOMOVEMENT AND ITS ASPECTS

To indicate a new kind of description appropriate for giving primary relevance to implicate order, let us consider once again the key feature of the functioning of the hologram; i.e. in each region of space, the order of a whole illuminated structure is 'folded up' and 'carried' in the movement of light. Something similar happens with a signal that modulates a radio wave (see *Figure 10*). In all cases, the content or meaning that is 'folded up'

Figure 10

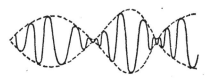

and 'carried' is primarily an order and a measure, permitting the development of a structure. With the radio wave, this structure can be that of a verbal communication, a visual image, etc., but with the hologram, far more subtle structures can be involved in this way (notably three-dimensional structures, visible from many points of view).

More generally, such order and measure can be 'folded up' and 'carried' not only in electromagnetic waves, but also in other ways (by electron beams, sound, and in other countless forms of movement). To generalize so as to emphasize undivided wholeness, we shall say that what 'carries' any implicate order is *the holomovement*, which is an unbroken and undivided totality. In certain cases we can abstract particular aspects of the holomovement (e.g. light, electrons, sound, etc.). But more generally, all forms of the holomovement merge and are inseparable. Thus, in its totality, the holomovement is not limited in any specifiable way at all. It is not required to conform to any particular order, or to be bounded by any particular measure. Thus, *the holomovement is undefinable and immeasurable.*

To give primary significance to the indefinable and immeasurable holomovement implies that it has no meaning to talk of a *fundamental* theory, on which *all* of physics could find a *permanent* basis, or to which *all* the phenomena of physics could ultimately be reduced. Rather, each theory will abstract a certain aspect that is *relevant* only in some limited context, which is indicated by some appropriate measure.

In discussing how attention is to be called to such aspects, it is useful to note that the word 'relevant' is derived from a verb 'to relevate', which has dropped out of common usage, and which means 'to lift up' (as in 'elevate'). We can thus say that in a particular context that may be under consideration, the general modes of description that belong to a given theory serve to *relevate* a certain content, i.e. to lift it into attention so that it stands out 'in relief'. If this content is pertinent in the context under discussion, it is said to be *relevant*, and otherwise *irrelevant*.

To illustrate what it means to relevate certain aspects of the implicate order in the holomovement, it is useful to consider once again the example of the mechanical device for stirring a viscous fluid, as described in the previous section. Suppose that we first put in a droplet of dye and turn the stirring mechanism *n* times. We could then place another droplet of dye nearby and stir once again through *n* turns. We could repeat this process indefinitely, with a long series of droplets, arranged more or less along a line, as shown in *Figure 11*:

Figure 11

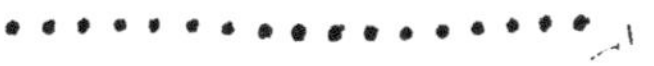

• • • • • • • • • • • • • • • • • ˎ˺

Suppose then that after thus 'folding up' a large number of drop-lets we turn the stirring device in a reverse direction, but so rapidly that the individual droplets are not resolved in perception. Then we will see what appears to be a 'solid' object (e.g. a particle) moving continuously through space. This form of a moving object appears in immediate perception, primarily because the eye is not sensitive to concentrations of dye lower than a certain mini-mum, so that one does not directly see the 'whole movement' of the dye. Rather, such perception *relevates a certain aspect*. That is to say, it makes this aspect stand out 'in relief', while the rest of the fluid is seen only as a 'grey background', within which the related 'object' seems to be moving.

But, of course, such an aspect has little interest *in itself*, i.e. apart from its *broader meaning*. Thus, in the present example, one possible meaning is that there *actually is* an autonomous object moving through the fluid. This would signify, of course, that the whole order of movement is to be regarded as similar to that in the immediately perceived aspect. In some contexts, such a meaning is pertinent and adequate (e.g. if we are dealing in the ordinary level of experience with a rock flying through the air). However, in the present context, a very different meaning is in-dicated, and this can be communicated only through a very differ-ent kind of description.

Such a description has to start by *conceptually* relevating certain broader orders of movement, going beyond any that are similar to those relevated in immediate perception. In doing this, one always begins with the holomovement, and then one abstracts out special aspects, which involve a totality broad enough for a proper description in the context under discussion. In the present ex-ample, this totality should include the whole movement of the fluid and the dye as determined by the mechanical stirring device, and the movement of the light, which enables us visually to perceive what is happening, along with the movement of the eye and nervous system, which determines the distinctions that can be perceived in the movement of the light.

It may then be said that the content relevated in immediate

perception (i.e. the 'moving object') is a kind of *intersection* between two orders. One of these is the order of movement that brings about the possibility of a direct perceptual contact (in this case that of the light, and the response of the nervous system to this light), and the other is an order of movement that determines the detailed content that is perceived (in this case, the order of movement of the dye in the fluid). Such a description in terms of intersection of orders is evidently very generally applicable.[5]

It has already been seen that, in general, the movement of *light* is to be described in terms of 'the folding and carrying' of implicate orders that are relevant to a whole structure, in which analysis into separate and autonomous parts is not applicable (though of course, in certain limited contexts, a description in terms of explicate orders will be adequate). But in the present example, it is also appropriate to describe the movement of *the dye* in similar terms. That is to say, in the movement, certain implicate orders (in the distribution of dye) become explicate, while explicate orders become implicate.

To specify this movement in more detail, it is useful here to introduce a new *measure*, i.e. an 'implication parameter', denoted by T. In the fluid, this would be the number of turns needed to bring a given droplet of dye into explicate form. The total structure of dye present at any moment can then be regarded as an ordered series of substructures, each corresponding to a single droplet, N, with its implication parameter, T_N.

Evidently, we have here a new notion of structure. For we no longer build structures solely as ordered and measured arrangements on which we join separate things, all of which are explicate together. Rather, we can now consider structures in which aspects of different degrees of implication (as measured by T) can be arranged in a certain order.

Such aspects can be quite complex. For example, we could implicate a 'whole picture' by turning the stirring device *n* times. We could then implicate a slightly different picture, and so on indefinitely. If the stirring device were turned rapidly in the reverse direction, we could see a 'three-dimensional scene', apparently consisting of a 'whole system' of objects in continuous movement and interaction.

In this movement, the 'picture' present at any given moment

would consist only of aspects that can be explicated together (i.e. aspects corresponding to a certain value of the implication parameter, T). As events happening at the same time are said to be *synchronous*, so aspects that can be explicated together can be called *synordinate*, while those that cannot be explicated together may then be called *a-synordinate*. Evidently, the new notions of structure under discussion here involve *a-synordinate* aspects, whereas previous notions involve only *synordinate* aspects.

It has to be emphasized here that the order of implication, as measured by the parameter, T, has no necessary relationship to the order of time (as measured by *another* parameter, t). These two parameters are only related in a *contingent* manner (in this case by the rate of turning of the stirring device). It is the T parameter that is directly relevant to the description of the implicate structure, and not the t parameter.

When a structure is *a-synordinate* (that is, constituted of aspects with different degrees of implication), then evidently the time order is not in general the primary one that is pertinent for the expression of law. Rather, as one can see by considering the previous examples, the *whole implicate order* is present at any moment, in such a way that the entire structure growing out of this implicate order can be described without giving any primary role to time. The law of the structure will then just be a law relating aspects with various degrees of implication. Such a law will, of course, not be deterministic *in time*. But, as has been indicated earlier, determinism in time is not the only form of ratio or reason. And as long as we can find ratio or reason in the orders that are primarily relevant, this is all that is needed for law.

One can see in the 'quantum context' a significant similarity to

Figure 12

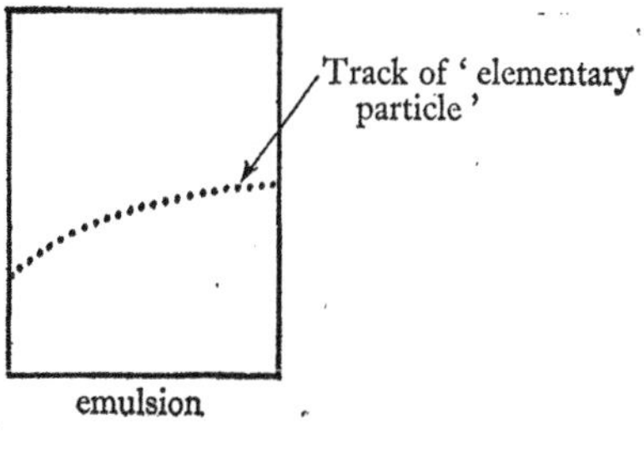

Track of ' elementary particle '

emulsion

the orders of movement that have been described in terms of the simple examples discussed above. Thus, as shown in *Figure 12*, 'elementary particles' are generally observed by means of tracks that they are supposed to make in detecting devices (photographic emulsions, bubble chambers, etc.).

Such a track is evidently to be regarded as no more than an *aspect* appearing in immediate perception (as was done with the moving sequence of droplets of dye indicated in *Figure 7*). To describe it as the track of a 'particle' is then to assume in addition that the primarily relevant order of movement is similar to that in the immediately perceived aspect.

However, the whole discussion of the new order implicit in the quantum theory shows that such a description cannot coherently be maintained. For example, the need to describe movement discontinuously, in terms of 'quantum jumps' implies that the notion of a well-defined orbit of a particle that connects the visible marks constituting the track cannot have any meaning. In any case, the wave–particle properties of matter show that the overall movement depends on the total experimental arrangement, in a way that is not consistent with the idea of autonomous motion of localized particles. And, of course, the discussion of the indeterminacy principle and the quantum of action indicates the relevance of a new order of undivided wholeness, in which it has no meaning to talk about an observed object, as if it were separate from the entire experimental situation in which observation takes place. So the use of the descriptive term 'particle' in this 'quantum' context is very misleading.

Evidently, we have here to do with something that is similar in certain important ways to the example of stirring a dye into a viscous fluid. In both cases, there appears in immediate perception an explicate order that cannot consistently be regarded as autonomous. In the example of the dye, the explicate order is determined as an intersection of the implicate order of 'the whole movement' of the fluid, and an implicate order of distinctions of density of dye, that are relevated in sense perception. In the 'quantum' context, there similarly will be an intersection of an implicate order of some 'whole movement' corresponding to what we have called, for example, 'the electron', and another implicate order of distinctions that are relevated (and recorded) by our instruments.

Thus, the word 'electron' should be regarded as no more than a name by which we call attention to a certain aspect of the holomovement, an aspect that can be discussed only by taking into account the entire experimental situation, and that cannot be specified in terms of localized objects moving autonomously through space. And, of course, every kind of 'particle', which in current physics is said to be a basic constituent of matter, will have to be discussed in the same sort of terms (so that such 'particles' are no longer considered as autonomous and separately existent). Thus, we come to a new general physical description, in which 'everything implicates everything', in an order of undivided wholeness.

As suggested earlier, it is now necessary to proceed carefully and patiently, to 'digest' and assimilate the whole of current physics into this new notion of order. Further work along these lines (including a mathematical discussion of how the essential content of relativity and quantum theory can be assimilated in this way) is now going on, and will be published in later papers.

NOTES AND REFERENCES

1 For a further discussion on this point, see BOHM, D. *Special Theory of Relativity*, New York, Benjamin, 1965, Chapter 18.
2 For a further discussion of this crisis, see BOHM, D. *Causality and Chance in Modern Physics*, London, Routledge & Kegan Paul, 1957.
3 For a very clear presentation of this view, see KUHN, T. S. *The Structure of Scientific Revolutions*, Chicago, University of Chicago Press, 1962.
4 PIAGET, J. *The Origin of Intelligence in the Child*, London, Routledge & Kegan Paul, 1956.
5 See BOHM, D., HILEY, B. and STUART, A. *International Journal of Theoretical Physics*, **3** (3), 1970, 171–83, where this description of a perceived content considered as the intersection of two orders is treated in a different context.

The Role of Discoveries
in Social Science

W. BALDAMUS

I. THE SERENDIPITY PROBLEM[1]

Traditionally, the advancement of scientific work is associated with the notion of 'discovery'. In so far as social sciences are based in some sense on pragmatic knowledge, it would seem probable that advancement towards new understanding is not entirely a function of scientifically formalized procedures. We should expect, in other words, that the discovery process extends into the realm of pragmatic experience. The present paper intends to follow up these clues. Most of it involved the breaking of new ground and is therefore extremely tentative.[2]

There are various ways of exploring this question methodologically. Perhaps the most obvious prospect lies in discussion of serendipity patterns. According to Robert Merton's celebrated definition, it refers to 'the fairly common experience of observing an *unanticipated, anomalous and strategic* datum which becomes the occasion of developing a new theory or for extending an existing theory'.[3] For all its striking plausibility, this formulation has never been quite convincing as far as the social sciences are concerned: it is hardly a 'fairly common experience'! Undoubtedly, what Merton had in mind was oriented by the discovery process of the natural rather than the social sciences. He had been taking his clue from a simple descriptive account of serendipity cases by the physiologist W. B. Cannon, reported in terms of chance discoveries chiefly in physiological and medical research.[4] In view of the fact that the popular stereotype of the scientist as a discoverer is derived from the spectacular recent history of the natural sciences,

276

it is understandable that social scientists, anxious to establish or to enhance the scientific nature of their work, like to believe that they, too, are engaged in discoveries. If we examine Merton's definition of serendipity in the light of Cannon's descriptive examples (such as the accidental discovery of penicillin) we can see why Merton places a special emphasis on 'strategic' data. 'Strategic' means that 'the unexpected fact . . . must permit of implications which bear upon generalized theory' and he adds that he refers here 'rather to what the observer brings to the datum than to the datum itself' (op. cit., p. 105). This idea occurs in Cannon's account only casually in so far as he talks about a 'prepared mind', 'sagacity', 'fresh insight', 'alert intelligence', etc. But this is not just a difference of emphasis. What happened most likely is that Merton started off by looking at the most striking unexpected discoveries in the *physical* sciences, and then cast his mind over the range of similar incidents in sociological research. He thus must have noticed, not only that it takes a good deal of searching around before one finds comparable incidents, but also that the few which seem to be relevant are curiously different. He realizes finally that what is new about new observations involves a great deal of interpretation and theorizing, an element, that is to say, which 'the observer brings to the datum'. It is obvious that this element weakens the whole idea of 'discovery', for what seems so impressive in the history of natural science is precisely the sheer force with which pure facts, in the sense of theoretically unadulterated events, have asserted themselves.

That the case of genuine serendipity in social science is noticeably weaker than one would hope is confirmed by the fact that Merton elaborates his definition by only one illustration from sociological research, one that is by no means particularly exciting: 'In the course of our research into the social organization of Craftown, . . . we observed that a large proportion of residents were affiliated with more civic, political and other voluntary organizations than had been the case in their previous places of residence. Quite incidentally, we noted further that this increase in group participation had occurred also among the parents of infants and young children. This finding was rather inconsistent with common-sense knowledge' (op. cit., p. 105). Obviously, to call this a 'discovery' would hardly be convincing. However, on two other occasions he does mention more startling cases; Lazarsfeld's and his associates' well-known work on voting behaviour (p. 96, footnote 18) and the concept of 'relative deprivation' developed in *The American Soldier* (p. 229, note 2, and p. 241, note 13). Although the word 'serendipity' is not explicitly mentioned, a possible third example might be the 'paradoxical' (and in that sense unanticipated) findings of the Western Electric Company experiments, which are discussed as an illustration of the 'discovery' of latent functions (p. 66 ff). That is all. Though there are so few examples, they are at any rate sufficient to show up the dominance of *theoretical* interpretation over the strictly accidental 'datum itself'.

In a more recent publication, Robert Merton followed up the serendipity problem under the aspect of 'multiple discoveries'.[5] The relevant passage is this: (the study of multiples will) 'help us to identify certain significant similarities and differences between the various branches of science. To the extent that the rate of multiples and the type of rediscoveries are much the same in the social and psychological sciences as in the physical and life sciences, we are led to similarities between them, just as differences in such rates and types alert us to differences between them. In short, the study of multiples can supplement the traditional notion of the *unity of all science* . . .' (my italics).[6] This suggests that the difference between the natural and the social sciences is a matter of degree only. Now the paper in which this statement occurs is dealing predominantly with multiple discoveries in astronomy, physics, chemistry, biology, and medicine, an important focus being reported disputes about 'priority'. As regards specifically the 'social and psychological sciences', the following scholars involved in such disputes are discussed: Saint-Simon, Comte, Ferguson, Adam Smith, Adam Robertson, Guizot, Le Bon, Sighele, Lester Ward, Albion Small, Herbert Spencer, Marx, Mosca, Freud, Jung, Adler, Moreno, Slavson, Sorokin (op. cit., p. 262). Now if we glance at these names, the question arises: what exactly is the nature of the discoveries which led to priority quarrels? Are they really comparable to what was at stake when Newton, Galileo, Laplace, or Darwin got involved in such disputes? Merton does not provide us with an explicit definition of the terms 'discovery' or 'multiple discoveries' or 'rediscovery'. In the context of the natural sciences he seems to allude to the 'repeated discovery of the same facts' (p. 238), but when he discusses social scientists and psychologists, he includes '*new ideas*', and in dealing with what he calls the 'eureka syndrome' he talks about the 'socially reinforced elation that comes with having arrived at a new and true scientific idea or result' (p. 270). In this latter context he discusses, side by side, Kepler's third planetary law, Gay-Lussac's discoveries in the behaviour of gases, William James's 'idea of pragmatism', Joseph Henry's 'new way of constructing electro-magnets', and finally Freud's early discovery of staining nervous tissue with a solution of gold chloride, as well as a later occasion when Freud reminds Karl Abraham that they had gained the 'first insights'. Evidently, any attempt to include social scientists under the category of scientific discoverers is forced to shift, once again, the emphasis from 'new facts' to 'new ideas'. Simultaneously the difficulty arises that somehow one has to be sure that the new ideas are 'true' or 'genuine' discoveries. Clearly, it would require quite an elaborate and controversial undertaking to determine exactly to what extent and in which sense Freud's insights represent a genuine scientific discovery, notwithstanding their tremendous influence on modern social science. This difficulty will be felt even more acutely if we exclude from the social sciences economics and such approaches to psychology which remain more or less closely linked to biology, physiology, or clinical psychiatry.

No doubt one of the most impressive features of the history of the natural sciences is the occurrence of multiple discoveries. Nothing else can demonstrate so convincingly the 'objectivity' of scientific procedure than the observation that one and the same 'fact' is found independently by two or more investigators. But the suggestion that social science is equally objective and scientific because here, too, discoveries – including multiple discoveries – are a typical occurrence is likely to defeat its own purpose. I think if one sets one's mind to it, one could make quite a good case by arguing that there are no clear cases of multiple discoveries at all. Even so, the questions that emerge from this matter are important. Not only do they indicate that there seems to be something odd about the nature of the 'facts' with which the social scientist is concerned. They also prompt us to look at the ways and means by which the kind of new results are brought about that we would like to call discoveries though we know they are not quite the real thing.

For this reason the next step is indicated by the need to obtain a better understanding of the nature of interpreted facts within the social sciences. It is at this juncture that the role of pragmatic knowledge appears to be particularly significant. For there is sufficient evidence to assume that it is the universe of pragmatic knowledge which functions, as it were, as an intervening medium between the results of systematically controlled inquiry, on the one hand, and the experience of uninterpreted reality, on the other. Obviously this universe is of great importance to specifically sociological work. For the sociologist's observations – all that goes into codified responses, fourfold tables, and zero-order correlations – are already the products of common conceptualizations in everyday life.

Seen from this vantage point, the social scientist's 'data' are merely derived observations, based on secondary sources. This important aspect is easily overlooked when we talk about 'common-sense data' in a casual manner. The conventional implications and meanings of the term are vague and variable, but a frequent connotation points towards unreliable, untested, non-scientific or even non-rational beliefs. Now, if we replace this term by 'common *knowledge*' or 'practical *knowledge*', we shall move in a different direction altogether. We realize that there is more to it than simply untested beliefs. The emphasis now is on experiences which have a *cognitive* dimension, which contain observations that are in some sense valid and relevant. It should be noted that ordinarily in social research this possibility is never seriously envisaged. Whether or not the answers to a questionnaire express an element of truth is simply not taken into consideration: the aim is, rather, to obtain honest and sincere answers, no matter whether they are true or false in their own right.

As soon as we start to identify our raw material as knowledge that could be more or less accurate, valid, or true, we seem to depart so radically from the conventional scientific approach, that it takes some effort to assimilate the idea. The main difficulty is that we can hardly imagine what sort of methodological consequences we would have to face. As a first step to understand such consequences, we might point to one conspicuous advantage that arises from a recognition of the cognitive attributes of practical knowledge. This is that it explains at once the puzzle of the 'obstinate' or 'active' facts. If we realize that our raw data – our observations on elements of practical knowledge – have potentially a validity of their own, deriving from the pragmatic contexts of everyday life, we can understand how it is possible that mere observational facts have a power to assert themselves. They perpetually generate *theoretical* interpretations of the world that compete, as it were, with the researchers' own theories, hypotheses, concepts, and analyses.

But although we can see now what it is that makes facts obstinate and self-assertive, on that basis it would seem even more difficult to comprehend the formal methods that we conventionally associate with social research and theory. According to thoroughly established practice, the procedural rules prescribe a unidirectional sequence of axiomatic theory, hypothesis formation, observation, testing, and conclusion; there is no other way to gain verified knowledge. Obviously, if the third step – the observations themselves – tend to generate valid knowledge on their own, the sequence is broken and the procedure seems pointless.

In trying to overcome this formidable difficulty we have to look at the facts. And 'the facts' in this case are the practices and techniques actually used in the doing of scientific work. Possibly, even here, the facts exhibit an assertive power of their own.

In a sense this would amount to attempting an empirical study of the available products of social science. In the course of it we would expect to come across certain bits and pieces of pragmatic knowledge: the 'knowhow' of social scientists that is acquired through constant practice and that appears to have obtained some degree of validity on account of its pragmatic usefulness in producing scientific results. In other words, we would have to presume that side by side with the official methodology that one finds in the textbooks on systematic theory, formal logic, statistical methods, survey design or interviewing procedure, there exists a reservoir of *unofficial*, non-formalized techniques of inquiry. Evidently this kind of phenomenon is not easily got hold of. While there is a well-established sociology of science, no systematic research has been done specifically on what would have to be called the 'sociology of social science'. It is surprisingly easy, nevertheless, to

visualize the nature of unofficial techniques. What comes to mind
is, for example, the exchange of personal experience, of 'gim-
micks' and lucky 'hunches', of frustrations and unexpected
insights, between researchers or theorists when they meet pri-
vately, at conferences or in staff commonrooms. In addition, one
could draw on the occasional autobiographical remarks in the
preface to published works and, of course, on one's own accumulated experience distilled from memory and introspection.

It would, however, be premature to expect that we have now
found a major difference between the nature of discovery in the
physical and the social sciences. Such a conclusion might be
suggested by the impression that the serendipity pattern in the
physical world originates from a different sort of unanticipated
events: events that occur *independently* of the theorizing, inter-
pretating, defining, conceptualizing investigator (or, in the case
of pragmatic knowledge, administrator). Vitamin K exists, one
would think, even if it should remain undiscovered. The newly
discovered fact is a physical thing that cannot generate by its own
power a meaningful theoretical interpretation; it would seem to
be 'obstinate' only in so far as the investigator's preconceived
theory is obstinate and unyielding. On the face of it, the difference
appears to be supported by the curious phenomenon that, while
serendipity in the natural sciences has very often taken the form
of simultaneous discovery – two or more observers stumbling
upon the same anomalous fact independently of each other – such
cases are not easily identified in the non-experimental sciences.

Unavoidably I have to touch here briefly on certain recent
developments in the philosophy of science. One of the approaches
that has become prominent in recent years suggests the view, to
put it very briefly, that scientific investigation (in the natural
sciences) involves a continual interaction of theory with fact.
There are no 'facts' as such, independent of a pre-existing theoretical framework.[7] Hence the discovery of an 'anomalous' event is
possible only if and in so far as a new theory has been created
which defines it as anomalous. On this basis, therefore, the
position in the natural sciences appears to be not markedly different from that in our own fields of inquiry. I shall have to revise
this conclusion at a later stage, but first I want to add a few more
details.

The approach of Toulmin (and others) has obtained considerable support from the work of Thomas Kuhn[8] which is centred on empirical–historical observations on the development of modern science, rather than being directly concerned with the theory of knowledge. This may explain, incidentally, why Kuhn's contributions have made a considerable impact even outside the circle of professional philosophers. What he has done is to examine closely and systematically the concrete processes by which scientific discoveries have come about. His interest was aroused by coming across, accidentally, an obscure monograph by a German physician, Ludwig Fleck's 'Entstehung und Entwicklung einer wissenschaftlichen Tatsache', published 1935. He refers to it as 'an essay that anticipates many of my own ideas' (p. ix). Fleck's study is devoted to a careful and detailed examination of one outstanding case, the discovery of the famous Wassermann-test as a means of diagnosing syphilis. In the centre of his analysis is the concept of *kollektiver Denkstil* by virtue of which he demonstrates that a 'scientific fact' is unthinkable without presupposing a theoretical framework, and that, moreover, such theoretical orientations (in the natural sciences) are the product of collectively maintained schools or paradigms of thought. The 'discovery' of a new event, therefore, can only occur through a change in the collective style of interpretation dominant at a given time. The discovery of syphilis depended on the gradual historical emergence of a new style of thinking about the nature of venereal diseases. Discoveries are, as he puts it brilliantly, the product of *gerichtete Wahrnehmung*: directional perception. To the sociologist it may be of interest to add here that Fleck's fundamental concept of the collective thought-style is virtually identical with Karl Mannheim's collective 'thought-model' developed a few years earlier, which is remarkable because Fleck's essay shows no traces of any acquaintance with sociological sources. As far as our own problem is concerned, Kuhn's work goes much further than Fleck's pioneering effort. He accumulates powerful historical evidence that the changing collective 'paradigms' which organize the manner in which scientists define their problems and their relevant facts are systems which have a logic (as well as a vocabulary and a worldview) of their own. Different paradigms are thus incommensurate. To choose a telling example: Einstein's physics is in no way comparable with Newtonian physics; the basic vocabulary of such terms as 'mass', 'movement', 'space', 'time', etc. has altogether different meanings in the two systems. To quote from a characteristic passage: 'Paradigms gain their status because they are more successful than their competitors in solving a few problems that the group of practitioners has come to recognize as acute. To be more successful is not, however, to be either completely successful with a single problem or notably successful with any large number. The success of a paradigm – whether Aristotle's analysis of motion, Ptolemy's computations of planetary position, Lavoisier's application of the balance, or Maxwell's mathematization of the electromagnetic field – is at the start largely a promise of success discoverable in selected and still incomplete examples' (op. cit., p. 24). This idea of pragmatic 'success' is further elaborated as a form of 'correspondence' between facts and prediction: 'Normal science consists in the actualization of that promise, an actualization achieved by extending the knowledge of those facts that the paradigm displays as particularly revealing, by increasing the extent of the match between those facts and the paradigm's predictions, and by further articulation of the paradigm itself' (ibid. and passim). The relevant point is here the assurance that apparently the absence of pure, uninterpreted facts is not typical of the social sciences alone; it appears to be a general affliction of scientific inquiry.

II. THE ACTIVITY OF THEORIZING

I propose to examine the problem of 'theory-determined facts', in the context of scientific discovery, by questioning the conventionally alleged formal connection between 'theory', 'hypothesis', and 'observation'. Accordingly I shall look at the *unofficial* techniques of work that condition or cut across the rules of formal methodology. I shall argue that the elements of the social scientist's work should be analysed behaviouristically, that is to say, as a type of prolonged and variable activity and hence as a process through time. As may be expected, however, it is as yet very difficult to maintain this approach: there is no sharp demarcation line between the formal and the informal, the published and the preparatory, the perceived and the real process of scientific discovery.

It may be recalled that for a number of reasons we were driven to the conclusion that the popular notion of a profound difference between natural and social science is misleading. As far as the discovery of facts – especially the discovery of obstinate facts – is concerned, there does not seem to be a decisive difference. Apparently the facts are, in both areas, always theory-determined. To pursue the question beyond this point would easily lead away from the main objective of the present essay. It would force us to inquire into the logical foundations of theory-building. We would want to know, for example, whether the sort of theory which is typically used (or believed to be used) in the social sciences is essentially different from the theories of the experimental sciences. In turn this question could not be tackled without getting involved in the controversy between positivistic and anti-positivistic (phenomenological) schools of thought.[9]

The whole problem may look very different on taking into account the informal processes out of which systematic theory is produced. As pointed out in an earlier discussion paper, the informal aspect of theorizing refers to the inarticulated techniques, devices, and practices which are customarily employed during the preparatory stages in the production of formal theories.[10] Ideally this can only be investigated by inquiring into the behavioural basis of sociological theorists at work, chiefly by means of suitably designed interviews of theoretical writers. The technical difficulties of such a method are numerous, but I do not think insuperable. However this may be, in the present context I am mentioning this possibility in order to show that the size of the gap in our knowledge of theorizing is unexpectedly large. While there is an extensive and ever-growing specialization concerned with the formal logic of theory in social science, its informal–behavioural side has virtually remained untouched. We simply do not know how in fact formal–theoretical works are brought about. It is even hard to imagine what kind of interview questions one would have to try out. It is difficult to understand why – considering the vastness of the available theoretical literature – so little has been done to identify the techniques and the skills which are normally employed in the production of theoretical writings. Partly, no doubt, the explanation is that the theorists themselves have very rarely seen the need to provide their readers with clues as to how they operate.[11]

Another reason is the peculiar manner in which statements of systematic theory are customarily presented: it takes the form of a sequence of *suggestions* which are offered without ostentive justification in terms of theoretical axioms. As A. Rapoport has pointed out, from a formalistic point of view, the initial stage of theory-building is particularly revealing in so far as it seems to involve a high degree of arbitrary selection. 'The stuff from which human relations and social structure are made is not evident intuitively. It must somehow be distilled, or abstracted from innumerable "events", and the selection of these events depends to a great extent on one's experiences, cultural background, and biases'.[12] The question whether this is inevitable because of the unique logical properties inherent in the subject-matter of social science does not concern us here. From our point of view, the crucial work in the above quotation is the word '*somehow*'. The fact that the style of theoretical argumentation is cast in a distinctive mould may serve as a clue. If we take Parsons's *The Social System* as the most sophisticated type of modern sociological theory, it may be significant that all its fundamental concepts are stated without formal definitions. The reader is introduced to such concepts usually by suggesting some combination of several, more or less interchangeable expressions which in turn merely suggest certain commonly known but technically undefined associations. Let us look for example at the familiar pattern variable of 'affectivity versus affective neutrality'. Neither of these or the associated equivalent terms 'gratification' (versus 'discipline') and 'expressive' (versus 'evaluative') interests etc. are specified by explicit definition. It is obvious throughout the book that the omission is intentional. Another aspect comes into view when one tries to locate the origin of the conceptual components. There are practically no footnotes in *The Social System* containing references to particular sources. It is evident, however, that the principal source is the accumulated body of abstract concepts available from current usage in social science generally. The use of specific references would be cumbersome and indeed misplaced, because it is always only a broad, and frequently merely a temporary, association with current usage that is required. The important thing is to keep within the hard core of consistent meaning of a given vocabulary. And this is all that is possible. For none of the constituent terms of a theoretical framework could be traced back to a precise formal definition at its primary source: all of them are, as we have seen, 'constructed constructs' distilled from pragmatic knowledge.[13]

So far, then, the relatively most tangible characteristic of theorizing points to a process through time that can best be described as sustained '*articulation*': an initially vague and vacillating image of a complex framework is perpetually redefined so as to produce an increasingly definite and stable structure. The most penetrating description of conceptual articulation I have come across has been presented by Michael Polanyi. Though primarily directed towards a clarification of the role of conceptualization in the natural sciences, certain aspects of his analysis are relevant to our problem. Very briefly, his point of departure is the kind of progressively structured behaviour that is known from the dynamics of animal and child learning, commonly associated with the rudimentary trial-and-error type of problem-solving. He then proceeds from this kind of 'inarticulate learning' to the role of articulate language, the crucial basis of which devolves on the creation of 'interpretative frameworks'. Still further along this dimension Polanyi refers to the articulation process which governs certain logical operations on the level of scientific conceptualization. Omitting here the technical details of the subsequent steps of Polanyi's exposition, of special interest to the analysis of sociological theorizing is the following statement which is adapted from G. Polya's introspective account of mathematical problem-solving: 'This (casting about for a solution) we do by performing two operations which must always be tried jointly. We must (1) set out the problem in suitable symbols and continuously reorganize its representation with a view to eliciting some new suggestive aspects of it, and concurrently (2) ransack our memory for any similar problem of which the solution is known. The scope of these two operations will usually be limited by the student's technical facility for transforming the given data in different ways, and by the range of germane theorems with which he is acquainted.'[14] I am quoting this at length because of the obvious, if unexpected similarity between the highly formalized articulation in mathematical problem-solving and the apparently crude process of sociological conceptualization.

Applied to sociological theorizing, the essence of the first operation is reflected in the perpetual reorganization, the unceasing restructuring, of symbols; whereby the 'symbols' consist in this case of the core meaning of existing conceptual elements (such as 'affective', 'gratification', 'expressive', in the example mentioned earlier on). The second operation – searching one's memory for similar problems with a known solution – reappears in the sociologist's endeavour to utilize available conceptual frameworks that have proved to be clarifying in other contexts or have become established by usage. To strengthen the comparison, I would suggest that the phrase 'known solution' of a mathematical problem might be replaced, without serious distortion, by 'other mathematical operations that have proved to be effective'. The difference, however, between the articulation process of mathematical problem-solving and sociological theorizing should not be overlooked.

The decisive difference is founded upon the paramount importance of communication. Each step in the building-up of successively more sophisticated conceptual frameworks is severely limited by the prerequisite of uninterrupted communication within the community of social scientists as it exists at a given stage of development. Thus, as is well known, most of Parsons's writings move closely along the extreme limit of comprehensibility in terms of current sociological usage. This has often been attributed, erroneously, to lack of skill in his personal style of writing. But it should be clear from the foregoing that the difficulty of communication is largely inherent in the very process of progressive articulation. The available conceptual raw material can be precise only to the extent that the core meaning of the relevant symbols has already become institutionalized in the prevailing culture of the scientific community. The importance of communication to institutionalized scientific work in general has been clearly established by the study of Kuhn, mentioned earlier, and need not be elaborated here. Unsolved, however, is still the problem of the special conditions that derive from the lack of precision of sociocultural concepts. Evidently these conditions pertain to the nature of the symbols required to handle sociocultural phenomena.

III. CONCEPTUAL INNOVATIONS AND ECLECTIC
DISCOVERIES

In the foregoing discussion I have suggested certain apparent similarities as well as differences between intuitive mathematical problem-solving and informal sociological theorizing. It involves, by all appearances, an unceasing manipulation of both the content and the relation of particular symbols. What has to be explained next is the purpose of these operations. If this were to be done by studying the contemporary literature on the logic (or lack of logic) of social inquiry, we would be faced with a very difficult and some-what dreary undertaking. In what follows I shall attempt a short-cut that will take us directly into the medium of unofficial practices.

This shortcut is based on the assumption that the activity of theorizing is not confined to manifestly theoretical works. Some form of theorizing also takes place in the execution of *empirical* studies. The advantage of using empirical work as our source rests on the fact that in such a perspective the technique of theory-building seems to be somewhat out of place: it appears to be an unofficial activity and it is thus more conspicuous and more tangible than in the case of overtly theoretical operations.

An invaluable source here is the collection of autobiographical reports presented in P. E. Hammond's *Sociologists at Work*,[15] in which we find a modest beginning towards a potentially systematic, comparative study of the unofficial practices of research. The contributors (among them a few outstandingly successful researchers) were asked to portray their own research activity 'as it was experienced during some *specific* investigation' and to report the actual sequence of events and ideas in the mind of the investigator, so as to 'let the reader in on the *sub rosa* phases of contemporary research' (op. cit., Introduction, p. 3). At first sight the result of this endeavour seems curiously disappointing. The reader who expects useful information about the most effective techniques that generate research discoveries finds hardly anything worth recording. Throughout these pages there is a striking contrast between the obvious success of these authors in terms of previously published works and the highly insecure, frequently trivial, and unaccountably erratic descriptions of their unofficial methods. More specifically, the following two features deserve particular attention:

(a) the preoccupation with theory, and (b) the absence of discoveries.

(a) Although the chronicles are concerned with empirical works only, all the contributors are extensively engaged in theorizing or theoretical problems of one kind or another. This is remarkable because on the basis of published works, no effective interaction between theory and research seems to exist. Apparently, then, the theoretical activities take place during the preparatory (unpublished) stages only. They appear to be a private, more or less illegitimate, occupation. This curious attitude pervades the bulk of the chronicles and is indeed its most puzzling feature. To understand it we must first bear in mind that the author's conception of 'theory' does not easily fit into any of the established categories of conventional methodology. For example, this conception could not be described by any of the many types of social science theory that are presented in R. Brown's *Explanation in Social Science*.[16] The way in which the word 'theory' is used here informally and loosely suggests a sort of continuous speculation without a definitive purpose. It has neither a recognizable beginning nor an end. It certainly does not yield a theory, a specifiable end-product that can be used to design a set of hypotheses (which subsequently would be 'tested' by observation or experiment). More aptly, therefore, we should speak of 'theorizing', a word that is actually employed a great deal in these reports. The ongoing nature of the process is well expressed, for example, by Stanley H. Udy: 'During this phase of the work, I "theorized" . . . during the afternoon, read my data and checked it against the afternoon's result during the evening, slept on the outcome, and tried proposing hypotheses in the morning' (op. cit., p. 177). Another aspect, equally frequent, is the notion that informal theorizing is a highly personal experience. It comes about by organizing one's general ideas around a 'central theme', by steering the investigation into a certain direction. The process appears to be propelled by the desire to obtain in the end such observations as may confirm the investigator's preconceived ideas. Thus we find an unceasing search for an 'integrating principle' (Blanche Geer), 'a new theoretical amalgam' (David Riesman and Jeanne Watson), 'a basic conceptual framework' (Robert N. Bellah), 'an organization or synthesis which provides the essential structure into which the pieces of analysis fit' (James S. Coleman), 'a crucial insight' (Peter M. Blau), 'a major idea' (James A. Davis), 'a relevant typology' (Stanley H. Udy), and so forth.

Several of the writers describe this technique of 'theorizing' alternatively as 'hypothesizing'. It is, however, quite clear from the context that the word is used either to ridicule or at least to throw doubt on the conventional concept of a rigorous hypothesis that is testable. For example: 'The research was not preceded by consciously elaborated hypotheses but grew vaguely out of my confusion and irritations. . . . This was a kind of implicit hypothesizing that gave more freedom of thought and more rapid movement from hunch to hunch than initial preoccupation with formal hypothesizing about limited facts would have allowed' (Dalton, p. 63; similarly Blau, p. 19 f; Riesman and Watson, p. 305, Coleman, p. 202; Bellah, p. 159); 'Since I had reached my "hypotheses" by a combination of verbal reasoning and ex post facto induction (sic!), the appropriate method in most cases appeared to me to be to array frequencies in fourfold tables, with controls as appropriate. This I did, proceeding from one hypothesis to another through a verbal chain of reasoning' (Udy, p. 181). – All this of course makes nonsense of hypothesis construction in the accepted sense. Yet this remarkable idea of informal theorizing or hypothesizing is expressed and elaborated by the various authors with such consistency that it requires some explanation. Why, for example, does it remain an unofficial, normally unreported activity?

(b) Once again it needs to be emphasized that none of the eleven contributors could be called a theoretician. The intensive preoccupation with theory takes place in the midst of empirical (including statistical) works: it appears to be an integral element throughout the process of collecting data. On that basis, however, the method of informal theorizing appears to be even more perplexing. It flatly contradicts the whole idea of scientific testing. Indeed, what really goes on here amounts to a process of falsification. The investigator pursues a selected 'central theme', a pet theory that he wants to drive home; he looks around for observable facts that fit his theme; then, and only then, does he fabricate a hypothesis that fits the facts. This reversal of scientific procedure goes so much against the grain that several of the authors acutely feel the need to offer some form of apology or justification for it. It is found in what may be called the 'abundance' dilemma. 'There are so many questions which might be asked, so many correlations which can be run, so many ways in which the findings can be organized, and so few rules or precedents for making these choices that a thousand different studies could come out of the same data' (Davis, p. 232); 'How did I know that this classification would be better than some other scheme, that is, that I could predict more about organization structure by using it than some alternative taxonomy? I did not. One never does, for in principle there exists an infinite number of ways of classifying anything' (Udy, p. 176; similarly Bellah, p. 159; Dalton, p. 54; Riesman and Watson, p. 307 and passim).

It is obvious, however, that the abundance dilemma, though it explains why *some* choice has to be made, cannot justify the selection of data to fit a particular preconceived theme. Moreover, it contradicts the canons of scientific objectivity in yet another point. Observations which are selected deliberately so as to make sense in the light of pre-existing knowledge are the precise opposite of empirical discoveries – of 'unanticipated, anomalous and strategic data', in Robert Merton's terms. And, indeed, as soon as one looks at the chronicles from this angle, one is struck by the total absence of genuine discoveries. As my interest in this book was initially aroused by the editor's announcement that it deals with the 'context of discovery' (Introduction, p. 3), I went through it page by page to look for them. I found none.

So once again the substance of 'discovery' seems to evaporate on closer inquiry. Perhaps these investigators just happened to be unlucky? In following up this – admittedly somewhat unrealistic – possibility, I came to notice one element supporting it. Throughout the chronicles one finds an attitude that manifests an *expectation* of discovery: everybody is searching, casting around, exploring. In fact the word 'exploratory' stage is among the most frequently used terms to describe the informal processes. Now, supposing we take this expression literally, we would arrive at a concept of 'discovery' that is distinctively different from our previous notion. For we could say then that the kind of discoveries that the researchers are after are in the nature of 'territorial' discoveries: the exploration of uncharted areas of sociocultural entities which are relatively unknown or unfamiliar. The resultant findings would be anomalous and unanticipated, but, and this is important, they would not be strategic. The word 'discovery' is therefore ambiguous in this context. At the most we could speak here only of 'sociographic discoveries'.

The relevance of this interpretation of the chronicles obtains further support if they are seen in their connection with the official monographs or projects to which they refer. The subject-matter of these is always the descriptive exploration of a special field, a new territory, an unusual situation: Blau's study of the behaviour of officials in a particular kind of bureaucratic agency, Dalton's equally specific description of the motives, aspirations, informal activities, 'out-of-role' adaptations of a selected group of supervisors and foremen, Lipset's inquiry into the 'deviant case' of the ITU, Wright's and Hyman's investigation into the effectiveness of training methods used by institutes of the Encampment for Citizenship, Bellah's research on the Tokugawa religion, and so on.

The predominance of sociographic specialization explains a great deal. Not only does it account for the undaunted spirit of discovery of the explorers, it also explains the obsessive preoccupation with theorizing, conceptualizing, 'hypothesizing', etc. Obviously, any kind of highly situational descriptive exploration is bound to produce numerous findings that are 'new' – in the sense of observations which have not been made before in exactly the same manner. But, of course, if these can be called 'discoveries' at all, they are merely in the nature of trivial, eclectic, or peripheral data. They are in direct contrast to those which would be of central importance to the fundamental properties of society at large. Hence it becomes all the more important to theorize. In other words, it is necessary constantly to reinterpret the accumulating new findings until they finally appear in some sense to be strategically relevant to general, centrally important problems.

We have now reached a position which takes us back to the broader aspects of the serendipity problem. I think it is a safe assumption that Hammond's chronicles are fairly typical in so far as the bulk of contemporary social research produces merely eclectic sociographic discoveries. This means our data are pecu-

liarly deficient on account of their triviality and speciality. Hence
the need to theorize is a universal prerequisite. Earlier on I
described, provisionally, the activity of theorizing as a trial-and-
error process by which conceptual frameworks become progressively more articulate. Although we do not know exactly how this
is done, it is evident that the process involves a large element of
inventiveness and creativity. The perpetual restructuring of
concepts around their core meanings is essentially a matter of
theoretical innovations. To see the importance of this we have only
to recall a few sociological concepts that became characteristically
incisive through the work of individual thinkers, e.g. alienation,
anomie, conspicuous consumption, bureaucracy, oligarchy, ideology, latent function, social system, pattern variables, reference
group, other-directness, power elite.

These innovations manifest a sharp contrast to the observational
data. Whereas the empirical findings are insignificant details of
sociographic description, the conceptual frameworks are implicitly
aimed at centrally important phenomena: values, ideologies, social
change. Furthermore, while the data are derived from verifiabled
observations, the concepts are the product of the sociologist's mind.
In the last analysis, it is the inevitable triviality of social observations, the absence of genuine discoveries, which is responsible for
the precarious situation of social science. There are many sociologists who, quite naturally, would not like to admit this openly.
They pursue their laborious efforts in the hope that by some lucky
hit they may yet stumble upon one statistical correlation that
transcends the narrow triviality of sociographic data. Frequently
this hope is fostered by the example of strategic statistical discoveries in economics, such as Juglar's, Pareto's, or Bowley's. Now
and then a fresh effort is made to prove that Durkheim's analysis
of suicide rates *did* produce a discovery of general theoretical
significance. It did nothing of the sort. The very essence of social
observations, statistical or interpretative, precludes the possibility
of yielding a 'general law'.

IV. DOUBLE FITTING

While many of the unofficial activities remain obscure, we have
come some way towards recognizing their wider implications. I

think we can be reasonably sure that informal theorizing is a large and indispensable element of all empirical research. Furthermore, my earlier assumption, that the researcher's theoretical activities are essentially akin to the theoretician's endeavours seems fairly plausible in view of the importance of conceptual innovations. What is still puzzling is the curious repetitiveness of the process: its outstanding feature is the interminable *re*structuring, *re*defining, *re*interpreting, *re*formulating of conceptual frameworks. Linked with this is the extraordinary wastefulness of the process. Apparently a very large amount of the results of informal theorizing is unusable and therefore unsuitable to be included in the final published work. It remains hidden away in notebooks, research files, and preliminary drafts. It is this element of apparent wastefulness that more than anything else conflicts with the official notion of systematic scientific work presented in most methodological texts.

In attempting to reduce this contradiction I propose to supplement our first approximation to the trial-and-error process of 'articulation' (see p. 291) as follows. Informal theorizing (henceforth simply called 'theorizing' as opposed to formal theory-construction) involves a continuous restructuring of conceptual frameworks whereby a specific technique of reciprocal or *double fitting* is employed. This may be envisaged by imagining a carpenter alternately altering the shape of a door *and* the shape of the door-frame to obtain a better fit, or a locksmith adjusting successively *both* the keyhole and the key. In one sense such a technique looks like deliberate falsification: the investigator simultaneously manipulates the thing he wants to explain as well as his explanatory framework. In a strictly scientific context it would mean 'cooking the facts'.

As theorizing in the shape of double fitting is evidently not defensible in terms of official procedures, its rationale is difficult to identify. It should be noted, in the first place, that the direction of the process is indeterminate. On the face of it there is merely an interminable sequence of alternating changes of a framework and its content. If so, what would be the purpose? To simplify the matter, we may argue that the final adjustment is done either to the framework or to the content (the keyhole or the key). In the practice of scientific work this would mean that an investigator's chief interest is centred either on problems of conceptualization or on empirical observations. Thus, although double fitting takes place all the time, the process as a whole may be conceived in two ways: it can be either dominantly theoretical or dominantly empirical.

Theorizing then reveals that kind of double fitting which is *dominantly* oriented towards inventing and articulating conceptual frameworks. Here the process starts, arbitrarily, with some cluster of observations and it ends with a framework. At the beginning there is only a vague notion of some observed but unfamiliar or puzzling phenomenon (whereby it is of no importance at present whether the data have been arrived at by pragmatic knowledge or quantitative methods). This first notion virtually amounts to a crude interpretative innovation. It is gradually articulated by trying to 'fit' it into a succession of combined criteria (which may be simple, dichotomous, or multidimensional). The bulk of such criteria is usually chosen from the reservoir of generally known and accepted concepts. But while one knows what they mean if taken separately, their combination may nevertheless produce new meanings that might eventually illuminate the original unfamiliar phenomenon from which the process set out.

The importance of theorizing (by means of double fitting) in empirical work is a consequence of the triviality of eclectic sociographic discoveries. The unique process which we have identified as theorizing corresponds to what the autobiographical chronicles variously and uncertainly describe as the search for the central theme, the synthesis, the integrating principle, and so on. But theorizing is not the only method of organizing an investigation. We have seen already that the articulation process of double fitting may be directed dominantly towards empirical instead of theoretical tasks. We must now look at this other possibility. I shall call it 'hypothesizing'.

As before, the substance of this technique is again an interminable sequence of alternately modifying frameworks and their contents. But this time the investigator's interest is dominantly 'empirical'. The arbitrary point of departure is now an interpretative framework, a more or less articulate theoretical statement or simply a vague generalization that is barely more than a hunch. The focus of interest, however, is located in empirical observations. The theoretical framework is merely a means to an end, namely to discover the existence of some regularity, some recurrent features among certain data, or some invariant relationship between factual observations. As a rule the expected findings are in the nature of causal relations, notably so in the context of sociographic discoveries. Like all causal relationships, even trivial (non-strategic) data may suitably be treated in the light of a 'hypothesis'. But there is no need for it to be explicitly formulated. As usually employed in the practice of research, the term 'simply' means that some causal connection between certain classes of events may possibly be found to exist. The best illustration for this notion is the trial run on an IBM. Similarly, instead of actually carrying out a series of trial runs, it is often expedient simply to reflect upon the most promising possibilities. Or one may search the literature of past research for comparable cases that suggest a lead. All these informal activities may be conveniently classified as 'hypothesizing'. They have in common with theorizing the informal, improvising disposition of a trial-and-error process.

The suggestion that theorizing and hypothesizing are but two versions of one and the same process provides a partial answer to the question: what is the rationale of double fitting? It is a sort of psychological answer, not a description of the logical structure of the process. The answer points to the kind of satisfactions or the goals that are attached to sociological work. One type of satisfaction is grounded in the need for theorizing, for projecting some order into the multitude of eclectic data by relating them to major problems, basic political issues, central values, etc. To be fulfilled, this need requires value-commitments. The other type, concerned with hypothesizing, stems from the striving for detachment, verification, scientific certainty. It relies on the assertive power of obstinate facts. Since both needs are deeply institutionalized in contemporary society, it is not surprising that the two corresponding activities are occurring side by side in any given piece of work. As regards individual scholars, the relative strength of the two motives will vary. Some are more theoretically minded, others more interested in empirical observations. The important thing is that either of the two specializations has to use both operations.

But the motivational aspect cannot fully explain the unique nature of double fitting. I shall add therefore one further characteristic. It is evident from the chronicles and similar sources that the interlocking of theorizing and hypothesizing is spread over the whole exploratory process. The interaction is continuous. Somehow it does not seem possible to specialize on the one or the other operation for any length of time. Apparently, in a concrete study one cannot engage solely in theorizing for, say, one month, then change over to pure hypothesizing for the next month, return to another month of theorizing, and so on. In practice the two modes of double fitting are nearly simultaneous. This is clearly emphasized in the reports by the recurring phrase of 'constantly moving back and forth'. We must assume therefore that double fitting, no matter in which form it manifests itself, contains a directional element. It is not an activity that goes on in a random fashion for ever. Rather, I believe, it is gradually *progressing* in a uniform direction; there is some sort of progress, some advancement, some kind of product, that is gradually emerging from the innumerable trial-and-error actions. To get hold of this element, the process might properly be called *'progressive'* double fitting. To look at it from another angle, we should recall here the conspicuous wastefulness of these techniques. If there is so much wasted effort, there must also be certain positive residuals, however small their amount.

As regards that part of double fitting which I called 'theorizing', the potential positive net effect is fairly obvious. It consists of a gradually rising level of abstraction. Starting from a relatively narrow cluster of observations, there is a trend which moves towards more and more comprehensive conceptual frameworks. The net effect of hypothesizing is more illusive. It is particularly difficult to identify it if one looks at any one brief period. But if we take sufficiently long periods, comparing the position at the beginning and the end, it appears that progress comes about by way of relatively increasing *complexity*: keeping the level of abstraction constant, the number of variables or phenomena that have been found to be causally (or otherwise) related to each other is larger at the end of the period than at the beginning. To be more precise about this, we would need a systematic inquiry into the actual development of concrete sociological studies during their preparatory stages. The question of how to measure the net effect of increasing complexity will certainly depend a great deal on the type of investigation. Moreover, any further elaboration of this matter would lead away from the behaviouristic approach into the problems of formal logic (set theory, etc.).

What is more important in the present stage is to realize that theorizing and hypothesizing are always interdependent. Hence the overall 'progress' of the total process must involve simultaneously a relative rise in the level of abstraction as well as a relative increase in the degree of complexity. Taken together, the two effects bring about a gradual improvement in the stability of the total process. That is to say, both the emerging conceptual frameworks and the clusters of eclectic discoveries will appear in the end less arbitrary, less fluctuating, more established, and more structured than they did initially. Obviously this kind of increasing stability can only be relative. *Some* amount of subjectivity will always adhere to the theoretical frameworks, and *some* degree of arbitrariness regarding the selection of data will still be present in the finally published product. It should be noted that I am describing here only an idealized picture of the process. In a concrete case, there will be many ups and downs before a measure of stabilization is reached that warrants the publication of the results. And of course it is possible that it is never reached at all (e.g. the case of the project-failure reported by Riesman and Watt in Hammond's chronicles). I have also neglected the further complication that even a small-scale study will always be following several lines so that at any given moment there will be floating around side by side several unrelated frameworks and accordingly several unconnected clusters of data. But in principle we can treat each line of actual or potential inquiry as a single current of double fittings.

The particular advantage of this analysis appears to me in the possibility of treating theorizing and hypothesizing by a single analytical device. Since both represent a recurrent activity of double fitting, it is possible to see them as operations that are capable of interaction. At the same time it will thus be realized that this sort of interaction can only materialize as an ongoing process through time, a process that is at any given moment precarious and highly unstable, and does not produce a specifiable end-product. It can certainly not be seen by looking at the finalized published version of a given study. It must be remembered the problem is not *whether* there exists such interaction between theory and research. That it does exist in the practice of sociological work has hardly ever been doubted. The real question is: how can

it be possible, considering that theory is concerned with interpretative innovations and empirical research with causal discoveries? The general process of progressive double fitting is also
relevant to a number of other points that are well known but rarely
seen in their bearing on the uniqueness of social inquiry. I would
mention the notorious difficulty of the arbitrary starting-point of
any piece of work (do we start with 'concepts' or 'facts'?). Then
there is the familiar dilemma of value-determined theory, the
vagueness of concepts, and the related fact of the lack of genuine
replication. Equally characteristic is the insoluble question of when
to 'terminate' a given theoretical or empirical study. Questions of
this sort will seem to be of minor importance when we consider
that the technique of progressive double fitting is an activity *sui
generis*, and that there is no other way of doing sociological work.

V. CONCLUSION

To round off this inquiry into unofficial techniques I shall try to
connect it with a few aspects of formal methodology that seem to
me of general interest. The topic of 'discoveries' was chosen as
my main theme because the term reflects an attitude that is very
common among social scientists. It acts as a symbol of scientific
objectivity and it derives from the belief that, apart from certain
difficulties connected chiefly with the problem of values, social
science could be just as rigorous as physical science. This attitude
is often reinforced by the assumption that such imperfections are
merely temporal, they are characteristic only of the 'present stage'
of social science. As a consequence of this dependence on the
experimental sciences, it seems to be overlooked that meanwhile
an increasing amount of evidence is accumulating that suggests
that the procedures actually used in the praxis of social research
and theory may well turn out to be of a unique, unprecedented
type. This important development started only some fifteen years
ago. An incisive impulse in that direction came from the work of
Merton, in his insistence on the need for investigating the social
research behaviouristically.[17] But at that time the ideal of the logic
of the physical sciences was still so deeply ingrained in our minds,
as for example the preoccupation with 'discoveries' demonstrates,
that it blocked the view to the *sui generis* features of our methods.

Somewhat similar, in the same period, was the situation in which Lazarsfeld and his pupils started to analyse and codify the most important formal techniques of specifically sociological research. It was then already noticed that explicit hypothesis-testing was not the only legitimate method: the most typical techniques were recognized as revealing a distinctively different pattern, tentatively called 'elaboration'.[18]

I realize that my argument implies that theorizing and hypothesizing are epistemologically incommensurable. I have no answer to that. But in realizing that the two operations have at least one basic element in common, the trial-and-error process of recurrent double fitting, we may be one step further in understanding the interdependence of theory and research. What we know about it so far suggests a type of interdependence that is unique to social science and therefore wholly out of reach to any positivistic theory of knowledge derived from the physical sciences.

NOTES AND REFERENCES

1 This is an abbreviated version of an essay first published as an informal discussion paper in 1965. Apart from the correction of minor inaccuracies in the presentation, my position has remained unchanged. Indeed, I have come to believe that the technique of 'progressive double-fitting' is even more typical of sociological work than I thought at the time. This can now be seen by recognizing the basic similarity between such apparently incommensurable works as MORRIS ROSENBERG'S *The Logic of Survey Analysis*, 1968 and FLORIAN ZNANIECKI'S *Social Actions*, New York, Farrar & Rinehart, 1936.

2 The main topic emerged from methodological discussions with colleagues and students; I am especially indebted to Vic Allen, William M. Evan, Peter Gleichmann, Julian Nagel, Peter Rickman, and Michael M. Walker. I also wish to thank Dietrich Goldschmidt, Wolfgang Lempert, and Burkhard Lutz for giving me the opportunity to act as a participant observer in a large-scale survey project at present being carried out in Germany.

3 ROBERT K. MERTON, *Social Theory and Social Structure*, 2nd ed., Glencoe, Free Press, 1957, p. 104. In taking this work as a point of departure, it should be noted that my criticism involves only minor points. As a matter of fact, it is Merton's concept of latent function that forms the basis of my analysis.

4 WALTER B. CANNON, *The Way of an Investigator*, New York, 1945, pp. 68 ff.

5 ROBERT K. MERTON, 'Resistance to the Study of Multiple Discoveries', *Archives européennes de sociologie*, **4**, 1963, pp. 237–82.
6 op. cit., p. 243.
7 STEPHEN TOULMIN, *Foresight and Understanding*, Indiana University Press, 1961, p. 95.
8 THOMAS S. KUHN, *The Structure of Scientific Revolutions*, Chicago and London, University of Chicago Press, 1962.
9 WALTER BUCKLEY, 'Structural-Functional Analysis in Modern Sociology', in H. Becker and A. Boskoff (eds.), *Modern Sociological Theory*, New York, Dryden, 1957.
10 The Category of Pragmatic Knowledge in Sociological Analysis, *Archives for Philosophy of Law and Social Philosophy*, **53**, 1967, pp. 31–51.
11 Cp. TALCOTT PARSONS, "The Point of View of the Author', in Max Black (ed.), *The Social Theories of Talcott Parsons*. Englewood Cliffs, Prentice-Hall, 1961, pp. 268–88.
12 A. RAPOPORT, 'Uses and Limitations of Mathematical Models in Social Science', in L. GROSS, *Symposium on Sociological Theory*, Evanston, Ill., Row Peterson, 1959, p. 351.
13 The Category of Pragmatic Knowledge, op. cit., pp. 10–14.
14 MICHAEL POLANYI, *Personal Knowledge*, London, Routledge, 1958, p. 128.
15 PHILLIP E. HAMMOND (ed.), *Sociologists at Work*, New York, Basic Books, 1964.
16 op. cit., pp. 165–93.
17 Merton, op. cit., pp. 19, 100–17.
18 PAUL F. LAZARSFELD and MORRIS ROSENBERG, *The Language of Social Research*, Glencoe, Ill., Free Press, 1955, pp. 121–5; the latest contribution from this school, M. ROSENBERG'S *Logic of Survey Analysis*, N.Y., Basic Books, 1968, reveals even more the specifically 'analytical' processes of hypothesizing (including double-fitting) throughout the methodology of survey research.

Praxis:
the controversial
culture–society paradigm

ZYGMUNT BAUMAN

Theorizing means ordering, structuring; as such it is an iso-morphic correlate of material practice, its *'alter ego'* in the Janus-faced human existence. Exactly like the productive activity, theorizing consists in modelling reality. Theories *are* models. Any segment of universe we isolate in order to formulate its regularities presents itself to us as a cybernetic black box: a pro-cessual going concern with only two points – inputs and outputs – open to the investigator's inspection. If we are experimenting, we can manipulate the input values; if we only observe a 'natural' phenomenon, we have to confine ourselves to registering only their oscillations. In both cases we record additionally the changing values of output. We conclude the empirical stage of investigation with two sets of recordings in hand. If we decide to proceed to the theoretical stage, the only way open to us is to try to devise a mechanism which behaves in the way the 'real' phenomenon does, e.g. responds by the same output values to related input. With this performational requisite the affinity between our model and the 'real' phenomenon begins and ends at the same time. We do not and would not know what 'really' happens between input and output of the black box we put to test. It does not matter to us, anyhow, as the only task we are interested in is to discover – or, rather, to articulate – the repetitive and predictable regularity of the investigated object's behaviour. The aim is to arrive at an equation of $O = f/I$/type, in which output values can be depicted as correlates of input. The trouble is that this hardly ever can be achieved in such a simplified form, as the relation between isolated input factors and behavioural outcomes is seldom

303

reducible to a neat one-to-one correspondence. That is why our model takes usually a more intricate shape of a $O = f/I, v_i/$ equation, in which v_i stands for one or more 'intervening variables' which we introduce and define to account for variability of input–output relations. The procedure is most transparent in behaviour-ist psychology and its numerous offshoots, learning theory in-cluded. A very elaborate example of how intervening variables with little if any empirical references can serve to relate empirical observations into a theory can be found in C. L. Hull's 'law of primary reinforcement'.[1] Reflecting on the scholarly conduct of modern psychologists, Melvin H. Marx drew the obvious con-clusions from what has been in most cases an unreflexive activity: 'Any behaviour obviously must be mediated by some sort of psychological function; to ignore the fact is quite legitimate, but it does not deny that *some* process or mechanism *exists* for the intervening variable. The important point is that none is *specified*; the present preference for handling the problem is to think of the intervening variables in terms of "whatever process is needed to mediate the S–R relations".'[2]

The procedure consciously or, more often than not, uncon-sciously applied by students of social relations makes no exception to the general rule. The difference between a psychologist's and a socio- or culturo-logist's cognitive activity is not located in its inherent logic. It is reducible entirely to the initial decision as to what kind of empirically ascertainable data are to be defined as the input and output values of the black box the respective scholar deals with. Both study human behaviour, but each allocates differently the set of relationships he intends to model. Let *Figure 1* represent a section of the human interaction string; let *s* stand for an initial stimulus acting upon individual A, to which R represents

Figure 1

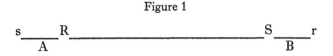

A's response; let S stand for a stimulus leading to an individual B's response, r; then the psychologists' black box appears on our figure twice, on both its extremes—s,S stand for its input and

R, r for its output. But the social scientist's black box covers the mysterious section stretching from R to S: for what all sociology and all 'culturology' are about *is how the response of an A turns into the stimulus for a B*. What we do observe empirically is that the actual or potential behaviour of some As eliminates the possibility of certain conduct for some Bs and increases the probability of their behaving in some other ways (that is what we call by the shorthand term of 'relationship'). All the rest is a matter of theory, e.g. modelling or introducing some intervening variables whose only checking limits are provided by the need to relate intellectually what Bs and As do in the same way as they correspond to each other in empirical records.

Now, both sociologist and 'culturologist' share the same sets of input/output data as empirical foundations for their theoretical models – the circumstance which seems to be responsible for many a misunderstanding as well as for most of the unnecessary feudal warfare between two disciplines. The first names his model a 'social structure', while stressing in most cases the limits enforced on Bs by As' actual performance and potentiality of manœuvre. The second is interested primarily in how Bs come to know what their limits are and names the results of his modelling endeavours a 'cultural system'. The fact that concepts like 'power', 'norm', 'value', 'role' are employed interchangeably as intervening variables in both types of model is indicative of the general confusion, which is exactly what one could expect from the notorious unwillingness of both disciplines to reflect on the nature of the creative, and not just the recording side of their activity.

We leave aside the moot problem of how the sociologists' and the culturologists' models are and how they pretend to be related. What we try to find in the first place is the general nature of the model the two owners of the R–S black box (and other scientists as well) strive to arrive at. What distinguishes these models at first sight is their ordered, system-like character; to denote this crucial feature, we say that models are 'structured' or possess structure. Now, the structure we think of and describe is always an attribute of the model itself and not of the reality modelled. 'The term "social structure" has nothing to do with empirical reality but with models which are built up after it',[3] says Claude Lévi-Strauss, and the statement is logically invulnerable whatever one may think of this thinker's philosophical bent. It is true that empirical evidence foists on the theoretician's imagination limitations no conscientious scholar can dispose of. But inside empirical limits any theoretician will find plenty of loose rope to choose freely between alternative models accounting for impenetrable causal links between the two sets of recorded data. Reflecting on the famed formulation of Roland Barthes[4] ('structure is an *image* of the object, but a controlled image, subordinated to some interest – as the imitated object reveals something heretofore invisible or unsensible in the object in its natural form'; the new element added by the structuring imagination being the object's intelligibility: 'the image is reason attached to an object'), Leszek Kolakowski pointed out that no structure construction can ever achieve its final form, because 'since the structure consists in reconstructing, from the fragments supplied by the "nature" . . . of a meaningful object . . . not only the meaning-bestowing ordering activity, but the choice of fragment as well are not determined by empirical data'.[5]

It is order we pursue when engaging in theorizing, modelling activity. It is order that constitutes the state of the reality meaningful to us – contrary to chaos, in which nothing is impossible and everything can happen. The 'structure' is intelligible to us precisely because, as Jean Piaget defines it, 'the elements are being united in a whole which by itself is characterized by certain properties and the properties of the elements depend, totally or in part, on the characteristics of the whole'.[6] We replace the chaotic flow of sensory perceptions by an ordered hierarchy of connected and mutually determined links. To achieve this, we seek to cleanse the data of our experience of everything accidental and fortuitous; as a matter of fact we cleanse it of its qualitative peculiarity, selecting the stable essence of the pure form; 'To understand the exchanges which rule birth, marriage, initiation, or death we have to pluck them of their qualitative features, reduce them to their nature as operations.'[7]

This casual remark by C. Lefort contains an understanding of structure as modern as it is – unfortunately – unusual in most of the standard sociological treatises. It should be clear by now – from the very way in which the notion of structure was introduced – that this term relates not to a particular spatial ordering of beings, as is frequently assumed in equating 'social structure' with an ordered field of social identities,[8] contrary to the understanding in Ralph Linton's definition of status as polar positions in a 'pattern of reciprocal behaviour',[9] but to a set of rules which define the limits and degrees of freedom of the elements of the 'structured' aggregate. According to Danesh and Hausenblas,[10] to exhaust the notion of structured system we should take into account both means of action admitted by the system and the rules which determine how these means should be used. In other words, we cannot conclude for sure from the structural model what the conduct of elements in some particular circumstances will be. The only thing we want to know when constructing the model is what are the options open to acting elements – what is their 'acting power' as determined by the structure itself. Instead of clinging to deterministic habits we shall do better if we allow ourselves to be inspired by the cyberneticians' approach to the concept of structure as a system of limitations.[11]

SEARCH FOR ORDER

One can hardly imagine anything as cruel and stupid as a nature that provided its creatures with logic alone; no living organisms need to decipher all the secrets of the world they live in – not even those vital to their survival; the basic qualities of their world – and basic means unchangeable in time-spans commensurable with the duration of their life – are built into their own structure; from the painful process of evolution, surviving species emerge with salutary disregard for countless highly improbable states of the world; as a matter of fact, they manage somehow to make the best out of their world only because they have been made to its measure. . . .

That is a modern version of Kant's time-honoured conjecture, that the basic structure of perceiving the world is given to cognitive mind *a priori*. It was brought to the attention of the participants of the University of Illinois Symposium on Self-Organization in June 1961 by George W. Zopf Jr.[12] Other members of this unusually insightful congregation were equally outspoken and revealing in disposing of the relics of the Lockean 'empty cabinet' fallacy and doing away with the behaviourists' fad of the limitless blessing of unlimited learning. W. Ross Ashby has pointed out incisively that the capacity for learning and above all its functional prerequisite – the art of memorizing – endowed with critical adaptive value in an organized world (i.e. in a world in which some events are much more probable than others, so that the eventual outcomes of present interaction can be grasped on the basis of a less-than-limitless amount of information) can easily turn into a suicidal device if something goes wrong with the expected orderliness of the universe. A rat, relying on its memory in learning that fat served regularly in a particular part of the sewage system is harmless, falls the easiest victim of the man who masters the skill of injecting irregularity into an otherwise repetitive fragment of the universe. To cut a long story short – a living organism coming of age (phylo- and onto-genetically) in an ordered world acquired a vested interest in maintaining the regularity and orderliness of its environment. The greater the role played by learning in shaping its behavioural repertoire – the more significant the need for order. Learning presumes ordering; the more learning, the greater the role of organizing activity.

Were the lower animals able to think and inclined to speculate on the condition of living creatures, they would probably decide that the world they lived in (i.e. the aspects that matter to them) is far more comfortable and cosy than that of humans. Just like all other living beings, they owe their survival to attaching proper responses to proper signals. But the very meagre number of their very generalized behavioural patterns corresponds to the only few signs they have to distinguish. The begging response of a young herring gull is elicited by a red spot on the mother's beak – a beak without a colour-spot elicits no response at all; a stickleback assumes a fighting attitude towards any object of any shape that has a red 'belly'; a dummy dragged over a pond with its shorter 'neck' first makes young ducks and geese escape in panic; the same dummy dragged the other way – i.e. with its long 'neck' first – is viewed with complete equanimity.[13] Well, there are no mother herring gulls without colour-spots on their beaks; no red-belly-less body can turn into a competitor for the nest-building site of a stickleback; and no long-necked bird predators threaten the well-being of duck youngsters. The world all these animals live in consists of very few bricks indeed – but in its contracted realm it is a clear, secure, transparent world, built up according

to the yes-or-no principle, leaving no room for ambiguity, oper-
able with a handful of bipositional switches. Where only the most
extemporal, the least changeable aspects of reality play the role
of response-releasing signs – instinctual equipment is enough to
administer the entire life-cycle of the animal. An individual does
not order his world; he inherits the world ordered. Is this why
we find it so difficult to refer to those lower vertebrates as
'individuals'?

It is not by chance that the increase in amount of significant
oppositions a species was able to distinguish (i.e. to differentiate
its responses accordingly) went side by side with the parallel
increase in the ratio of learned patterns to inherited stereotypes.
Fine hair-splitting distinctions just cannot depend on inert immutable attributes of the universe in the way the cruder and more
sketchy discriminations did. More and more potentially percept-
ible features of reality acquire semiotic significance – and more
and more flexible the individual's behaviour becomes while
responding to the now perceived and significant variability of the
outer world. This flexibility is achievable only by learning, and
learning means the organism entering into a reciprocal relationship
with its environment, in which both sides are active, both shape
each other, both augment the regularity and repeatability of the
other side. A misleading, deceitful world playing erratically with
the meanings of the signs, would make futile the learning effort
of the organism. Even worse – it would turn it into a lethal
suicidal weapon.

The world conforming to the pattern presupposed by the learning capacity is an ordered world: a world, the probable future
shape of which one can grasp by treating its present state as a
system of signs – i.e. visible events, unimportant in themselves,
but referring to some still invisible events of real importance to
the organism that makes the reading. Prompt perception of a
wolf's smell is important to a hare not because of the rapture of
olfactory sensations. And not for aesthetic joys does the motorist
switch on his headlights at nightfall.

Now, to possess and to convey any meaning at all, signs need
company. 'A single-term object has no meaning. . . . We perceive
differences and thanks to this perception the world "acquires
shape before us and for us".'[14] It is not the sign itself that has

meaning but its presence or absence, its appearance or its substitution by another object. The 'contrastive function' is one of the
two only properties any potential sign must have to convey any
meaning at all (the other being the combinatorial faculty).[15] The
expressive (*signifiant*, according to Saussure)[16] plane of any sign
system consists of distinct, discrete, contrasting units. And so
we come to the most important point of all: according to John
Lyons's formulation of one of the focal statements of structural
linguistics, 'there must be some "safety margin" between the
range of sounds which realizes one [unit of meaning] and the
range of sounds which realizes another'.[17] It is not enough for
signs to be distinct from each other. They must be separated,
drawn far apart to the opposite poles of the perceptual spectrum.
Otherwise it would be difficult to decipher their genuine and
exact meaning, the content of the message might be lost, there
would be too much 'noise' in the communication channels. If the
orderliness of the world is secured and communicated by un-
ambiguity of the semiotic code – then haziness of signs is tanta-
mount to opacity of the world's order. It can perhaps be ascertained just how much blurring of semiotic frontiers, or overlapping
of semiotically distinct units, is necessary to turn the learning
capacity of a living being from a miracle weapon into a curse.
The darkness phobia is one of the few fears innate in infants;
everything is possible in darkness, because no contour is sharp
enough to distinguish one thing from another. Pavlov brought
about severe neurosis in his dogs simply by converging two signs
to which the animals had been taught to respond differently.

In the artificial man-made human world of cultural conventions
these two things: orderliness (i.e. predictability, *ergo* manipul-
ability) of the external reality and unequivocality of semiotic
oppositions fuse into one matter. In their semiotic capacity cultural items convey, by opposing each other, vital information on
the significant differentiations in the realm of social structure
(this function is best illustrated by the diversity of distinctions
among army ranks or the technically inexplicable variety of dress
employed to denote the various roles of a single human being;
but it is illustrated as well by placing a warning 'No way through'
on one side of the door only, by allowing the high priest alone
to pronounce the 'real' name of God, or by forbidding the Jews

to eat pork, which all other human beings around enjoy). While transmitting this information, perceived cultural items shape and structure the perceptual–behavioural (input–output) field of every member of a given cultural community (i.e. any being understanding and obeying the given cultural code). But do they not by the same token create the very social structure they are supposed to reflect? The headlights I switch on inform passers-by that my car is approaching. But do they not, by doing just this, shape the structure of events on the road ahead? If so, does not turbidity of cultural signs turn social order into chaos? Motorist, how are you going to react to red and green lights signalling simultaneously at the crossroads, or to white and red lights on the same side of a car in front of you?

In an essay much too little referred to, Edmund Leach[18] elaborates on the intimate bond between the need for a clear, functional system of concepts and the need to repress the 'boundary percepts'. Owing to the character of the volume, discussion is limited to 'verbal concepts', but there is nothing to distinguish between linguistic terms and other, non-language, cultural items in their communicative function. You can convey the same information on a fragment of the social structure by a meaningful phrase or by an equally meaningful specialized behaviour pattern, and we can hardly expect different standards of clarity for each of the two interchangeable or complementary ways; the standards stem not from the nature of the semiotic code but from the superior need for order. If we tried to pluck Leach's argument from its accidental linguistic garment, we would probably be able to set forth the main ideas in the following way.

We secure an ordered character of the world we live and move in by selecting some percepts particularly indicative of events which for different reasons are important to us ('reading the natural code of the universe'); grouping these percepts into syndromes, usually appearing together, and so splitting the indiscrete world into discrete categories; attaching to each category a particular response pattern or interaction etiquette; only at this moment does the 'existence' of separate categories begin; they have no existence except through human praxis, they are separated not 'by themselves' but by the conventional differentiation of human behaviour. That is why 'keeping the borders sharp' is so important a matter. As if losing our way because of irregular entanglement of signs belonging to different syndromes were not enough; what is at stake is the very existence of the comprehensible universe (and that is the only form in which the universe is of any importance to us). In fighting incoherent border monsters, we defend our own integrity and the very existence of our socially created world.

TOOLS OF ORDERING

How do we fight them? Anthropologists borrowed from Polynesians the word 'taboo' to denote this peculiar intricate mixture of awe and fear, attachment and hatred, curiosity and escape drive, which characterized attitudes usually expressed towards everything ambiguous, equivocal, blurred to the point of indefinability. The exotic name suggests that the phenomenon of taboo is limited indeed to the 'primitives',[19] a corollary of magical practices, pre-scientific beliefs, and weird pre-religious ceremonies. Only recently anthropologists began to disentangle the basic culturological concepts, the concept of taboo among them, from the comfortably remote 'primitive' scenery where they were left and kept by the Frazerian tradition. The feeling of dissent began to mature long ago, but it was due to the effects of structuralists like Claude Lévi-Strauss in France, Stanner in Australia, and Edmund Leach and Mary Douglas in England that the discovery of common and universal thought patterns became finally possible and what was considered heretofore a manifestation of the immaturity of the savage mind could be comprehended as another form of proclivities and performances well known to us from our immediate neighbourhood. Maoris see menstrual blood quite properly as a human being unfinished and incomplete; it could turn into a person, but did not, thus destroying a life yet unborn; it is therefore an exemplary manifestation of ambiguity, as only the death of something which never lived can be; Maoris consider menstrual blood a very dangerous, threatening substance and use it eagerly in magical procedure.[20] Now Malinowski and Boas were right that this belief belongs historically and functionally with a relatively closed and complete cultural system together with special ceremonies attached to launching a canoe, initiation rites, etc. But it is at least as true that, logically and psychologically, this belief belongs – with abstention from treating domestic animals as meat, the cult of a human God-Mother, and suspicious anxiety aroused by marginal people – to the same class of manifestations of identical rule, structuring the human world-ordering praxis. It is a universal requirement of any coherent cultural system that the no-man's land between culturally discriminated positions in the social structure be tabooed. It is of minor importance whether the border monsters take the shape of 'ubi leones' or tricephalous Cerberus, are christened a saint or a witch. Both saints and witches guard the only thing that is to be guarded indeed – the secure unequivocality of culturally separated categories.

The specific sociocultural way of ordering-through-limitation is intimately correlated with one paramount characteristic of the human condition: the link between an individual's position inside the group and his biological, 'natural' equipment is mediated. Which means that the 'social' status of any individual is not determined unambiguously, if at all, by his natural attributes in general, and his physical powers and prowess in particular. Which means in its turn that the inherited or developed, but in both cases biological, indices of the individual's quality in the framework of *nature* become *socially* irrelevant if not misleading. The impressive brawn of a dock worker would surely guarantee him a most respected status were he a member of a herd of deer or of a birds' pecking order. They are, however, utterly misleading as signs of his position in a human society.

The mediation began with the production of tools. Ever since, human beings have surrounded themselves with artifacts not to be found in natural conditions, products of their modelling activity. Once created and appropriated, these artifacts destroyed the previous homology between the natural and the social order by changing entirely the action-capacity of individuals and so creating a new arrangement of environmental opportunities and probabilities. Thus a decisive adaptive value was conferred on the ordering of and orienting in the web of specifically social (which in this context means primarily 'non-natural') relations.

Life – whether social or pre-social – always consists in reversing the second law of thermodynamics in the 'living' entity: in retaining and/or increasing the level of 'negentropy' (Schrödinger's expression) in some part of a world tending to unlimited increase of entropy, i.e. to an ultimately disorderly, amorphous, undifferentiated state. Now this process can be analysed (and indeed is in cybernetics) into two aspects: energy and information. The first refers to the ability of the system to perform its job; the second is related to what the job is about, e.g. the degree of orderliness, predictability, differentiation already achieved or striven for. The living, but pre-social, organisms suck their energy directly from nature; whether they will succeed in continuing their life processes depends on their ability to decipher the 'natural' order, or rather that part of it which is relevant to the availability of the kind of energy they are after. This situation, however, changes dramatically with the emergence of a supra-organic living entity known under the name of human society.

Since the advent of tools and production, the human need for energy is only indirectly satisfied by natural sources. Between human beings and natural resources, between the refined needs of a socialized person and the alienating coarseness of raw natural stuff, mounts a new, mediating system of the producing and distributing society. Like any self-regulating (living) machine, this system possesses its ordered channels of energy transmission, which are usually talked about under the heading of the social structure: in the last instance everything which has been said so far and can be said in future on social structure is related to differentiated, i.e. preferential or disprivileged, access to the various kinds of energy (goods). But the system also possesses a code, e.g. a device whereby a message can be articulated, conveyed, read, and so eventually release a desired energy-transmission. This code is what the term 'culture' is about. Its knowledge, shared by the members of a cultural community is – through the process of socialization – ingrained into human minds much in the way the knowledge of grammatical rules is ingrained into the minds of the members of a linguistic community. Few members, if asked, would be able to articulate consciously the systemness of the code; but they owe their ability to communicate and to interact with each other, to achieve their portion of energy and to supply some to their partners, precisely to the generative rules that constitute the substance of the code. In other words, the social structure of any society lives and is lived, exists and develops, through isomorphism between energy – and information – flows, and this isomorphism is made possible (though by no means determined; the grammar decides how any sentence has to be built to convey whatever message one wants to convey, but it does not determine the content of the message) by the shared code of a cultural system. The so called 'culturally patterned' behaviour that provides the 'material stuff' for the social structure is related to the cultural system in the same way as utterances are to the grammar.

Thus substituting an artificial environment for the natural one means that an artificial (not natural, not created independently of human activity) order is substituted for the natural one. 'Order' is a graded notion: the level of orderliness is measured by the degree of predictability, e.g. by the discrepancy between the probability indices of events admitted by the system and those which the system is attempting to eliminate. In other words, ordering means dividing the universe of abstractly possible events into two subsets of – respectively – events whose occurrence is highly probable and those which can hardly be expected at all. Ordering dissipates a certain incertitude as to the expected course of events, which existed heretofore. It cannot be accomplished except by selecting, choosing a limited number of 'legalized' options from an unlimited multitude of sequences. This understanding of the way the orderliness of a system is achieved stands behind the classic, though forgotten, remarks of Boas on the intimate link between the statistical and moral meanings of the 'norm' in the order-generating and order-maintaining process.[21] Let us turn our attention to the fact that Boas does not distinguish between order-establishing and orientating-in-order faculties, probably assuming tacitly that we somehow like and evaluate favourably the habitual and expectable while disliking and rejecting the unusual and sudden (a conjecture which was granted a full corroboration by psychologists); and that this single human capacity accounts for both the need for order and the efficiency of the culture's guiding function. A single vehicle is enough to achieve both aims – since ordering (structuring) means making the ordered sector meaningful, e.g. arriving at a situation in which some concrete events usually follow a particular condition, and some beings to *whom* the sector is meaningful know that these

events do indeed follow it. In other words, the sector is meaningful to those to whom it is if and only if they possess some information on its dynamic tendencies. The discrepancy between the
information actually needed to determine the sector completely,
and the amount of information which would be necessary were
the sector entirely 'unorganized', is a measure of its degree of
'meaningfulness'.

The distinction made by Saussure between *signifiant* and
'*signifié*' (translated into English in many ways, of which 'signifier'
and 'signified' seem to be the most preferable) is one of the best-
known basic concepts of structural linguistics. As we know, Saussure
protested against hypostatizing the two concepts; they are more
aspects than ingredients of the physically single and indivisible
phenomenon-sign. As we know also, one of the fundamental
axioms of Saussure's theory was the absence of any necessarily
determined link between *signifié* and *signifiant*: the form of a sign
was, according to his strongly held opinion, totally undeter-
mined by its content – by the nature of the information it conveys.

It was Émile Benveniste[22] who stressed, on the contrary, the
intimate and indissoluble link between the two aspects of a sign.
The two aspects of a sign are not only brought together conventionally; they do not exist in isolation, they always occur in each
other's company; they cannot be evoked or exist in any imaginable
form (the mental including) without each other. What is told by a
sign is not only 'expressed' by it; it is created at the moment the
sign appears. The message is not only conveyed by the semiotic
act, he would say: it exists due to this act and through it.

From quite a different realm the famous assertion of W. I.
Thomas on the creative role of human 'beliefs' leads to the same
mode of thinking: if humans define a situation as real, it becomes
real. In its classic formulation the statement does not go far
beyond the not very exciting, though time-honoured, conflict
between 'idealism' and 'materialism'. Nevertheless we can,
neglecting the initial context and subjective intentions of the
great scholar, reformulate his assertion more in the spirit of
information theory: while attaching labels, defining, distinguishing, etc. and in this way making the situation 'meaningful' (i.e.
ordered), people create the situation itself, shape it, bring it into
being. It is no use quarrelling about whether behavioural patterns

or human social identities are primary. They are both introduced simultaneously, like *signifiant* and *signifié* in the semiotic act.

The third, also totally independent, tradition, suggestive of the modern solution of the culture/social-structure paradigm, is that of the 'activist', non-positivist branch of Marxism, which has found its most outspoken representative in Antonio Gramsci. Gramsci defined the Marxian world-view as 'philosophy of praxis', locating the category of praxis in the very centre of his social theory. Gramsci ridiculed those who like to consider 'reality as such', 'in itself'; we contact the world only through and in action, and there is no knowing what the world would be if left to itself and looked upon in a detached, 'objective' manner (the problem is that this point of view is simply unachievable). Social reality exists through constant encounter between a set of chances and possibilities and human forces able to transform (or unable to for that matter) these chances into facts, to actualize them. If a certain view of the social world meets a matching set of chances, a 'historical block' results, which leads – through praxis – to reshaping the state of things and opening up new, broader, and more far-reaching options. All aspects of the human world, the social structure and cultural systems included, exist only through human praxis.

We deal here only with those aspects of the above traditions, which are directly related to the nature of the semiotic act in general and the two faces of one cultural sign in particular. Let us notice that most of the modern sign-theoreticians, contrary to what most epistemologists of the past used to do, stress the active, stimulating, and organizing role of the sign much more than its expressive, signalling function. This approach is not connected with any particular school – we can take it as representative of modern semiotics as such, represented by writers as different as the Norwegian Ragnar Rommetweit,[23] the Chilean Louis Y Prieto,[24] the Ukrainian N. V. Popovitch, [25] and the Russian A. A. Zinoviev.[26]

In all these authors the notion of sign and semiotic act appear in a context reminiscent rather of the lights switched on by a motorist at dusk than of a stiff 'outer reality' which a human being must decipher and submit himself to in order to survive. Switching on the lights we make use of established, readable means to organize the space in front of us, to impose on it a meaningful, i.e. manageable and predictable, order. We warn the other motorists that we are approaching; by this we create a situation in which we can reasonably expect that there is high probability of their behaving in a way we are able to previse, and to adjust ourselves to, in advance. What is socially determined beforehand is not the exact allocation of cars along the road, their velocity and time of arrival at different places, this being solely a matter of coincidence between mutually independent actions governed by separate sets of variables. The only thing determined socially is the code structure, which each motorist uses to signal his own intentions, and to obtain optimal conditions for their implementation.

This example proves to be quite helpful in an effort to elucidate the relationship between culture and social structure as seen from the dual perspective of the theory of signs and the concept of *praxis*. The location of cars along the road (with some positions more favourable for a quick and efficient ride, others much less so) may be compared to the social structure as it is described in most cases in sociological textbooks; the code the motorists use to obtain specific positions in the above structure corresponds to the cultural system. By virtue of belonging to and being made meaningful by this system, the specific cultural items-signs both express the existing social structure and create it; they are at the same time operative in achieving relative durability and its dynamic fluidity. So the two spurious, ill-famed 'contradictions' between 'thought' and 'reality' and between 'statics' and 'dynamics' are overcome at one stroke. The opinion of this author is that the two fallacies can be overcome either together or not at all.

Hjelmslev distinguished in 1942 three possible points of view from which language can be studied. The first is the *schema*, or the pattern due to which the elements become meaningful at all; the second is the *usage*, or the set of habits which are formed in a particular language as to the application of the schema; and the third, the *norm*, or what the members of a specific linguistic community think proper to use. Using the Hjelmslev's terms, we can say that 'the butterfly collectors'[27] and – as a matter of fact – most anthropologists and comparative sociologists until relatively recent times were concerned exclusively with the study of norm (sometimes called 'culture') and usage (sometimes called 'social structure') but they hardly ever went so far as to ask about the schema prior to both usage and norm and not reducible to mere similar points of different usages and norms accepted by different communities.

It was generally accepted to identify the problem of universals with Murdock's idea of institutionalized fields of human usages, derivable as easily from 'cultural comparisons' as from any classified telephone directory. It was as if a linguist tried to establish linguistic universals by enumerating themata which appear in the recorded texts of all known communities. The task consists now in descending from the very high level of application – that of 'tests' and 'utterances' – to the 'deep-seated regularities' which govern the formation of any text and utterance, whatever the material and purpose they are applied to. This descent will mean a shift from the stage of description to the phases of theoretical analysis. The aim is to arrive at a kind of 'generative grammar' of culture as a semiotic system.

'If, as we believe to be the case,' says Claude Lévi-Strauss, 'the unconscious activity of the mind consists in imposing forms upon content, and if these forms are fundamentally the same for all minds – ancient and modern, primitive and civilized (as the study of the symbolic function, expressed in language, so strikingly indicates) – it is necessary and sufficient to grasp the unconscious structure underlying each institution and each custom, in order to obtain a principle of interpretation valid for other institutions and other customs, provided of course that the analysis is carried far enough.'[28]

NOTES AND REFERENCES

1 Cf. HULL, C. L. *A Behavior System*, New Haven, Yale U.P., 1952, p. 5 ff.

2 'The General Notion of Theory Construction', in *Theories in Contemporary Psychology*, ed. by Melvin H. Marx, New York, Collier-Macmillan, 1963, p. 25.

3 CLAUDE LÉVI-STRAUSS, *Structural Anthropology*, New York, Basic Books, 1967, p. 271. Translated by Claire Jacobson and Brooke Grundfest Schoepf.

4 ROLAND BARTHES, 'L'activité structuraliste', *Les Lettres Nouvelles*, 1963. **32.**

5 *Swiadomść Religijna i Wieź Kościelna*, Warszawa, 1965, p. 39.
6 JEAN PIAGET, *Éléments d'épistémologie génétique*, Paris, Presses Universitaires de France, 1950, vol. II, p. 34.
7 C. LEFORT, 'L'échange et la lutte des hommes', *Les Temps modernes*, 1951, **64**.
8 Cf. WARD H. GOODENOUGH, 'Rethinking "Structure" and "Role" ', in *Cognitive Anthropology*, ed. by Stephen A. Tyler, Holt, Rinehart, and Winston, 1969, p. 311–29.
9 RALPH LINTON, *The Study of Man*, New York, Appleton Century, 1936, p. 114.
10 Cf. DANESH, F. and HAUSENBLAS, K. 'Problematika urovnej s tochki zrenja struktury wyskasyvanii i sistemy iazykovych sredstv', in *Edinicy rasnych urovnej grammaticheskovo stroja iazyka i ich vzaimodejstvie*, Moscow, Nauka, 1969, pp. 11–12.
11 Cf., for example, ASHBY, W. R. 'The Principles of self-Organization', in *Principles of Self-Organization*, ed. by Heinz von Foerster and George W. Zopf, Jr., London, Pergamon Press, 1962.
12 Cf. *Principles of Self-Organization*, ed. by Heinz von Foerster and George W. Zopf, Jr., London, Pergamon Press, 1962.
13 The modern view of animal behaviour was founded by the classic studies of LORENZ, K. Z. *King Solomon's Ring*, New York, Crowell, 1952; TINBERGEN, N. *The Study of Instinct*, Oxford, Clarendon Press, 1951; *Social Behaviour in Animals*, London, Methuen, 1953, THORPE, W. H. *Learning and Instinct in Animals*, Cambridge, Mass., Harvard University Press, 1956.
14 GREIMAS, A. J. *Sémantique structurale*, Paris, Librairie Larousse, 1966, p. 19.
15 Cf. JOHN LYONS, *Introduction to Theoretical Linguistics*, London, Cambridge University Press, 1969, p. 67.
16 *Cours de linguistique générale*, Paris, 1916.
17 John Lyons, op. cit., p. 68.
18 'Anthropological Aspects of Language; Animal Categories and Verbal Abuse', in *New Directions in the Study of Language*, ed. by Eric H. Lenneberg, Chicago, University of Chicago Press, 1964. The essay has not been listed even in Mary Douglas, *Purity and Danger*, London, Routledge and Kegan Paul, 1966, devoted almost in full to a basically identical subject. Mrs Douglas strives to arrive at generalizations already stated by Leach, in many cases with more success.
19 'So entrenched have our beliefs become concerning the ortholinear evolution of man that our conceptions of "progress", "development", and "evolution" have rendered the assumption automatic that what developed later in time must therefore be more "advanced" or more "evolved" than that which developed earlier. From this "logical" inference followed that what was less developed must be earlier than that which was more developed, and therefore the earlier was the more "primitive" and the later

more "advanced".' I could not refuse myself the pleasure of quoting here ASHLEY MONTAGU'S (*The Concept of Primitive*, New York, The Free Press, 1968, p. 2) insight into the peculiar logical fallacy supporting the time-honoured conceptual structure.

20 Cf. LUCIEN LÉVY-BRUHL, *La Mentalité primitive*, Paris, 1922.

21 Introduction to the Handbook of American Indian Languages, Smithsonian Institution, 1911; reprinted in *Classics in Linguistics*, ed. by DONALD E. HAYDEN *et al.*, New York, Philosophical Library, 1967, p. 220.

22 ÉMILE BENVENISTE, 'Nature de signé linguistique', *Acta linguistica*, 1939.

23 RAGNAR ROMMETVEIT, *Words, Meanings, and Messages: Theory and Experiments in Psycholinguistics*, Oslo, Universitetsforlaget, 1968, p. 9–10.

24 LUIS Y PRIETO, *Messages et signaux*, Paris, Presses Universitaires de France, 1966, p. 6.

25 POPOVITCH, M. V. *O filosofskom analize jazyka nauki*, Kiev, 'Naukovaja dumka', 1966, pp. 50–1.

26 ZINOVIEV, A. A. *Osnovy logitcheskoj teorii nauchnych znanij*, Moscow, 'Nauka', 1967, pp. 16–17.

Systems, Structures, and Consciousness: the social psychology of meaning

ARTHUR BRITTAN

The perennial discussion of the objective–subjective dichotomy in the social sciences is never resolved because it is always posed in terms of categories which owe their potency to a continuous dialogue with the ghost of Descartes. Man's 'inner' and 'outer' worlds are conceived of as being in some form of timeless opposition. Ever since Descartes first posed the problem, Western thought has been engaged in a heroic attempt to bridge the gap, but never with complete success. With the advent of linguistic philosophy, and its insistence on the strict application of technical criteria in the analysis of meaning, there has been an attempt to put the dispute into cold storage. It has been officially declared as being a non-problem. We have all been seduced by language. This seduction is believed to have gone a long way in the social sciences, particularly in sociology, where language unfortunately seems to obtain an autonomy of its own.

It is not my purpose to chart the objective–subjective controversy in the social sciences – this is well documented in the literature and to a certain extent has been placed in perspective by Michael Polanyi's seminal analysis of the role of valuation in science.[1] Certainly since Weber's time, sociologists have been aware that claims about the objective and neutral nature of the scientific enterprise are in fact claims about certain forms of commitment – one chooses science from a sense of commitment just as one chooses art. Arguments for objectivity often turn out to be statements about ways of measuring aspects of the phenomenal world. As Hampden-Turner has put it, objectivity is a plea for consensus. It is really nothing more 'than a consensus among investigators as to how a phenomenon is to be regarded and measured. Here calls for objectivity are like calls for consensus politics – they affirm the most obvious and least controversial.'[2]

In the social sciences, in spite of our pretensions about the unmasking functions of social research, we still suffer from the delusion that social science itself is sufficiently aware of its contextual and historical underpinning – we still believe that the sociology of knowledge is peripheral to the mainstream of sociological activity. At the back of the sociological mind, there is the hidden assumption that sociology has a privileged status which exempts it from self-analysis. This assumption goes hand in hand with the ideology of objectivity and the assertion that sociology is a science. In this respect, the recent attention that some sociologists have devoted to the 'sociology of sociology' is an index of the disquiet that they feel about sociology's continuous flirtation with the natural-science model. It has become increasingly obvious that the sociologist's self-image enters into his sociological work as a constitutive element of the process. Thus a plea for objectivity turns out to be a plea for an acceptance of the sociologist's image of himself as a scientist – and this image, as Friedrichs reminds us, is very reminiscent of the image of the priest. Consequently the sociologist begins to see himself as the arbiter of truth, the interpreter of reality, to whom the layman turns in order to understand both himself and the social world he lives in: 'The liturgy of the priestly mode in contemporary sociology holds – that scientists as scientists make no value judgements and that because sociology is a natural science, sociologists are likewise exempted. It is a position that is always hedged by the phrase "*qua* sociologist", even though the segmentation of man's activity into roles is itself a product of a sociological perspective and thus begs the question."[3]

Even though the worst excesses of behaviourism and positivism are apparently behind us, there is still implicit in some of the newer systems models so popular in the social sciences, the hope that 'given time', the social sciences will approximate to the condition of the natural sciences in which the subjective aspects of social action can be neutralized by the employment of 'intervening variables' to designate what occurs within the little black box. However, this view of man and society has been under severe attack from a variety of quarters. The hidden, submerged, and sometimes irrational dimensions of human behaviour have emerged under new sponsorship. Linguistics, anthropology, and philosophy have provided suitable rallying-points for the counterattack against an oversocialized conception of man. In addition, biological models of animal behaviour have emphasized the importance of biological structure. This has spilled over into the study of man. The social sciences have not remained immune from these attacks – this is particularly true of sociology and social psychology. The 'coming crisis of Western sociology' is not necessarily to be construed as being primarily a confrontation between consensus and conflict theory, but is also a confrontation between the Lockean tradition and the Leibnizian tradition.

I. THE LEIBNIZIAN INSURGENCY

'A specter is haunting the academic halls of the "Lockean Establishment" in psychology – the specter of "Leibnizian Insurgency".'[4]

The image of man as a *tabula rasa* on which experience imprints itself has had a long and successful run in Western thought. It has also, since Locke's time, provided psychology with its associational underpinning. Most contemporary stimulus–response theories in experimental psychology can trace their lineage to the Lockean tradition. Until recently (in the United States particularly) except for the flowering of Freudian psychology outside the portals of the academic establishment, there has been a prolonged commitment to a variety of learning perspectives. Although alternatives were allowed to encroach in certain areas, especially some versions of gestalt and field theory, the stimulus–response paradigm is still the dominant one in both American and British psychology. The important psychologies that grew up on the Continent and placed great emphasis on cognition and the 'little black box' took a long time to infiltrate the Anglo-Saxon empiricist stronghold. The long-drawn-out reaction against introspection has remained a constant feature of the psychological scene. It has been only recently that cognitive psychology has begun to make incisive inroads into American psychology – major figures like Bruner have managed decisively to break the spell that neo-behaviourism cast over the study of perceptual and learning processes. In addition, Piaget has finally managed to break out of Europe and become part of the psychological establishment. At the same time, there is evidence that this process has not been one-way. G. H. Mead has been neglected and ignored by European social scientists – unfortunately he has been labelled a social behaviourist, and this means that his unique contribution to the study of the relationship between self and social matrix has until recently remained part of the American context. A cursory examination of the works of Sartre, Lévi-Strauss, Merleau-Ponty, Foucault, and others fails to indicate that any of these theorists have ever even read Mead. This is strange, particularly when it is remembered that pragmatism enjoyed quite a vogue in Europe, especially in the works of Peirce, James, and Dewey.

In the main, the Lockean position, in spite of being subject to heavy attack, has remained relatively inviolable. (Even Chomsky's blast against behaviourism has not dislodged reinforcement psychology from its strategic pinnacles. Instincts were relegated to the intellectual rubbish heap, and, anyway, psychoanalysis was beyond the pale – it was attacked for being non-scientific.) With the emergence of the 'new instinct theory' deriving from the work of ethologists like Tinbergen and Lorenz, there has been a marginal breach in the hegemony of the ruling paradigm, but the breach has been effected in the field of animal behaviour, not in human psychology, despite the dubious efforts of popularizers like Desmond Morris and Robert Ardrey. It was only when the academic establishment was attacked from unexpected quarters that the Leibnizian insurgency got under way. The Leibnizian insurgency is not a conscious and deliberate attack on behaviourist psychology and empirical social science. It is composed of diverse strands whose common theme seems to be the rejection of simple, directly observable stimulus–response linkages, and the substitution instead of some form of internal schemata or structure. For some, the reaction was centred on the elevation of consciousness to the position it once held in philosophy and the cultural sciences. Here the position of existential phenomenology and intepretative sociology are of critical importance, especially in their approach to meaning. For others, the reaction came from the so-called new linguistics and its rediscovery of deep structures and their expression in a universal grammar. Chomsky's reaction against empiricism is not to be seen as a simple return to the tradition of Descartes and Leibniz, but arises directly out of his conviction 'that innate properties of mind provide a schematism that determines what counts as experience, and that restricts the knowledge (in our case, the grammar) that is based on experience'.[5] For others, the reaction derived from French anthropology and its apogee in the person of Lévi-Strauss and his advocacy of structuralism. Structure in this sense is no longer a concept in the natural sciences which was translated by Durkheim and Radcliffe-Brown and others into the language of sociology in order to describe patterns of recurrent relationships in a society. It now becomes a code which is, first, a method for deciphering social relationships and myths, and, second, a cognitive universalism.

The Leibnizian insurgency, then, is made up of strange bedfellows who would not recognize themselves in that role. At one end of the scale 'consciousness' is seen to be the most crucial problem in the human sciences, and at the other end the problem is posed in terms of the assumption 'that there may be certain cognitive capacities for forming kinds of schemata that are neurologically "wired into" all human beings, are genetically determined, and are presumably a product of evolution'.[6] However, no matter what the reaction is, it is not an insignificant fact that both language and consciousness are firmly at the centre of the field of interest.

It seems strange that the current debate on the nature of structuralism is partly premised on the hoary problem of the relationship between innate and situational variables. Neither Chomsky nor Lévi-Strauss is a naïve psychological or biological reductionist. But they have both reacted in their different ways to the dominant orthodoxy in the human and social sciences. This orthodoxy has assumed a view of man and society that left no place for the possibility of a viable alternative to man's being a plaything of vast impersonal sociocultural forces. Indeed, the Lockean position leads directly to the most blatant sociological determinism. In a sense, contempory theorizing in both sociology and social psychology has been very much committed to what A. F. C. Wallace has called the 'Microcosmic Metaphor'. The

'Microcosmic Metaphor' assumes the complete submergence of the individual in society. It is the sociological equivalent of the 'Hegelian State' with the metaphysics left out. In other words, the emphasis is on man as an infinitely pliable and plastic actor who continuously takes on the shape and content of the society in which he lives. Thus the social sciences have, in the main, tended to concentrate on content at the expense of form. If men were empty vessels, then it followed that the only thing that could give them substance was the impress of the culture into which they were born.

As a direct consequence of this state of affairs, both sociology and social psychology have paid a great deal of attention to the socialization process, particularly those aspects of the process which lead to standardized social behaviour. In social psychology the emphasis has been on the study of conformity – this being particularly true of the discipline in the United States. Socialization was considered to be the means whereby a social system maintained itself by inculcating its norms, values, attitudes, etc. into the incoming generation. Unfortunately, as we have already indicated, this approach meant that the individual disappeared under the weight of social imperatives. In a sense, therefore, we are left with the distinct impression that the social sciences unconsciously assume that man is a victim of mass society. The notion of victimage leaves the individual without the means of countering the sheer overwhelming power of the social world. This left very little scope for alternative formulations. It was not only a question of determinism versus voluntarism; it also involved a fundamental denial of subjectivity as witnessed by individual actors, and the denial of autonomous motivation. If all motives were socially induced, then, obviously, reflexive subjectivity was merely an illusion. The alternatives to sociological determinism were in the main some form of watered-down instinct theory. Although many social scientists embraced psychoanalysis, they did so from the perspective of Neo-Freudianism rather than from orthodox Freudianism. As Dennis Wrong and others have demonstrated, what emerged was a strangely emasculated version of the original theory of the dynamic nature of the unconscious. Social theory found it very difficult to come to terms with the idea that behaviour could be influenced by non-sociogenic factors. The idea of the irrational was anathema to believers in the fundamental ubiquity of social determinants. In addition, academic psychologists found the idea of the unconscious as unpalatable as some social scientists did. This is not the time and place to get involved in a lengthy discussion on the concept of the unconscious. What is important from our point of view is the way in which the unconscious has now emerged under different intellectual banners. In the new version, we are no longer expected to adhere to Freudian topology, but rather to a cognitive unconscious. Motivation and emotion are now subsumed under the aegis of mediational processes which often operate below the level of awareness. However, this does mean to imply that the new Leibnizian position regards the individual in terms of atomistic 'windowless monads'. This would be a gross distortion of a perspective which endeavours to place cognition back in its rightful place in the social sciences.

It is of course true that the cognitive structures that we are considering are not empirically available, just as the Freudian unconscious is not empirically available. But there is certainly enough evidence originating from structural anthropology, linguistics, and interpretative sociology to lend support to the cognitive revolution in social psychology. The surprising thing is that so few practitioners attempt to make the necessary linkages with similar work in complementary disciplines. Ultimately as I have already proposed, the new look is focused on language, meaning, and consciousness.

II. THE ISOMORPHISM BETWEEN THOUGHT AND THE WORLD

'The isomorphism of thought and the world is a familiar pre-occupation of philosophy: to the Wittgenstein of the *Tractatus* just as much as to Lévi-Strauss the fundamental categories of human thought mirror the structure of the world although not directly asserting anything about it. The role of logic in the epistemology of the early Wittgenstein is not unlike the role of myth in the epistemology of Lévi-Strauss, and in a sense this is only to be expected, since it is part of Lévi-Strauss's purpose to show that the kind of logic in mythical thought is as rigorous as that of modern science. But having said that the fundamental categories of human thought, whether revealed by ethnography or by introspection are somehow isomorphic to the world, how are we ever to demonstrate either the nature or the cause of this connection without lapsing into a regress?'[7]

Structuralism and Cognitive Universalism

Lévi-Strauss's proposal that social structure is a construct or model which the anthropologist can apply to concrete social reality is not startling, nor is his insistence that the model (social structure) is a category in the mind of the anthropologist really revolutionary. As a cognitive model, it serves the heuristic function of ordering social relationships in a logical manner – it provides a map whereby social relationships can be deciphered. But this is only a superficial rendering of Lévi-Strauss's subtleties. There is explicit in his work the belief that social structure does not exist at the level of the 'conscious' models of social relations which men employ to conceptualize the social reality in which they are en-meshed. For Lévi-Strauss, social structure is based on a pattern of order that remains hidden behind the surface of the phenomenal world – it is an 'unconscious' order, disguised and only approach-able by assuming some form of isomorphism between the structure of thought and the hidden structure of social relationships and myth. The relationship between conscious and unconscious models (structures) is basically similar to that between the mundane usage that everyday speech is put to, and the rules of syntax that govern this speech. If we manage to construct this syntax (unconscious model), then what we have really done is to have placed some internal image of the structure in some kind of relationship with the structure – in other words, cognitive categories are translated into social categories. There is, of course, a fundamental paradox and contradiction involved here. In this connection David Schneider comments – 'there is the notion that structure inheres not in the concrete constitution of any particular society, but rather in the model or the construct which may be developed by the anthropologist in order to understand that society, yet the structural principles which are at work so to speak, are somehow real, existent, substantive and are expressed in the social definitions, the social conventions, the social rules of a particular society'.[8]

The model exists, therefore, both as a cognitive structure and as a simultaneous reality in the society which is being studied. Social structures are not only constructs – they are constituted of the same coding as the constructs which are supposed to act as the codifying mechanism for the structures themselves – hence we can understand Runciman's complaint about the 'lapse into regress'.

The assumption of an internal structure which is isomorphic with external structure is an old theme in Western thought. In exploring social reality there is a tradition which conceptualizes experience in terms of systems and structures. Indeed, the systems model has been called the 'Procrustean model' by Paul Meadows.[9] The history of social thought is a graveyard of holistic models which have replaced each other in endless succession – machines, organisms, equilibrium states, etc. have served to provide men with frames of reference on which to hang their images of society. But more than this, it is asserted that these models tend to serve as expressions of the tendency of men to cognize their world in some form of patterned connexity, system, or structure. The structure of the mind is in this sense universal and timeless – it presupposes the psychic unity of the human race. If the mind is everywhere cognizing the world in the same fundamental way, then it follows that the mind's products can be deciphered by the cracking of the universal code, no matter how complex the code might be in different social contexts. There is, therefore, the implication in Lévi-Strauss's thought that the unconscious psychological structures – logical structures – are somehow prior to social structures, but that in the final analysis the way to understand these structures is to decipher the social structure. When it is asked how we are to study and locate these structures, then we find that the answers given by Lévi-Strauss are ambiguous. They are not to be found in associationist psychology, nor are they to be found in the intuition of phenomenological structures like the 'self'. Lévi-Strauss finds his cognitive universalism in the symbolizing capacity of the human mind which is everywhere the same. This universalizing symbolic capacity is demonstrated by certain universal features of language. But men as a rule are not aware of the rules of language – they are in fact hidden and unconscious. The anthropologist is not concerned with the contents of the mind, but only with the formal properties of the hidden structures.

Superficially, Lévi-Strauss's discussion of unconscious models is premised on the Freudian unconscious, but it is a strangely intellectualized unconscious. However, it is not to the Freudian 'unconscious' that we must turn to for an analysis of cognitive organization. This is provided by a number of emphases in contemporary psychology and social science which pay attention to schemata and internal structures, although not from the perspective of cognitive universalism. Despite the glamour of the structuralist apotheosis, other theorists have been working along complementary if not similar lines. It is to these we now briefly turn.

The Gestalt Approach

The gestalt school has been sadly neglected and criticized in recent years. The idea that our perceptual and cognitive capacities could be construed in terms of wholes was an elegantly simple oversimplification, but it served to counter the mechanical associative models which broke up experience into discrete components. Gestalt theorists argued that the flow of stimuli impinging on receptor mechanisms do not elicit single responses but energize total forms of organization. In other words, the organism radically modifies the stimulus. These wholes are somehow embedded in the neurological system, thereby allowing organisms to transform sense experience into forms of organization. This process is automatic and seems to be genetically determined. The reaction against gestalt psychology by learning theorists was made in terms of their basic counter-assumption that perceptual wholes could be explained in terms of stimulus–response contingencies. So extreme was this reaction, that all mediational activity was seen as being reducible to learning connections. However, from our point of view, the gestalt emphasis on wholes and structures is not under debate. I think we can assert that such structures have consequences for human conduct – all the evidence seems to point to the reality of cognitive organization, but that their genesis is not necessarily to be construed as being innate in the sense of some prior Platonic essence. Nor, for that matter, can they be explained by the positing of a process of psychological accretion whereby they are built up step by step, so that the whole is considered to be the sum of its parts. What is missing from gestalt psychology is an adequate treatment of communicative processes, especially language and other symbolic forms. The configurations that seem to be psychological 'givens' are far more problematic than was realized by early gestalt theorists. Contemporary cognitive psychology has moved beyond these models by taking both culture and social structure into account in its discussion of internal structuring. This leads me to the constructionist approach.

The Constructionist Approach

By the constructionist approach I am thinking of two very different traditions: one deriving from Piaget and his associates, and the other from the American symbolic interactionists, of whom such figures as G. H. Mead and Herbert Blumer are the most typical representatives. In many ways these traditions have developed independently of each other, but they both treat structures not as if they were innate or predetermined codes, but rather as processes involving the interaction and collaboration of internal and external factors, which together construct knowledge and identity structures.

Piaget, for example, argues that there are three ways of conceiving of and understanding the genesis of structures: (1) preformation, that is either the attribution of innate characteristics of a genetic kind or, philosophically, the assumption of Platonic 'forms'; (2) contingent emergence – which Piaget believes is not really compatible with the concept of structure in spite of Michel Foucault's eloquent plea for the ubiquity of the inexplicable; and, finally, (3) constructivist accounts. The constructivist approach, in Piaget's view, simply asserts that structures are only intelligible when they are seen as part of an adaptive process between an organism and its environment. The organism does not simply respond to a stimulus, but responds in a way that is compatible with the essential structure of the organism. The stimulus is never pristine, but is used by the organism to construct its own responses. Ultimately, these structures are dependent on the continuous exchange between environmental inputs and the manner in which the organism assimilates these inputs. In human terms, the structures that Piaget is concerned with are knowledge structures which are intimately related to the cultural environment and whose development is therefore inconceivable outside that environment. Constructionism implies a specific attitude towards objectivity. Things exist in the world, but knowledge is not built up by subjectively emulating that world; it is constructed out of that world. Structures are then not timeless essences – they are always in process of 'becoming'. This runs directly counter to some of the ahistorical aspects of Lévi-Strauss's structuralism. Piaget's discussion of the genesis of structures seems to be eminently reasonable. He writes – 'in areas where genesis obtrudes on everyday observations, as in the psychology of intelligence, one cannot help but become aware that structure and genesis are necessarily interdependent. Genesis is simply transition from one structure to another, nothing more; but this transition always leads from a 'weaker' to a 'stronger' structure; it is a 'formative' transition. Structure is simply a system of transformations, but its roots are operational; it depends therefore on a prior formation of the instruments of transformation – transformation rules or laws.'[10]

Of course it is precisely these transformation rules that generate so much heat in the discussion of structures. Construction allows for the generation of meaning in the interaction between environment and the human organism. This meaning is not automatically attached to inputs but depends on the way in which both the individual and the environment simultaneously construct symbolic modes in order to prepare the individual for further elaboration of his cognitive structures. Hence, from an entirely different standpoint, Piaget delineates knowledge structures in much the same way that Mead conceptualizes the genesis and function of the self in social processes. Mead, as is well known, argued that objects are *constructed* out of the consummation of acts. Whatever else we may say about man, he is primarily a social animal, and social behaviour implies the construction of social objects. The stimulus is never directly given to the experiencer, but only becomes an object if it is of relevance to the individual – the criterion of relevance being governed by the meaning the object or stimulus condition has for the individual. Social objects are constructed objects – their significance being defined by the symbols employed to generate meaning out an infinite number of possible permutations and combinations of stimuli. By himself the solitary individual would not be able to cope with this stimulus bombardment – the presence of others is essential for the realization of the self as a social object. It is only through the indications of others that the individual can conceive of himself both as a part of, and as separate from, the social context in which he is enmeshed. For Mead the 'self' is a social product, but a social product that has been constructed in communicative acts, that is, in symbolic interaction between men. Symbols and language, in this sense, can be said to be constitutive of self and society. By constitutive we do not mean to imply the creation of and the determination of individual and social processes. This would obviously be absurd – indeed, this is completely contrary to the notion of the 'act' being built up or constructed – it is contrary to the assumption of reflexivity as a dialogue between self and others.

Both in Mead's discussion of the self and in Piaget's notion of the 'epistemic subject' the traditional distinctions between subjectivity and objectivity fall away because they are treated as being aspects of the same process. Organism and environment, self and other, are reciprocal processes, each in a state of continuous interchange with the other, involving the mutual construction of each. However, reflexivity must not be construed in terms of mirror-image representation of the object in the 'epistemic subject'. The self is a process, but it is a *structured process.*

What do we mean by a structured process? Ever since Bartlett suggested that an organism is capable of reflexively observing its own schemata,[9] there has been a wealth of theorizing on the nature of cognition as a reflexive mode – cognitive psychology rediscovered the self-concept by admitting that the only way we can become aware of our schemata is by symbolizing them to ourselves. In some cases, these schemata have been described as being unconscious, and hence our knowledge of them has been inferred by the decoding of fantasy, myths, and dreams, etc. Unconscious structures belong to psychodynamic theories of motivation and to certain forms of structuralism. Their presence can never be made explicit, but in principle they can be decoded. Whether conscious or unconscious, schemata are not static structures dependent on mechanical stimulation – they tend to be dynamic; they are an orientation or set which allows for an active interpretation of the meaning of the incoming stimulus. A schema generates an expectation of what to focus on in the stimulus field.

Sociologically, a schema is equivalent but not identical to the 'individual's definition of the situation'. The definition of the situation implies a situated activity, which, as Eugene Weinstein has suggested, is a 'kind of shorthand summary of all the internal processes mediating between the impinging of situational stimuli and the selection and evocation of responsive lines of action'.[11] It is the 'individual's best guess as to the nature of the reality with which he is concurrently engaged'.[12] But this guess as to the nature of the ongoing reality in which he is engaged is dependent on the 'epistemic subject', on the saliency of the schema which the individual brings into play in a specific situation. In this connection, it is interesting to note that a number of computer and simulation techniques have been responsible for a broadening of the meaning of schemata to include both cognitive maps (images in Kenneth Boulding's sense)[13] and 'plans'. Plans involve the translation of the image into projected future actions. Miller, Galanter, and Pribram, for example, conceive of plans as being analogous to computer programs in which the individual is hierarchically organized to behave in certain ways in certain situations. These hierarchical structures are discoverable at both the neurological and the behavioural level. They are continuously being modified by experience and new encounters.[14] Translated into sociological language, we can say that plans imply what Blumer calls the process of self-indication. As he says:

'We must recognize that the activity of human beings consists of meeting a flow of situations in which they have to act and that their action is built on the basis of what they note, how they assess and interpret what they note.'[15]

The interpretation of the situation is always dynamic in that images and plans are not determinants of behaviour, but are reflexively related to the interpretations of others. It follows that the internal frame of reference is not to be understood as a static structure or frozen schema. We can agree with George Kelly in his belief that psychological processes are always structured in order to anticipate future events – the future is always a datum of the present; images merge into plans and are restructured by new situations, which in turn are reinterpreted and restructured. 'We assume that all our present interpretations of the universe are subject to revision and replacement.'[16] We also assume that, without some sort of structuring, there would not be any continuity in the experience of the 'self', and consequently no possibility of meaningful communication between social actors. Schemata, identities, attitudes, motives, plans, images, cognitive maps, etc. presuppose structural organization, but it is not necessary to demonstrate that these structures can be found empirically at the biological level, or, even if they can be discovered, that biological structures can be translated into symbolic structures. *Human behaviour involves both the structuring and the breaking-down of structures.* Schemata are relatively persistent, but they are modifiable by experience, albeit this modification is always in terms of the prior state of the organism and the way in which the schemata are hierarchically organized. Whether we call these schemata 'cell assemblies' and 'phase sequences' in the physiological language that Hebb uses,[17] or whether we conceive of them as 'information-retrieval systems' in the language of information and communication theory, there can be no doubt that they exercise a considerable influence on the course of human interaction.

Even if we demonstrate the ubiquity of the structuring process, and even if we establish that we think in structures, this does not mean we can draw the conclusion that the world is patterned on structures existing at the mental level. This certainly would be the ultimate regress into 'idealism'. However, if we argue that only cultural objects are reducible to mental structures, then we are arguing for the primacy of psychology in the social and cultural sciences. But this is precisely what we cannot do, because, as we have tried to show, structures are meaningless outside social interaction. All we can do is to indicate that the relationship between culture and schemata is not one in which the 'epistemic subject' is ranged up against an overwhelming objective reality (culture, society). The subjective–objective dichotomy falls away because both mind and society are twin born in the dialogue between selves and others. Structures are meaningless outside symbolic contexts.

What we really need is a concept that simultaneously handles both schema and symbolic context. Parsons and other sociologists speak in terms of the internalization of norms and values, but this tends to boil down to cultural determinism. In this case internal schemata reflect the master patterns of society and man is relegated to the status of a *tabula rasa*. This is not the time and place to enter into a discussion about the relative autonomy of the normative system, but it does seem to me absolutely imperative that we handle both cultural and psychological facts simultaneously, in order to construct a model of social relationships that is not a mere repetition of stimulus–response psychology, on the one hand, and Leibniz's solitary windowless monads, on the other. Nor, for that matter, can we be satisfied with a formal structuralism that relegates meaning to a secondary place. The decoding of structures is an essential and valuable instrument for the generation of structural isomorphies, but structure devoid of meaning is like food without taste.

What this all means is that structures are not circuits that are predetermined. The scientific enterprise as applied to man does not necessarily lead us to an image of human nature that excludes self-knowledge – in which social structure is merely the codification of cerebral categories. Recently, some social scientists have turned to cybernetics and modern systems theory for concepts and methodological tools which they hope will allow them to handle objective–subjective categories simultaneously. Let us look briefly at this approach.

Systems and Consciousness

In both psychological and sociological theory, the systems concept is tied up to concepts relating to equilibrium and homeostasis, thus indicating its association with mechanical and organic models. Perhaps more significantly, modern systems theory utilizes a computer analogy—psychological processes being treated as if they were in fact comparable to input–output programming. The trouble here is that the analogy is sometimes extended to a belief in the ubiquity of feedback mechanisms, not only as a model for the construction of a theory, but as exemplifying the processes themselves. What starts off as an analogy becomes the process. Modern systems theory is openly theoretical in that it is concerned with the nature of systems themselves. It asserts that all systems show structural similarities and isomorphies. 'Thus there exist models, principles, and laws that apply to

generalized systems or their subclasses, irrespective of their
particular kind, the nature of their component elements, and the
relations of "forces" between them. It seems legitimate to ask for a
theory of systems of a more or less special kind, but of universal
principles applying to systems in general.'[18] Thus, at the formal
level at least, modern systems theory makes the same sort of
statements about the isomorphy between levels as does structuralism, but in conceiving of systems as being the units of analysis
special attention is devoted to the key concept 'organization'. It is
organization that seems to be immanent in nature, whereas in the
structuralist position, organization is isomorphic to the structures
of the mind, especially those structures which are man-made
(social structure, language system, mythologies, art, religion, etc.).
Supporting the systems model are the mathematical equations
which legitimate a number of contemporary approaches, such as
information and communication theory, and which are essential
for the understanding and manipulation of computers. One
advantage that systems theory has over gestalt theory, for example,
is that it allows for information interchange and the subsequent
construction of symbolic systems which are a necessary basis for
the understanding of consciousness.

The axioms of information theory enmeshed in a compound of
propositions derived from neurology and communications
engineering provided the impetus for the development of cybernetics, and hence modern systems theory. These models were
taken over, sometimes without due care, by both psychologists
and sociologists, who saw in them a possible solution to the thorny
problem of the relationship between subjectivity and objectivity.
Consciousness could now be defined in terms of the feedback
mechanisms which are supposed to guide both individuals and
organizations in their relations with the environment. Indeed Karl
Deutsch defines consciousness 'as a collection of internal feedbacks
of secondary messages'.[19] Walter Buckley has argued that the
modern systems perspective is of value to the social sciences
because it does away with the artificial distinctions between
psychological and sociological explanation. He expresses the
utopian hope that it will:
First generate a common vocabulary which cuts across disciplinary
isolation; *second* allow a methodology to develop which encom-

passes both micro- and macro-processes simultaneously; *third* counter the tendency to treat human conduct atomistically and in so doing will conceive of social relationships as dynamically organized in a field or context; *fourth* pay due regard to the socio-cultural matrix in which social interaction is enmeshed with particular reference to communication nets and the coding of messages in social structures; *fifth* allow structures to be viewed as a set of relationships between events rather than entities. This would enable it to treat rules of transformation as processes rather than the relationship between atomistic units and, *sixth*, allow for the introduction of purposiveness, consciousness, and symbolic processes into the study of the individual and society.[20]

(In this respect it is of interest to note that Lévi-Strauss pays equal attention to mathematical and linguistic rules of transformation which derive from information and communication theory.[21] Structures, in this sense, are decoded in qualitative rather than in quantitative terms. Similarly, structuralism corresponds to systems theory in its insistence that it is not only a theoretical programme but also a methodology.)

In its view of cognitive processes and the relationship between the inner and outer worlds, modern systems theory elevates the two principles of organization and communication to the status of master processes which are constantly transforming structures into newer levels. Consciousness is seen as not merely the reflection of the empirical world, but as partly responsible for, and constitutive of, that world. The key element here is the reciprocal interaction between men and other men in their construction of models of 'individuality' and 'social structure'. (These models have logical properties, but in the first instance they are constructed by men as part and parcel of their everyday concerns in the everyday world. It is only later that they are codified in social and psychological theory.) The great distinction between systems theory and structuralism is the latter's insistence that the appropriate rules of transformation are analogous to the decoding of structures, whereas systems theory does not give priority to structure in any one domain but insists on the mutuality of subjectivity and objectivity. In structuralism the subjective–objective dichotomy disappears when all structures are treated as being isomorphic to thought, whereas in systems theory both consciousness and social structure are envisaged as communicative processes without any priority being attributed to any one domain.

Whatever its merits, systems theory suffers from the primary defect when applied to sociocultural phenomena of utilizing a battery of concepts which owe their efficacy to mathematical applications in engineering and other applied sciences. The assumption of conceptual neutrality is a false one. In this sense, it is limited like all attempts to construct models of psychological and social phenomena in terms of a highly technical language; the language tends to achieve an autonomy of its own. Ultimately the world is not a differential equation, nor is it pure form. There is nothing intrinsically wrong in borrowing concepts from game, communication, and information theory provided one realizes that the translation from one frame of reference to another is only of value when the translation is recognized for its heuristic value rather than for its isomorphic correspondences. To use the organic metaphor is one thing, to construe society as an organism is another. To construe schemata purely in terms of computer programming has its attractions, but it leaves out and ignores a great deal: 'If a computer can serve as a model for a theory of the human brain this has nothing to do with the fact that they both work by electric impulses nor does it in the least justify the assertion that the brain is nothing other than a computer or that the artifact is nothing other than a thinking machine.'[22]

In our examination of some of the elements in the resurgence of interest in cognitive structuring we have assumed that structures are not static entities, but are somehow open to the world. With Piaget we have argued for a constructionist approach to the study of schemata and whatever our reservations about systems theory, we have assented to its insistence on the crucial importance of consciousness and communication in a theory of individual and social action. Similarly, I think we can accept Lévi-Strauss's structuralism without assenting to the proposition that 'content' is not the focus of inquiry in the social sciences or that social structure is isomorphic to thought processes. What we have really been doing, by implication, is reinstate the cardinal importance of some of the preconditioned aspects of social behaviour as expressed both in symbolic interaction and also in the construction of systems of meaning. We have avoided discussion of Chomsky's deep structures because by definition this would involve us in a detailed analysis of the formal structure of generative grammar. However, our interest in Chomsky is precisely in his rationalism and in his apparent commitment to nativism. Here the difficulty is how to describe and account for innate schemata. The answer is obviously one that only biologists can give, but as Piaget has argued: 'Contrary to the too facile explanations by conditioning, which imply that language acquisition starts as early as the second month, the acquisition of language presupposes the prior formation of sensori-motor intelligence, which goes to justify Chomsky's ideas concerning the necessity of a prelinguistic substrate akin to rationality. *But this intelligence which antedates speech is very far from preformed from the beginning; we can see it grow step by step out of the gradual coordination of assimilation schemes.*'[23] Piaget is of course arguing for a constructionist account of language acquisition, but he does not directly challenge Chomsky's prelinguistic substrate. Chomsky himself has argued against the 'indefinite plasticity' thesis implicit in so much contemporary learning theory. He believes that the neurological basis of learning is just as obscure and misunderstood as the apparent obscurity of a universal grammar. In general terms the whole question of preconditioned models is still very open, especially the whole question relating to their manifestation in symbolic contexts. Without doubt, it is Lévi-Strauss who has done most to pose the problem in social structural terms, even though we cannot accept his cognitive universalism.

There is another level of analysis which explicitly acknowledges the operation of implicit and unstated models and assumptions about man and society. We turn to this level of analysis in the final part of this paper.

III. PHENOMENOLOGY AND INTERPRETATIVE SOCIOLOGY

'Man is biologically predestined to construct and to inhabit a world with others. This world becomes for him the dominant and definite reality. Its limits are set by nature, but, once constructed, this world acts back upon nature. In the dialectic between nature and the socially constructed world the human organism itself is transformed. In this same dialectic man produces reality and thereby produces himself.'[24]

While Lévi-Strauss and Sartre have been on opposite sides of the fence in the debate about the role of the dialectical method in philosophy and history, this debate was conducted in the belief that the old categories of the Cartesian formula are no longer valid. For Lévi-Strauss they are meaningless anyway because structuralism is only concerned with formal analysis of schemata – content is a secondary consideration. In rejecting Cartesian dualism, structuralism reasserts the unity of science in the study of man and society. In this view man and his history have no privileged status and therefore are not the *subject* of science, nor do they have any meaning in any phenomenological sense. From an entirely different stance existential phenomenology also discards Cartesian dualism by insisting on relational facts, that is, it stresses that what is out there in the 'objective world' is only meaningful if it is a datum of human consciousness. In the social sciences this assumption is shared by those theorists who emphasize the ubiquity of the actor's definition of the situation. Peter Berger, for example, has tried to assimilate both the sociological and the phenomenological traditions in his attempt to construct a sociology of knowledge which reflects the continuous 'world-building activities' of men in interaction. Men create their own objects and in turn these objects create men – thus man is both in society and society is in man. It is precisely this insistence on meaning as being the pivot of social experience that is anathema to the structuralist position. However, when I say it is anathema to structuralism, I am aware that Merleau-Ponty does not altogether ignore structure or meaning, and that, despite his identification with phenomenology, he is not unresponsive to structuralism. Indeed, structure for Merleau-Ponty is precisely what we ascribe meaning to at the perceptual (phenomenal) level. He conceptualizes structures in three different ways, namely, the physical, the vital, and the human.[25] The physical corresponds to behavioural constancies as expressed in stimulus–response contingencies, the vital implies instinctual organismic needs, and the human involves 'signification' or the construction of meaning structures. All three structural levels are discoverable in human behaviour, but they are not reducible to each other. His critique of contemporary psychology and social science is that it tends to remain in the first two orders without really taking the human order seriously. It is in this respect that he prefers Weber to Durkheim because of the former's ability to interweave the themes of historical and human action in such a way that they are not reducible to each other.[26] Merleau-Ponty's treatment of social phenomena is reminiscent of the similar approach in 'interpretative sociology' deriving from the German school and symbolic interactionism. In this respect I think we can agree with Rabil that, in comparison with theorists like Husserl, Marcel, Heidegger, and Sartre, Merleau-Ponty conceives of the social world in terms of intersubjectivity rather than in a dynamic confrontation between subject and object. 'His is, in short, a social philosophy, a philosophy of intersubjectivity.'[27]

We can therefore look at the problem of submerged or hidden models at the level of phenomenological distortion. Currently, American sociology has been hit by a wave of theories emphasizing the precariousness of the 'of course world' in everyday interaction. Since Goffman[28] introduced his dramaturgical model in terms of the masking activities of actors trying to maintain 'fronts' at all costs, there has been a tendency to see all social conduct as a performance which is legitimated before audiences. Audiences evaluate and applaud certain performances – they attach labels to the performance. Ultimately all conduct is reduced to labelling and the attribution of motives. In addition, 'ethnomethodology' tears aside the veils of 'common sense' and finds that the constitutive rules of human interaction are not at all those believed in by the official definers, but rather that they are operational at the level of mundane everyday behaviour. The hidden models that social scientists attribute to men in society are therefore merely constructs that the social scientist employs to order his perceptions, they do not exist for men in the trivial encounters and episodes that they engage in. Hence the assumption of 'motives' which are hidden from the investigator is only plausible when we can demonstrate that they are not mere inventions to legitimate a research methodology or a conceptual scheme. The sociological-phenomenological reduction involves the sociologist in the literal abandonment of his concepts and a voyage of discovery into the 'common-sense world'. Sociologists are encouraged to undertake this voyage of discovery by losing their 'false consciousness' of their roles as official definers of the social world. Only then, presumably, will they be capable of teasing out the constitutive rules of interaction.[29]

IV. CONCLUSION

I have briefly examined some of the psychological, sociological, and philosophical components of the current resurgence of interest in structures, particularly those structures that are presumed *not* to be dependent on the stimulus–response paradigm. The kindling of interest in the black box in the social sciences is, of course, not unexpected, after the years in which both behaviourism and its operational ideology seemed to hold the citadels of academic social science. I have implied that, although heuristically it is still useful to categorize certain elements of experience in terms of the objective–subjective dichotomy, in the last analysis, such a distinction seems to be useless in the social sciences, in which men ascribe meaning to the world. However, it is precisely because they define the world symbolically that we can conceive of the mutuality of the experiencer and the experienced. For Lévi-Strauss it is *form* that is all-important, particularly those forms which are expressed in grammars and thus can be codified into social structures. The notion of the empty box is of course completely absent, and Locke's *tabula rasa* is just as inappropriate for structuralism as it is for existential phenomenology. The development of a sophisticated modern systems approach has tried to incorporate the mathematical theory of communication and game theory to reinstate consciousness in the social sciences. At the moment this remains a hope, not an accomplished fact. Its importance lies precisely in the attempt to relate structure to behaviour via the medium of language, but unfortunately language is lost in the process, it remains a mechanism and is not constitutive of social order. Perhaps Piaget's constructionism comes nearer than most attempts to bridging the gap between structures and process, but again this seems to me to be at the expense of meaning. The family of associated constructs such as schemata, attitudes, motives, images, plans, all point to the urgency of the search for a secure basis for cognitive psychology and sociology. In this connection it seems to me that the meeting of the European tradition (in the form of certain aspects of existential phenomenology and structuralism) and the American social-psychological tradition (in the form of symbolic interactionism) offers a possible resolution of the debate between the Lockean and Leibnizian positions.

REFERENCES

1 POLANYI, M. *Personal Knowledge: Toward a Post Critical Philosophy*, Chicago, University of Chicago Press, 1958.
2 HAMPDEN-TURNER, C. *Radical Man*, New York, Schenkman Publishing, 1970, p. 27.
3 FRIEDRICHS, R. *A Sociology of Sociology*, New York, The Free Press, 1970, p. 135.
4 TIRYAKIAN, C. A. 'The Existential Self and The Person' in *The Self in Social Interaction* edited Gordon, C. & Gergen, K. J. New York, Wiley, 1968.
5 CHOMSKY, N. 'Problems of Explanation in Linguistics', pp. 462–7 in *Explanations in the Behavioral Sciences*, edited Borger, R. & F. Cioffi, London, Cambridge University Press, 1970.
6 WALLACE, A. F. C. *Culture & Personality*, New York, Random House, 1970, p. 78.
7 RUNCIMAN, W. G. 'What is Structuralism', *Brit. J. Sociol.*, **20**, 1969.
8 SCHNEIDER, D. M. 'Some Muddles in the Models', p. 32 in *The Relevance of Models in Social Anthropology*, edited by Banton, M. London, Tavistock Publications, 1965.
9 MEADOWS, P. 'Models, Systems & Science', *American Sociological Review*, 1957.
10 PIAGET, J. *Structuralism*, pp. 140–1, London, Routledge & Kegan Paul, 1971.
11 WEINSTEIN, E. 'The Development of Interpersonal Competence', p. 755, in *Handbook of Socialization Theory and Research*, edited D. A. Goslin, New York, Rand McNally, 1969.
12 WEINSTEIN, E. op. cit.
13 BOULDING, K. *The Image*, University of Michigan, 1956.
14 MILLER, G. A., GALANTER, E., & PRIBRAM, K. H. *Plans and the Structure of Behaviour*, New York, Holt Dryden, 1960.
15 BLUMER, H. *Symbolic Interactionism*, New York, Prentice-Hall, 1969, p. 16.
16 KELLY, G. *The Psychology of Personal Constructs*, vol. 1, New York, Norton, 1955.
17 HEBB, D. O. *The Organization of Behavior*, New York, Wiley, 1949.
18 VON BERTALANFFY, L. 'General System Theory', p. 116 in *System, Change and Conflict* edited Demerath, M. J. & Peterson, R. A., New York, Free Press, 1967.
19 DEUTSCH, K. *The Nerves of Government*, New York, Free Press, 1966, p. 98.

20 BUCKLEY, W. *Sociology & Modern Systems Theory*, New York, Prentice-Hall, 1967.

21 LÉVI-STRAUSS, C. *Structural Anthropology*, New York, Basic Books, 1963

22 KAPLAN, A. *The Conduct of Inquiry*, San Francisco, Chandler, 1964, p. 258.

23 PIAGET, J. *Structuralism*, London, Routledge & Kegan Paul, 1971, p. 91.

24 BERGER, P. L. & LUCKMANN, T. *The Social Construction of Reality*, Allen Lane, the Penguin Press, 1967, p. 204.

25 MERLEAU-PONTY, M. *The Structure of Behaviour*, London, Methuen, 1965.

26 MERLEAU-PONTY, M. op. cit.

27 RABIL, A. *Merleau-Ponty*, Columbia University Press, 1967.

28 GOFFMAN, E. *The Presentation of Self in Everyday Life*. New York, Doubleday, 1959; London, Allen Lane.

29 GARFINKEL, H. *Studies in Ethnomethodology*, New York, Prentice-Hall, 1967.

The Social Sciences and their Impact on Society[1]

GUNNAR MYRDAL

I

The sociology of science and technology in general, and that of social science and social engineering in particular, is an under-developed discipline. In the almost total absence of research in this field, all we can do is to speculate, trying to put in some systematic order the impressions we have from our work and its practical impact on society. While this obviously entails the risk of going totally wrong or, at best, of only reaching conclusions that are less specific and determinate than the standards we ordinarily try to attain in our work, such speculation is nevertheless the beginning of the search for knowledge: it raises questions and formulates hypotheses for research.

Quite aside from this rationale, we who are professionally engaged in social sciences and technology – and who are not naïve about the meaning of what we are doing (that is, however, not unusual in our profession) – can hardly avoid speculating on the topic stated in the title I have chosen. Speaking for myself, this complex of problems has been a major preoccupation of my mind since my early youth, when curiosity about society and the urge to improve it first led me to the study of social facts and relationships. It has remained so for almost a lifetime of work in the field, interrupted even by brief excursions into the political arena, where the translation of ideas and knowledge into action for the welfare of society is supposed to take place. And I strongly believe that we social scientists and social engineers should ask ourselves this question: what difference does it make to policies and developments in our countries and in the world, if we can increase knowledge about society and liberate men's ideas from ignorance and irrational inhibitions? I should perhaps make clear before I begin that I will be speaking mainly as an economist, though trying to keep in mind the situation of my colleagues in the other social disciplines.

II

As social scientists we share with all fairly educated people in the world a general disturbing understanding that in our field of study progress is very much slower than in the natural sciences. It is their discoveries and inventions which are compelling radical changes in society, while ours, up till now, have been very much less consequential. There is spreading a creeping anxiety about the dangerous hiatus inherent in this contrast. While man's power over nature is increasing fast and, indeed, acceleratingly fast, man's control over society, which means in the first place over his own attitudes and institutions, is lagging far behind. In part, at least, this is due to a slower pace in the advance of our knowledge about man and his society, the knowledge that should be translated into action for social reform.

Let me, therefore, start out by raising the more fundamental question of why advance in the social sciences is so much slower than in the natural sciences. One possible explanation would be that the students of natural phenomena are brighter than we who labour in the social sciences. In the total absence of research on the selective processes by which people are channelled into one or the other field of research, we cannot exclude this possibility. Nothing succeeds like success, we know, and the very rapid advance in natural sciences, to which I also reckon medicine, definitely lends them prestige and glamour. Moreover, those who enter upon a career as students in those fields have the prospect of greater immaterial and material rewards, provided they have superior intelligence and are lucky.

The tremendous acceleration of advance in the natural sciences during the last two generations could, indeed, be expected to give rise to a vicious circle, in which ever smaller proportions of a nation's superlatively gifted young people entered the social sciences and ever larger proportions entered the natural sciences. As the inflow of genius in the natural sciences would rise, our intake of comparable quality would decline, and this would continually decrease further our chances of keeping pace with them.

I should not be honest with my audience if I did not confess that I have the impression that this is what has happened during my lifetime and is still happening. Our profession is swelling, even if not so fast as that of natural scientists and technologists; but it seems to recruit a rising share of mediocre students and, more important, attracts less of that small minority in every generation who are endowed with the rare combination of mental and physical stamina, will power, adventurousness, and high intelligence, that engenders radical departures from conventional approaches and produces great discoveries and inventions.

When I say this, I should add that it is merely a scientifically uncontrolled induction from the unassorted experiences gathered while living and working as a social scientist with many friends among the natural scientists. I might be wrong. Let me state that we don't need to be in doubt about the facts. Indeed, I consider it one of the many indications of the general dullness and relative absence of fresh departures in the pursuit of social sciences at present, that this important problem of the recruitment to the various sciences has not been investigated and, worse still, that the problem has usually not been recognized to exist.

I should also add that what I judge to be the present intellectual depression in the social sciences might be a passing conjuncture. The threatening trends of change in human affairs – I am thinking, for instance, of the nuclear and the less publicized chemical and biological armament race, of the pending hunger crisis in the underdeveloped countries, and in a country like the United States the rapid physical and moral deterioration of the cities and the rising temperature in interracial relations – might again attract more students of the adventurous, independent-minded, and highly intelligent type, whom we need in order to make radically new departures and generally to raise standards in our research.

III

But our less fortunate recruitment opportunities – if my hunch is correct – cannot be the only reason why the social sciences are lagging. The problems we deal with are truly more difficult to solve than those in the natural sciences. For one thing, we don't have the constants which, for instance, permit a physicist like Albert Einstein and, indeed, the whole profession of physicists, to make fundamental discoveries at their writing desks by simply applying mathematical reasoning to a limited number of ascertained facts.

If we economists, for instance, establish by observation the income or price demand elasticity for, say, sugar, it is valid for only one social group of consumers in a single community at a particular date – not to mention the fact that the concept itself loses what I call adequacy to reality and thereby analytical usefulness in underdeveloped countries that have no markets or only very imperfect ones.

In recent times there has been a strenuous and strained effort by many of my colleagues to emulate the methods of the natural sciences, though in constructing their simplified models they usually require only the elementary type of mathematics taught in high schools, at least in European high schools. Indeed, this is now the fashion in economics and increasingly also in the other social sciences which, in their turn, seek to emulate economics.

Fashion changes in a cyclical way in our field of study. My first visit to the United States as a young man coincided with the appearance of what was then called the 'new economics', or the institutional school. I foresee that in ten or fifteen years from now the institutional approach will again be the new vogue, and that the recent attempts to emulate the methods of the simpler natural sciences will be recognized as a temporary aberration into superficiality and irrelevance.

My reason for making this forecast is that the study of social facts and relationships really must concern much more complex and fluid matters than facts and relationships in nature. That in social study we do not have constants similar to those of the natural sciences is an indication of the deeper truth, that in our field human institutions and attitudes are prominent in the causal relationships. These phenomena can only very partially be represented by parameters and variables in simplified models of causal relationships; indeed, they are much more difficult even to observe and measure as facts.

This is true even in the highly developed countries where there are fairly perfect markets in the sense the economists give this term, implying that attitudes and institutions have been rationalized to the extent of permitting us to assume that they give free passage for social change or that they rapidly adjust to such change. But even in a country like Sweden, where this process of rationalization has gone further even than in the United States, it has, for instance, been demonstrated that mobility in the labour market and, still more, the prices of labour are less exclusively and simply dominated by demand and supply than model thinking has to assume.

The abstraction from attitudes and institutions, and also modes and levels of living, in the economic analysis of underdeveloped countries carried out in the simple aggregative terms of incomes, savings, employment, investment, and output, which is the ordinary procedure, leads to grossly inadequate and seriously biased inferences. After working for nine years on a study of the development problems in South Asia, I feel to my dismay that it is very much open to doubt whether the aid to planning given by the economic profession has helped more than it has hurt these unfortunate poor and backward new nations. The contribution of the other social sciences has up until now mostly been irrelevant and of little practical importance.

More generally, when in emulating the methods of natural science, we exclude from consideration everything related to the fact that human beings have a soul – and, specifically, that people live in a complex of institutions which manifest sharply differentiated combinations of changeability and rigidity, according to the attitudes that have been moulded by, at the same time as they support or react against, these institutions – this has led to a particularly dangerous type of superficiality in approach, namely, an unawareness of the assumptions upon which the analysis is based. When scrutinized by logical criticism, the reasoning of the model-builders, which is proudly paraded as in a particular degree 'strict', and 'rigid', is in reality found to be lacking in logical consistency as well as in adequacy to reality.

In other words, it is simply loose and muddled thinking, disguised in a straitjacket of pretended exactitude. It represents an approach which is greatly assisted psychologically by a naïveté in regard to the sociology and the philosophy of knowledge that has always characterized the social scientists and, in particular, the economists and which, in turn, is related to the fact that our sciences once emerged as branches of the metaphysical philosophies of natural law and utilitarianism and the simplicist hedonistic psychology. In order to free itself from these damaging legacies the new institutional approach in the social sciences, the emergence of which I look forward to, will, in fact, have to make a major effort to clarify concepts and improve the logic we employ in the social sciences. In a true sense, it will have to be more strict and rigid.

When I drafted this paper, I was just finishing the last part of my book on South Asian development problems which deals with the qualitative aspects of the population problem, health, and education. The chapter on health can, on the whole, be quite straightforward and simple in its approach, because health is a biological phenomenon and because there exists a medical science and a medical technology that is valid for all people and, for the most part indeed, even for animals. But no such exact science and technology of education exists and cannot, for reasons I have alluded to, ever be expected to exist. When in recent years economists belatedly became interested in education as a factor in economic development and, in the typical fashion of present-day social science, constructed simplified models in terms of 'investment in man', the exercise turned out – in my view – to be not even a formulation of the real problems in education to be solved by us social scientists, if we want to take due consideration of education as an important development factor.

IV

Another cause of greater difficulties in social research is related to the role of value premises for that research. It is true that, in principle, all scientific and technological work has to be based on value premises. But in the field of natural phenomena, the value premises are simple and *a priori* evident. Basic research can branch off in every direction where knowledge can be advanced; applied research has the simple criterion of profitability or, as in medical technology, the prevention of death and, prior to that, the prevention and cure of disease. This is not so in the social field where valuations are immensely diversified and anything but self-evident. In order to avoid biases in research and to make it 'objective' in the true sense, we need explicit and concrete value premises, not only to draw meaningful and correct practical, that is to say technological, inferences, but already in order to ascertain relevant facts and factual relationships.

I am here touching on the main methodological problem of the social sciences. Without being able in this brief paper to give reasons, I have to restrict myself to the assertion that there can never be, and has never been, a 'disinterested' research in the social field as there can be in physics or other natural sciences. Valuations enter into our work from start to finish even if we manage to be unaware of it; and this is true however much it is directed upon simply observing and recording the facts. A study of Negro voting in the southern parts of the USA is, in the cultural and political milieu of that country, confined within the value-loaded concept of discrimination. The fault is not that our approach in research is determined by valuations but that we fail to make ourselves and our readers aware of them by stating them as clear and explicit premises of that research. For otherwise we are drawing inferences with one set of premises missing. The value premises should not be defined arbitrarily but must be relevant and significant in the society under study.

The metaphysical philosophies from which the social sciences stemmed actually asserted that the valuations could themselves be objective; this was, indeed, the metaphysical element in these philosophies. Traditional social sciences have not broken away from this legacy of false thinking, which, of course, also dominates popular thinking everywhere. What social scientists have done is to conceal the valuations so deep at the base of their theoretical structures – and in the very terminology they use – that they can happily remain unaware of them in their researches, and believe that their inferences are merely factual. This implies also that the hidden valuations remain non-concretized, vague, and general. Consequently, whenever they are then used in such a way as to imply that they have been given a definite meaning, this meaning and the inferences drawn are unfounded and arbitrary. This is what I mean by saying that social scientists are quite commonly working with one set of premises too few.

Among the social scientists, the economists have in their so-called welfare theory provided themselves with a vast and elaborate coverture for their escape from the responsibility to state, simply and straight-forwardly, their value premises – a 'monumentally unsuccessful exercise . . . which has preoccupied a whole generation of economists with a dead end, to the almost total neglect of the major problems of our age', to quote a recent statement by Kenneth E. Boulding.[2] It grows like a cancerous tumour; hundreds of books and articles are continuously produced every year on welfare economics, though the whole approach was proved to be misdirected and meaningless at least three decades ago. We should note that this recent flourishing of welfare economics is closely related to the growing predilection for hyper-abstract models: among their implicit and not sufficiently scrutinized assumptions, and sometimes even in their explicit superstructures, the objectified welfare conception almost always plays a major role.

An institutional approach, which gives due importance to people's attitudes and institutions, cannot so easily escape the valuations that are at the same time objects of research and implied as premises in research.

v

These main difficulties in social research – that it must concern attitudes and institutions which in a complex way combine changeability and rigidity, that we therefore have no constants as in the natural sciences, and that valuations enter into research from the beginning to the end – and the escapist ways we have tried to bypass these difficulties, are not unrelated to the fact that so very little stands out as undisputed truth in our findings. In regard to all problems there are schools of thought with different gospels, among which the politicians and the citizens at large can choose according to their predilections. It has even become a popular stereotype that economists never agree; if the same view is not so commonly expressed about the other social scientists, it is only because people apparently care less about what they are saying.

When more than sixty years ago Knut Wicksell, now recognized as the great economist of his time, gave his installation lecture on the occasion of his ascendancy to the chair in economics at Lund University, he began by stating that economics, 'like theology and for approximately the same reasons', had failed to arrive at generally accepted results. It is true, he pointed out, that the history of all sciences is a history of controversy. But in the natural sciences such warfare of ideas usually leads to a definite outcome. Theories are refuted, hypotheses become obsolete, the frontiers of knowledge are pushed forward.

'The Copernican idea of the universe, the Newtonian system, the theory of blood circulation, and the phlogiston theory in chemistry once found both adherents and opponents. Nowadays these theories are either universally believed or disbelieved – provided, in the latter instance, that they have not simply been forgotten.'[3] In economics, on the contrary, *all* doctrines live on persistently. No new theories ever completely supplant the old. He gave examples that are all equally relevant today.

Wicksell, as a faithful and almost religious believer in hedonistic psychology and utilitarian moral philosophy, saw the explanation for this unfortunate situation in the fact that we had not succeeded in measuring 'utility'. If such a thing existed I believe we should concede that he was right: by measuring it we would advance to the same situation as the natural sciences, have constants, and be able to solve all our difficulties in terms of the maximization of welfare.

But this is exactly what we have not been able to do and never will be able to do, because there is this inescapable logical defect in the very concepts of utility and welfare that 'pleasures' and 'pains' of people cannot be gauged by a single measuring rod. The only way of defending objectivity in research, avoiding biases and arbitrariness, and dissolving the irrational controversies, is to work with explicit, often alternative, specific value premises that are relevant and significant.

Another great economist in the past, Karl Menger, once pointed out, however, that, in a sense and to an extent, the gifted student is superior to his methods. Our situation in the social sciences would otherwise be much worse than it already is. In fact, we see all around us important findings of great practical importance being reached by students whose fundamental notions of methodology are faulty and confused. One of Wicksell's own contributions was, as we know, his early formulation, at the beginning of this century, of the theory we now refer to as Keynes's, which explains why we in Sweden, who had been exposed to that theory already in our undergraduate studies, were a little ahead of the rest of the world in regard to the methods of fighting the Great Depression in the thirties. That theory is one of the major examples of important ideas and knowledge that to our great advantage are now generally translated into action –·recently and, on the whole, with ever more important practical effects even in the United States.

Much more generally our knowledge of social facts and relationships *is* advancing, though not as rapidly as we would wish. The very fact that we are dealing with social data in the rational terms of cause and effect and means and ends implies, in so far as our ways of thinking through education and other media are influencing popular thinking, a gradual liberation of people's preparedness to take action in order to improve society.

VI

Not only is knowledge in the social field so much harder to acquire than in the natural sciences; its translation into action for the welfare of society is a much more cumbersome process. Usually the invention of a new production technology, often founded upon a discovery reached by basic research, can rather easily be evaluated in terms of costs or the saleability of improved or entirely new products or services. There are in the ordinary case private entrepreneurs eager to make a profit by exploiting the invention; when the state enters the field it evaluates an invention in the same simple and, in a sense, objective, way. Rather effortlessly advances in natural sciences and technologies thus become translated into action for the welfare of society. As a matter of fact, both private industries and the state are themselves active by initiating and financing research which they expect to exploit to their advantage.

Our discoveries and inventions in the social field must generally be applied by the collectivities, i.e. in the first place the state and subordinate public communities. They must become public policies, accepted by those who have the power to determine the actions or non-actions of these collectivities. Ordinarily these people have their preconceived ideas. No less ordinarily, these ideas are founded on what they experience as their interests, which might be shortsighted or even erroneous, aside from the fact that they do not necessarily or even commonly coincide with what would stand out as the public interest of ordinary people if they were all alert and rational; this is what we call 'vested interests'. And those in power have not the same respect for the social engineers as everybody has for the technical engineers. They all have their own social theories; and the fact that social scientists so often disagree among themselves increases the self-assurance of the policymakers and provides them, in addition, with the opportunity to quote authority to support their own preconceptions.

When we want our ideas and knowledge translated into action for the welfare of society we have therefore, first, to convince our colleagues, so that we can form a fairly united front and, second, to win enough support in the lay society for the social reforms that can embody our inventions. These special duties laid upon us social scientists and technologists have little or no correspondence in the field of the natural sciences and technologies. In the latter field unanimity about what is truth follows naturally and rapidly after discovery, and there is little need to convert people to the willingness of utilizing the inventions for their own benefit.

This special position of social scientists and technologists has, in the great tradition, particularly perhaps in economics, generally been accepted as a challenge. We have spared time to explain our main findings in simple terms that laymen can understand. We have formulated our practical policy conclusions in equally simple terms, and tried to impress them upon those forming policies. The final acceptance only in the sixties of the Wicksell-Keynes theory as guidance for United States economic policy demonstrates what a long struggle we have to wage in order to have our ideas and knowledge translated into action. But it also shows that that struggle can be won, even if it takes time and effort.

At this point I have to note with regret how in recent decades economists and social scientists generally have shown a tendency to abandon the tradition, adhered to through generations by even the greatest scholars, that they have a responsibility for the formation of public opinion. They are increasingly addressing only each other. Using knowledge to enlighten the people is not encouraged: young men learn that this might lower their standing and chances for advancement in the profession. They exhibit an unhealthy interest in research techniques for their own sake; they avoid taking up politically controversial issues for study; or they focus such studies on terminology, methods of measurement, and similar other-worldly problems.

Fundamentally this is escapism, even if they convince themselves and each other that it establishes them on a higher level of scientism. The price society pays is that the social scientists become less consequential. When that pattern once becomes established, it lays a wall of inhibition on those who win entrance to our profession, limiting not only their usefulness to society but even, I believe, their research horizon.

Thus, with a few exceptions, neither the professional economists nor the sociologists had much to do with the rather recent and belated raising to political importance of the issue of pathological poverty in the United States, the rapid deterioration of the cities, the threat of intensified racial conflicts, and other developments within the same complex of social maladjustments. Partly the trends were not seen and studied; partly those few students who saw the writing on the wall were not listened to, which, in turn, did not encourage them or the others to make these problems a major field of study.

Again, when the superstitious doctrine of budget-balancing was broken by political action, and when we now see many equally superstitious ideas related to that fatal metal, gold, gradually losing their grip over Congress and the people, publicists, enlightened businessmen, and politicians were in the end more important in causing the break with inherited faith than the many thousands of university economists in the United States.

I should make the qualification that even in our time there have been a few professors, like Alvin Hanson and Kenneth Galbraith, who have devoted time to enlightening the general public and then not evaded, but sought out, the issues of needed economic and social reforms. Undoubtedly their writings, and a general educational influence from the teaching of the social sciences in colleges and universities, has had importance both for activizing individuals in the categories mentioned who have been more directly pressing for the reforms and also for preparing the general public for their acceptance. But the reforms matured very much too slowly and are more imperfect, than would be needed in our society, which is changing with explosive rapidity, often in directions creating new and bigger maladjustments.[4]

NOTES AND REFERENCES

1 A shortened version of a lecture delivered at the occasion of the Fifteenth Anniversary Celebration of the School of Applied Social Sciences, Western Reserve University, Cleveland, Ohio, 29 September–1 October 1966.
2 'The Economics of Knowledge and the Knowledge of Economics', *American Economic Review, Papers and Proceedings*, **56**, (2), May 1966, p. 12.
3 *Ekonomisk Tidskrift*, 1904, pp. 457 ff.
4 In the subsequent deleted part, the article deals with the specific issue of the United States. A passage of a more general nature provided a more optimistic afternote to the bulk of the paper. 'When I observe from a distance the present trends of policy formation as well as public opinion in the United States, I feel that attitudes and institutions are now changing ever more rapidly, on the whole in the direction of reason and the inherited ideals I referred to, although there is much resistance and double-think. The social scientists and the social engineers have a role to play in this development and may be beginning to play it more effectively. If we are lagging far behind our colleagues in the field of the natural sciences and technology, we are equally far ahead of public opinion. With all the faults of our approach to social problems, which I have hinted at, we are in that sense rationalistic: we are, as I said, thinking in terms of cause and effect and of means and ends. As soon as we face a social problem, we are by logical necessity planners, producing plans for induced changes. We might not have many "inventions" in the narrow sense of that term to offer, but as spreaders of rationalism and, therefore, of the preparedness for planning, we play our role. And we will do it more effectively if we become less timid about tackling practical problems and less prone to escape into scientism.'

© *Gunnar Myrdal 1972*

Science and Alchemy

BRIAN GOODWIN

Few would now deny that we in the West have lost our sense of meaning; that the old symbols and ceremonies that once carried us into and beyond ourselves to a world of numinous significance no longer perform their function. This loss has been hailed by some as a liberation from delusion, by others as a tragic loss of sense of destiny. Scientists on the whole have seen the process as a release of man's consciousness from subservience to false gods and a turning towards the truth. The gods have been revealed as fraudulent because they are seen to be projections of man's psyche, not external beings at all. The truth can be discovered, according to current scientific consensus, only by a total withdrawal of all psychical projections on the world and a pure perception of natural phenomena, uncontaminated by psychological, subjective elements. Someone or something capable of pure perception of this kind defines the ideal scientific observer, the disinterested spectator, the witness of objective truth.

I believe that the concept of the disinterested human observer is a contradiction in terms; that it is a sterile foundation for the scientific enterprise and leads, because of its self-contradictory nature, to paradox; and that it is essentially amoral. However, there is a curious inevitablity about the development of this scientific ideal in Western thinking. Furthermore the essentially heretical nature of the concept, by carrying us to the brink of an abyss, releases the energy for a reaction that could carry us back towards a more adequate conception of the human being's search for understanding. This conception should restore man's sense of meaning and at the same time release science from an ultimately destructive inconsistency. In this essay I would like to explore some strands of thought discernible in the medieval science of alchemy which show interesting parallels to the present state of scientific metaphysics and also provide indications of how the contemporary dilemma, as I see it, might be resolved.

THE CONFLICT OF OPPOSITES

Two intertwined components of human endeavour lie at the centre of the dilemma that I would like to consider. In a philosophical context, these aspects of mind give rise to the epistemological problem on the one hand and the moral problem on the other. In more immediate terms, we may refer to them as the domains of knowledge and of meaning. Our heritage splits cleanly in two on these domains: the Greeks were very strong on knowledge, but weak on meaning; while the Hebrews had little time for epistemology, but filled the world with such a vision and sense of meaning that it is only now growing dim. Of course these aspects of mind are never separated from one another. But one can grow at the expense of the other, driving it underground, stifling it, as has now happened in our overdevelopnent of the Greek rationalist tradition. The endless human struggle is to keep them in balance and harmony so that they strengthen one another. Because of the extreme polarity inherent in our heritage, we have been presented with the dilemma in a particularly acute form. This conflict of opposites has resulted in the liberation of quite extraordinary amounts of physical and psychical energy in the West, a restlessness reflecting the failure to resolve and harmonize the strands of mental activity which has carried us with startling speed into a new age. This new age has dawned primarily as a result of the development of science. Since this age, with its new image of ourselves and the world, has grown out of a conflict, one might expect that the seeds of the resolution would be inherent in the present situation, the synthesis emerging from the dialectical confrontation of the opposites. I believe this to be the case, but it is of course exceedingly difficult to pick out relevant contemporary movements. That there is a general and growing disillusion with science and technology is evident; but where the resolution lies is not clear. It is easier to look for some historical antecedents and parallels, possibly picking up a thread that could help to unravel the present tangle and so release once again man's creative potential in a new synthesis of knowledge and meaning, a new understanding and vision.

THE ALCHEMICAL SYNTHESIS

The application of knowledge leads to power; the application of meaning leads to wisdom. One of these without the other is always dangerous. Use of power without wisdom is such a familiar abuse that little need be said about it. We are at the beginning of a debate on this issue in relation to the conflict between technological innovation and preservation of the natural order. Wisdom without power, on the other hand, is so unfamiliar to us that it often seems eminently desirable, and indeed it is enthusiastically embraced by the social out-groups who have renounced Western political and social institutions, the hippies being the most dramatic example. Total renunciation of power and absorption into a state of permanent vision, contemplation, and experience of meaning, is the image we have of Eastern, particularly Buddhist, wisdom. Believers in the Western way of life condemn this as irresponsible; and so, I believe, would the Jewish prophets, absorbed as they were with God's role in history as lawgiver and the problems of individual and social morality. Solomon was wise because he applied the law with insight and understanding. He would not have been regarded as wise if he had not applied his vision of meaning to the conduct of human affairs.

Essentially the same tension between power and wisdom is present in the alchemical tradition. The alchemist believed that the meaning of life was hidden, but could be perceived and experienced if one adopted the right attitude of mind and performed the right actions. The most singular and interesting aspect of this art is that the actions which the practitioner was called upon to perform were not simply moral exercises and ethical taboos such as one finds in most mystical cults; the alchemist was required to bring about transformation of the world, of matter and spirit, at the same time as he underwent moral transformation himself. He was called upon to participate in the changes of substance that took place in his retort; indeed, it was stated explicitly that unless he so participated in transformation, becoming himself more refined and pure as did his material, from oxide of mercury to gleaming silver metal and, ultimately, to gold, then the physical changes would not themselves take place. A passage in the *Musaeum Hermeticum* (1678) states that 'the mind must be in harmony with the work'. Another passage has it that to acquire the 'golden understanding one must keep the eyes of the mind and soul well open, observing and contemplating by means of that inner light which God has lit in nature and in our hearts from the beginning'. The essence of the alchemical process is thus quite clearly a two-way relationship between the adept and nature, both undergoing transformation together as occurs in a true dialogue. The basis of this relationship was the belief that nature has an innate tendency to seek a state of perfection, matter transforming into immortal, imperishable gold. Likewise man has a longing for perfection. He can thus learn from nature and at the same time assist her in her striving.

The contemporary image of the alchemist as one who was concerned solely with the use of magical formulae to turn lead, copper, iron, and other lower metals into gold, thus achieving riches and power, is a materialist travesty of the most extraordinary proportions. It is roughly equivalent to the view that the pinnacle of achievement of the scientific tradition was the development of the atomic bomb, the transformation of matter into energy, and its use in the destruction of Nagasaki and Hiroshima. The current misconception of alchemy is due to the fact that it was vigorously discredited as heretical by the Church throughout the Middle Ages and the Renaissance because, like all mystical cults, it believed that God should be experienced, not simply believed in by the faithful; and because of its own ultimate failure to resolve the tensions between knowledge and meaning, the tradition foundering under an accretion of ambiguous symbolism and virtually impenetrable jargon. Once a tradition fails, dies, and is discredited, it takes some devoted scholarship to rediscover its sources and significance. This has been provided in our time largely by the efforts and insights of C. G. Jung, who was led to the meaning of alchemical allegories via the analysis of dreams recorded by his patients, and through a comparative study of mythological and religious symbolism. His books *Psychology and Alchemy* and *Mysterium*

Coniunctionis (volumes 12 and 14 of his collected works, Bollingen Series XX) are masterpieces of inspired scholarship. Balanced accounts of the alchemical tradition can now be found in other volumes as well, such as Kurt Seligmann's *History of Magic* 1948). There is also a great deal of insight into the significance of Oriental alchemy and its influence in Eastern and Western thought in Needham's superb volumes on *Science and Civilization in China.*

The aspect of alchemy that is so central to the present inquiry is the fact that this tradition attempted to fuse knowledge and meaning by combining science (scientia, knowledge), the study of natural process, with morality, man's attempt to realize his own perfectibility and self-fulfilment, itself a continuous process. The difficulties inherent in such a fusion are legion. The use of alchemical knowledge without its transformational moral meaning resulted in the magical manipulation of nature for purposes of power, with the inevitable consequences of such perversion as described in the Faust legend. The pursuit of meaning, the experience of moral fulfilment, without application to the world and hence without the responsibility and compassion we recognize as manifestations of wisdom, resulted in total withdrawal from the human condition and a proliferation of elaborate, impenetrable symbolism and verbiage. Contemporary science has essentially chosen the course of knowledge and power, split off from meaning and morality because knowledge has become an end in itself. Scientists today do not expect to be morally transformed by their activities. They do not, in fact, participate in a relationship with the world that acknowledges the autonomy and the ultimate inviolability of natural processes, the condition for a dialogue with nature, which has now become something to be penetrated, known, and controlled. Participation in a process of mutual transformation is in fact expressly ruled out by the contemporary ideal of objective observation, preferably by a machine which cannot change its state except in response to the particular events which it is designed to record. The knowledge so obtained is regarded as neutral, without moral 'contaminants'. It can be used beneficently or malevolently, but it is always used to exercise control over the world, certainly not to transform oneself. Thus science as we know it today has largely opted to pursue the course of manipulation and power, drawing us inevitably into a Faustian crisis which arises from the irreconcilability of manipulation and wisdom. To manipulate wisely one must be wiser than nature, wiser than man, for both must be manipulated; hence one must be God. Faust found that only the Devil would play this game with him, tempt this hubris. The corruption arises with the decision to manipulate rather than to engage in a dialogue, the decision to be master rather than partner.

THE SCIENTIFIC HERESY

What, then is the alternative to the dominant contemporary attitude in science? How can one redefine the scientific enterprise so that it is coupled with the search for meaning and wisdom, not just the acquisition of knowledge and power? In what way is it possible for us to participate in this enterprise so that we may be transformed morally in the process of learning about the world? In seeking tentative answers to these questions it is instructive to try to follow the development of the essentially heretical concept of the objective observer, the amoral, non-participating agent, to its point of self-impalement on its own inconsistencies.

There is in fact a remnant of the ethical attitude in science which persists in the form of a commitment to the search for truth. However, this truth has become so refined in its meaning and significance, so intellectualized and divided from experience, that its moral force has been severely attenuated. To the alchemist the truth was revealed when he had achieved a union of soul and mind, of meaning and knowledge, and its symbol was gold, living gold, which he experienced within himself. Only then would he see in his crucible, the Hermetic vessel, gold emerging from the impure ingredients of the starting material as a sign that his own transformation had been achieved. There is no doubt that hallucinatory states and visions accompanied these experiences of transformation, visions that would be generally discounted now as highly subjective phenomena having not only nothing to contribute to scientific insight, but definitely detracting from it. And it is certainly true that the domain of trance and hallucination is dangerous in the extreme, bordering on total dissociation, a breaking of the dialogue. The proliferation of elaborate allegorical and

symbolic descriptions of psychical states and the extreme confusion and deliberate mystification found in many alchemical texts
is evidence that the Hermetic tradition was losing its way in the
psychological jungle, was not always finding the universal symbols
required for the communication of meaning. Despite some very
penetrating insights into the structure of physical inner space,
documented in detail by Jung in his volumes, alchemy was
ultimately overwhelmed by the richness and inherent difficulty of its
own subject-matter.

Empirical science in the seventeenth century turned its back
firmly on this most elusive domain of inquiry, regarding the insights as phantasmagoria and repudiating them as being without
value in the exploration of the world of 'fact' and 'reality'. Galileo's
science made extensive use of observation and experimental test,
providing criteria of universality that must have burst like a
revelation upon minds struggling with the interminable ramblings
of medieval scholasticism or the obscurities of alchemical allegories. There seemed to be nothing firm in these voyages of the
mind, no 'objectivity'. Lacking adequate procedures of classification and analysis, the exploration of inner space, of the psychological process, was first abandoned and then deliberately
excluded as a domain of scientific inquiry by the Galilean tradition,
which eliminated qualities from its world of investigation, retaining only quantifiable observables. Man's role in scientific discovery became that of the pure observer, distilling the truth in
ever more refined form from his observations and measurements.
Providing the correct procedure was followed, this truth would be
automatically revealed to man; he played no creative part in the
process. That is to say, what was revealed to the scientist was not
just human truth, but universal truth. The same truth would be
revealed to any other intelligence. Man could thus in effect step
right outside of nature and become the perfect observer, not inter-
fering in any way with natural process, much less participating
in it. In the past, only God was considered to be in a position to
do this if he chose. Small wonder the scientist felt himself to be
in a rather powerful position.

THE OBSERVER OBSERVED

This situation in science has now broken down for two reasons. The first has arisen within science itself. Observation *does* perturb microphysical states, because observation is perturbation. It is negligible only in macrophysical processes, where the mass and energy of the observed system is very much greater than that of the observing wave packet. This recognition gives us the uncertainty principle, satisfactory as far as it goes.

But there is within physics the unresolved problem how to describe the process of measurement itself: how microstates 'collapse' into unique, singular events in the macro-world. Classical or macrophysics did manage to describe the process of measurement in terms of a well-defined observer; but the situation in physics today is thoroughly unsatisfactory, with an arbitrary and so far unbridged gap between the micro- and the macroworlds.

Thus the postulate of the perfect observer has broken down within physics itself. But it has been under severe attack also in studies on the philosophy and psychology of science. The very notion of scientific truth as a unitary concept is disappearing. There are points of view and theories arising from them, defined by paradigms (Kuhn, 1962). Different points of view are in conflict at any one time, as illustrated for example in Kearney's (1971) recent study of the scientific revolution in the sixteenth and seventeenth centuries. Sometimes one view will dominate and eliminate another; or they may become fused in a unitary, higher-order theory, such as the wave–particle duality of modern physics. In the light of this dawning self-consciousness, the scientific enterprise may be about to enter an era of altogether greater sophistication, versatility, and creativity, with scientists becoming aware of the metaphysical assumptions which underlie the viewpoint they are holding at any moment in their development as scientists and as human beings. A similar rather dramatic increase in consciousness has occurred in the arts only in this century, with the development of what Malraux (1953) has called the museum without walls, the work of the art historian, which allows us to see works of art as a part of the panoramic unfolding of man's history. The Lascaux cave paintings or the Ashanti woodcarving can now be seen and experienced with every bit as much validity and meaning as work by Moore or Picasso. Science is about to cross this threshold as well, to be seen and understood in the context of cultural and intellectual history, as Collingwood (1945) predicted. The focus here is man's dialogue with his fellow men and with nature, his attempt to understand himself and his world.

The subjective element can thus return to science, but within a higher level of consciousness, the scientist becoming aware of the role he is playing in presenting or supporting one viewpoint rather than another. The objection to subjective factors in scientific work in the past has always been based upon the assumption that they were unconscious factors, hence distorting, irrational, i.e. they were unconscious projections. But if one is aware of one's viewpoint and the way it is moulding one's thinking and theorizing about a particular problem, this objection is largely overcome. Furthermore, this awareness allows one to transcend the limitations and constraints that accompany the belief in 'objective truth'. This belief can now be seen as a particular metaphysical commitment based upon a set of assumptions about the nature of observation and measurement, assumptions which themselves lead to unresolved paradoxes in physics. Axioms which lead to inconsistencies cease to be convincing or compelling. The recognition that the human being plays a central role in constructing an image of himself and his world and that these images or internal models or sets of hypotheses are conditioned both by internal (psychical) and by external factors provides a degree of freedom which could liberate human creative potential in a dramatic manner, as has occurred in the arts with the dropping of the representational norm, while simultaneously engaging his ethical responsibilities in relation to this freedom. At the same time this recognition might lead to the resolution of paradoxes which have arisen from the adoption of unnecessary assumptions about the nature of scientific investigation.

These must seem rather grandiose claims and need more detailed elaboration than can be provided in this essay. The contention is twofold: (1) The recognition of man as a creative agent who participates positively and with a degree of freedom in the construction of images of himself and the world imposes a responsibility upon him with respect to his reasons for choosing one image rather than another, and can thus lead to moral involvement in the scientific process; and (2) The realization that Man the Observer is in fact Man the Selector, seeing what he is prepared and able to see, conditioned as he is by his viewpoint, his hypotheses, eliminates the concept of the objective observer and so may lead to a more satisfactory account of the measurement process. The system observes what it is prepared to observe, in the same way that if one constructs a trap for a particle one catches a particle; if for a wave, one catches a wave. This is by no means an original suggestion, having been made and elaborated in some detail by Eddington many years ago, and developed more recently by Bastin & Kilmister (1954; see also Bastin, 1966) and others. I am not in the least competent to develop this argument, which has not yet succeeded in resolving the difficulties inherent in the relation between quantum theory and macrophysics. However, in a biological context, where I am somewhat more competent to assess the possible transforming power of new attitudes, the view of the organism as an hypothesis-generating and testing system is potentially very powerful. In the study of artificial intelligence there is currently an active investigation of the exact meaning which is to be assigned to the proposal that a primary function of mind is the generation of images, models, hypotheses about its environment, and the analysis of its consequences in epistemology and metaphysics. The exploration of the implications of looking upon all organisms as hypothesis-testing systems has not yet, however, begun. It could transform biology by placing model construction and observation at the centre of the biological process, not at the evolutionary periphery, the phenomenon of mind.

ORGANISM AND HYPOTHESIS

Let me elaborate this approach by a consideration of some of its consequences. I am particularly concerned to explore the possibility of resolving some classical antinomies and their modern counterparts by means of a change of context. One of the most celebrated of these conflicts was that between Aristotle and Hippocrates, an atomist, on the nature of the formative influences which are responsible for the generation of characteristic structure and behaviour in organisms. Hippocrates contended that the general similarity of static and dynamic form between parents and offspring was due to the transmission of specific substances from parental organs, carried by the seminal fluid, to the embryo. His position was clear, straightforward, and entirely materialistic: specific structure is transmitted by specific substances. The modern version of this theory is equally clear and unambiguous: the resemblance between parents and offspring arises in consequence of the transmission of specific genes, the hereditary units, from one generation to the next. It is the dominant view in biology today and preserves in remarkably pure form the traditional position of the Greek atomists. It appears so self-evident to the modern scientific mind that the difficulties of this position are often not even considered; or else these difficulties are dismissed in somewhat cavalier fashion by means of the additional principle that all one needs to add to it is the concept of interaction between the units, the genes, to complete the picture.

The fact that the same position in physics gave rise to the still unsolved many-body problem is not regarded as a warning of limitation; it is simply a hurdle to be jumped when necessary, with the help of a rather large computer presumably.

Aristotle's objections to the atomist position are both simple and cogent, but his own explanation presented some equally difficult problems. How, asked Aristotle, could a young man without a beard transmit to a son the substance required to grow a beard if that substance had to come from the beard itself? Or how could a man who had lost his hands in battle, say, nevertheless transmit the capacity to form hands in his offspring? The problem here is that between potential generative capacity and the realization of that potential. What substance can carry such potential? Aristotle contended that from substance alone one cannot make deductions about form; that knowing the composition of something is not sufficient to determine its structure, a position he inherited from Pythagoras. One must add to substance a principle of organization, which for Aristotle was a form or an idea, immanent in the process whereby order of a characteristic type emerges from disorder or lower order, as the embryo from the egg. Plato considered such ideas to be transcendental and autonomous, but for Aristotle the forms were sources of energy in matter striving to organize it in some perfect order which was the final goal, the telos, of the process.

What answer do we have today to this problem of the emergence of order, particularly that of creative, novel, order? As I have said, contemporary atomists ascribe the emergence of order to some principle of interaction between the parts of which the entity is made. This is a perfectly consistent and satisfactory idea as far as it goes. But so far it has yielded adequate solutions to simple interactions only, such as two-body problems, for example the motion of a planet around the sun; or to statistical regularities which arise from weak, uniform interactions between very many units, such as the ideal gas laws. This hardly seems a promising approach to the intricate organization of living systems, let alone their creative behaviour. But Aristotle fails us in this respect as well, for we want to know more about his forms or ideas. How are we to understand their nature and their operation?

To suggest that an answer to this problem may be inspired by studies on the nature and origin of scientific theories such as those of Kuhn may seem somewhat far-fetched, but let us consider where such a path may lead us. Suppose we regard living organisms as systems which generate and test hypotheses about their environment. At the psychological level this has fairly direct intuitive meaning. But what would it mean about a bacterium? It would mean that such a system has a set of hypotheses which are present in coded, symbolic form in order to satisfy our intuition about the nature of hypotheses; that these must be subject to variation and test in relation to an external world; and that there must be some principle of correspondence whereby 'good' hypotheses about this world can be retained and stored while 'bad' ones are discarded. It is probably evident to the reader that the obvious candidates for such hypotheses are the genes, or more generally the hereditary material of the bacterium.

This genetic information is in symbolic form; i.e. it cannot interact directly with the external 'world' of nutrients, salts, oxygen, etc., which define the environment of the bacterium. It has to be translated into another language, generally that of proteins, before interaction and testing can occur. A bacterium carrying the genetic information for the metabolic utilization of the sugar lactose, known as the lactose operon, may be said to carry the hypothesis that lactose is likely to be encountered in its world, and that this substance can be transformed in a particular way to provide energy and building blocks for growth. At a more complicated level, we may say that in the chromosomes of the egg there are hypotheses about the appropriate response of a cell in the ectoderm which is required to transform into part of the lens of the eye when it encounters a cell in the underlying optic cup.

Evidently by using the language of hypotheses and hypothesis-testing I am not providing any kind of an explanation for the phenomena under consideration. I am simply redescribing them, in a different context. However, the potential value of a new context is that it may virtually do away with old antinomies. It will certainly introduce new ones, but if the context is of value, these new dilemmas will occur at a higher level than the old. What possible value is there in regarding organisms as hypothesis-generating and testing systems? There are three consequences which occur to me immediately. The first is a suggested resolution of the atomist–idealist conflict. Hippocrates and Aristotle were both partly right, as they must have been for this argument to survive so long. Hippocrates and the atomists were correct to maintain that there are distinct substances which are transmitted from generation to generation and that the composition of the system is a very important aspect of its structure. Aristotle was correct to insist that something like formative 'ideas', different in some sense from ordinary physical matter, must guide the intricate and extraordinarily varied formative processes of organic nature. We now recognize this difference to lie in the symbolic nature of the genetic code and the remarkably elaborate system cells have for its translation. It is genetic symbolism that enables living matter to step outside of the constraints imposed by physical laws formulated in terms of minimal potential criteria. The primary structure of a protein is not, for example, determined by a condition of minimum free energy. It is determined by the sequence of bases in its corresponding gene or cistron. And this is determined by some organismic criterion of successful performance of the protein in interaction with its environment. The symbolic nature of the genetic material is what provides a virtually inexhaustible reservoir of potential genetic states for evolution, since symbols can be juxtaposed in very many different ways to provide new 'statements', new hypotheses, which can then be tested.

The second obvious result of looking at organisms in this way is the possibility of transcending a conflict that has arisen regarding the importance of genes in determining a process such as embryonic development. That the hereditary material is of the greatest significance no one will dispute. But it has been claimed that knowing the information in the genes is equivalent to knowing the embryological process, for example. Considering the hereditary material as a set of hypotheses immediately puts the genes in their proper place. For it is evident that a hypothesis is always considerably less than a total set of instructions for its interpretation and test, without which the hypothesis is useless. If a person says that he holds the hypothesis that there is life on Mars, then he is assuming a very great deal of knowledge on the part of the person to whom he is speaking. Quite apart from the basic assumption that the hearer is competent to interpret the sentence grammatically, extensive experience of the world is also taken for granted: that there is an actual entity located in a defined position known as Mars, that the hypothesis has some meaning, e.g. that there is some possible relationship between life and Mars; that there are ways of testing this meaning, etc. In like manner, the gene in the lactose operon which codes for the particular enzyme known as the lactose permease is taking for granted a great deal about the pre-existent structure and activity of the cell. If there were no cell surface, for example, no membrane, the genetic 'statement' would be meaningless, uninterpretable. So the hereditary material speaks to a competent hearer, and assumes that it can interpret and test the hypotheses it is presenting in some manner that will establish whether or not they have meaning.

And, third, this context provides a natural and immediate framework for comparison of different levels of organization of the biological process. It is intuitively evident that, at the level of mind, hypotheses are subject to continuous alterations as a result of experience, a testing of their relevance and meaning.

In contrast, within the lifespan of any single organism, genetic hypotheses cannot, according to current theory, be so altered or improved. An organism inherits a fixed set of hypotheses and its life may be viewed as an unfolding of strategies consistent with these constraints. The genetic hypotheses are subject to alteration from generation to generation, of course, by a process which neo-Darwinian theory ascribes to random mutation. Such alterations are not considered to be directed in any way, in contrast to mental hypotheses which are subject to criteria of improvement. Behaviour involving the cognitive processes can in fact be viewed as the continuous formulation, testing, and improvement of hypotheses according to criteria of behavioural success, whatever these may be. This context thus provides a natural framework within which to compare and contrast different levels of biological organization. There are finer comparisons than those mentioned, for example between levels of behaviour involving language, a distinctly human domain, and those involving cognitive processes without the linguistic facility.

These examples provide some indication of the potential value of a somewhat altered context for the description and interpretation of biological processes. Since the viewpoint is developed in terms of concepts which apply most naturally to high-level behaviour, the context does not run the risk of a reductionist treatment of these levels. Furthermore, it makes certain consequences self-evident. For example, the influence of a hypothesis or a model on the behaviour of an organism becomes axiomatic, since this is a basic determinant of the pattern which the organism follows in any given situation, from bacterium to man. Exactly how it enters as a determinant depends upon the level of organization one is considering, but in every one it is postulated as fundamental to the process observed. The hypothesis may be considered to specify certain basic constraints entering as contingent factors in the organic process, supplementing in a characteristically biological manner the 'laws of motion' of the organism seen as a physiochemical system. These constraints specify what the system can actually 'observe', how it can respond to its environment. Thus all organisms became observers conditioned by hypotheses. Whether or not this viewpoint can contribute anything constructive to the problem of observation and measurement in physics is far from clear; but, at the very least, the language is the same. This requires caution, since analogies can mislead; but it could also lead to clarification.

However, I am more concerned here with the consequences of

the breakdown of the concept of the objective observer in relation to the problem of meaning and wisdom, man's responsible participation in the world process. So long as man was regarded as a simple observer of nature, he could not be held responsible for what he observed. He could be held responsible for the way he used any power resulting from his observations, but the truth he deduced therefrom was considered to be as inevitable a consequence of the observations as the deductions of Euclidean theorems from the axioms. But if one is responsible for the axioms, then one is responsible for the theorems. This is the present situation, truth being as relative to viewpoint as theorems are to axioms. For example, the statement that psychological states are 'nothing but' the behavioural consequences of hormonal change is a perfectly correct deduction from particular assumptions, and has an indisputable element of validity. But a total commitment to an essentially reductionist view of this kind involves a value-judgement that needs examination. It is often associated with an essentially stoical attitude to the truth: e.g. human beings are very subject to romantic illusions about who and what they are, the 'truth' being that they are 'nothing but' this or that. The value-judgement is that it is good for people to face this 'reality', much as it is sometimes believed that good medicine must have a nasty taste.

It is often claimed in justification of a particular view or theory that it gives the best fit to the available data, and hence the criterion of choice is itself subject to objective measurement. When theories are in conflict, scientists ought therefore to choose the one which gives the most accurate predictions. However, it is quite clear from the history of science that this criterion is far from adequate to explain the choices that scientists have in fact made. As Kuhn (1957) has stated in his detailed study, *The Copernican Revolution* (p. 171): 'Judged on purely practical grounds, Copernicus' new planetary system was a failure; it was neither more accurate nor significantly simpler than its Ptolemaic predecessors . . . as Copernicus himself realized, the real appeal of sun-centred astronomy was aesthetic rather than pragmatic.' It is now widely recognized that the factors determining which of two competing theories will survive are not in the least obvious, and some eminent scientists such as Dirac and Schrödinger have been quite explicit about the importance of elegance, simplicity, and beauty in theories. These are undefined terms which need examination, but it is evident that they refer to values, not to objective criteria of measurement. Once again we are forced to recognize the two-way nature of the dialogue with nature: we can understand only what is intelligible to us; but at the same time, our questions must be intelligible to nature: they must, in some sense, be well-formed to generate a response.

Because there is a measure of freedom which scientists can exercise in choosing a particular viewpoint or theory or paradigm, they are in the same measure responsible for the viewpoints they adopt and should be prepared to justify them also on moral grounds. The image man has of himself and of the world is an exceedingly potent factor in conditioning his behaviour towards his fellow-men and his environment. We thus come full circle round to alchemy again, but displaced one step up the spiral staircase. The 'truth' we discover in the world is strongly conditioned by the image we hold of it (the world), our attitude towards it, as the alchemist believed. The difference lies in the fact that whereas the alchemist believed that one's attitude entered the natural process as a causal factor, we now see it entering as an interpretative factor. Our viewpoint probably doesn't alter the actual phenomenon observed (the 'probably' entering here to allow for the possibility of para-psychological phenomena): but it heavily conditions our understanding of the phenomenon; i.e. into what context we choose to fit it, to make it comprehensible. There is a context of understanding which involves man's commitment to a particular form of participation in the world. This context includes meaning as well as knowledge and can lead to wisdom as well as power. The exact form of this context is not at all clear, and untimately rests in the hands of each individual.

EMBRYOLOGY AND ETHICS

Since I am professionally engaged in the study of embryology the problem of ethical participation presents itself to me in this context. What can this mean in relation to activities such as vivisection, the mutilation of living organisms like Hydra or amphibian embryos, or the 'sacrifice' of mice and rats for the study of growth control in mammalian tissues? The usual way of justifying such interference with the integrity of organisms is to say that these studies are intended to lead ultimately to benefits in medical science, to the alleviation of human suffering and the improved health of mankind. I believe that to be both true and important, but it does not seem to me to be a sufficient justification for embryological research.

In order to approach an answer to this problem, let me ask another question. How can one justify the destruction of plants and animals to provide, say, wood for houses or food for oneself and for others? It is generally accepted that such actions are justified so long as basic human needs only are satisfied. Wanton destruction or slaughter is not condoned; it is unethical. Behind this attitude is the belief that humanity is part of a larger process of nature to which we should contribute in our own way. Our existence is justified only if we cooperate with this process, but not if we violate it. Each person has his own answer to the question what this process may be and how we fit into it. My own belief is that our contribution is to live our lives in as full and integrated a manner as possible, and in so doing to help others to do so. One of our characteristic attributes as human beings is the possession of consciousness. Fulfilment of human potential is possible only if we develop this attribute to the greatest extent we are capable of. This includes the discovery of knowledge, but knowledge must be developed within a context of meaning, not simply for power. In so far as our actions are dedicated to the enhancement of consciousness for the purpose of achieving wholeness and completion, for healing, making wholes out of parts, our actions are ethical and there will be an experience of meaning in creative participation. Thus the destructive interference with the nucleus of the atom or the developing embryo is justified if the knowledge so obtained is used to assist in the completion of integrated, cooperative relationships within and between individuals and with the world. This is creative activity which for human beings is inextricably associated with ever-increasing consciousness, involving a greater and greater sense of responsibility as one becomes more and more aware of the ways in which parts are and can be united into ever more extensive wholes.

Perhaps the most striking fact about embryos and creatures with regenerative powers like Hydra is their extraordinary capacity to make wholes out of parts, to realize themselves as complete entities despite various disturbances. There are, of course, limits: they are unable to recover from too severe a disturbance. But within these limits the developing or regenerating organism undergoes transformations which produce ordered, harmonious, and balanced relationships between their cells, tissues, and organs. They do this by the combined processes of differentiation of elements and their cooperative union into the whole which gives meaning to the elements. This is a very remarkable spectacle and not only brings one into a relationship of understanding with the developmental process, but also provides a metaphor for human and social transformations. Here, too, it is necessary to understand the specific functions of parts and how they may be cooperatively united into wholes. This metaphor is, of course, a very old one, a good bit older than the Greeks. And metaphors can be very misleading, so one should be exceedingly careful to avoid a simple identification of one process with another. Psychical and social transformations are potentially unending, new dialectical tensions constantly arising from previous resolutions, unlike the embryo which reaches a terminal state in the adult form. The contrast here is the same as that between ontogenetically fixed genetic hypotheses and free, non-terminating mental hypothesis construction, as previously described. The significance of the metaphor is to be found in the vision that inspires it, which is that man and nature are distinct but united. The world is both intelligible and meaningful because we reflect its basic structures and participate in its processes, much as the shape of a fish both reflects the hydrodynamic properties of the water in which it lives and also allows it to participate in water movements.

These simple observations clearly do not give any prescriptions for judging particular actions as ethical or unethical, since ethical choice becomes context-dependent rather than universal. Nor do they provide any automatic criterion of choice between competing scientific viewpoints or theories. However, there is obviously a very important dimension of value which can enter consciously into this choice so that science, far from necessarily destroying values, can itself become inextricably connected with the conscious exercise of ethical decision. Science could then become a transformed and transforming activity which engages man totally in responsible creativity, bringing knowledge and power into union with meaning and wisdom.

REFERENCES

1 BASTIN, E. W. 'On the origin of the scale constants of physics', *Studia Philosophica Gandensia*, **4**, 77–101, 1966.

2 BASTIN, E. W. & KILMISTER, C. W. *Proc. Camb. Phil. Soc.* **50**, 278–91, 1954.

3 COLLINGWOOD, R. G. *The Idea of Nature*, London, Oxford University Press, 1945.

4 JUNG, C. G. *Psychology and Alchemy*, 2nd edition. vol. 12 of *Collected Works*, ed. H. Read, London, Routledge and Kegan Paul, 1968.

5 JUNG, C. G. *Mysterium Coniunctionis*, vol. 14 of *Collected Works*, ed. H. Read, London, Routledge and Kegan Paul, 1963.

6 KEARNEY, H. *Science and Change 1500–1700*, London, World University Library, 1971.

7 KUHN, T. S. *The Structure of Scientific Revolutions*, Chicago, Chicago University Press, 1962.

8 KUHN, T. S. *The Copernican Revolution*, Cambridge, Mass., Harvard University Press, 1957.

9 MALRAUX, A. *The Voices of Silence*, New York, Doubleday, 1953.

10 *Musaeum Hermeticum* (Frankfurt), 1678. Translated by A. E. Waite: *The Hermetic Museum Restored and Enlarged*. London 1893, 2 volumes. Reprinted 1953.

11 SELIGMANN, K. *History of Magic*. New York, Pantheon, 1948.

Notes on Contributors
of Main Papers

WILHELM BALDAMUS. Professor of Sociology at the University of Birmingham. Main publication: *Efficiency and Effort*, and numerous papers on industrial sociology and the methodology of the social sciences.

MICHAEL BARRATT BROWN. Economist, Senior Lecturer in the Department of Extramural Studies, University of Sheffield. Main publications: *After Imperialism, What Economics is About*, and numerous articles.

ZYGMUNT BAUMAN. Professor of Sociology at the University of Leeds. (Previously at the universities of Warsaw and Tel-Aviv.) Main publications in English: *Between Class and Elite, Culture as Praxis* (in press) and articles. Numerous publications in Polish and other East European languages.

DAVID BOHM. Professor of Theoretical Physics at Birkbeck College, University of London. Main publications: *Quantum Theory, Causality and Chance in Modern Physics, Special Theory of Relativity*, and numerous articles.

ARTHUR BRITTAN. Lecturer in Sociology and Social Psychology at the University of York. Main publications: *Meanings and Situations* (in press) and articles.

PAUL M. CLARK. Lecturer in Physics at the Open University. (Previously at the University of Birmingham.) Articles on theoretical physics.

JOSEPH MARK GANI. Professor of Probability and Statistics at the University of Sheffield. Editor of the *Journal of Applied Probability* and others. Main publications: *The Conditions of Science in Australian Universities – A Statistical Survey 1939–1960, Stochastic Models of Bacteriophage*, and numerous articles.

BRIAN CAREY GOODWIN. Reader in Developmental Biology at the University of Sussex. Numerous articles on theoretical and experimental biology.

FREDERIC RAPHAEL JEVONS. Professor of Liberal Studies in Science at the University of Manchester. (Formerly biochemist.) Main publications: *The Biochemical Approach to Life*, *The Teaching of Science*, and (with others) *Wealth from Knowledge*; also numerous articles on biochemistry, the history of science, and science policy.

ARTHUR KOESTLER. Scientist by education and prolific author of political novels and essays, who has turned back since 1955 to history and the philosophy of science. Main publications since then: *The Sleepwalkers*, *The Lotus and the Robot*, *The Act of Creation*, *The Ghost in the Machine*, and numerous articles.

GORDON LEFF. Professor of History at the University of York. Main publications: *Medieval Thought*, *The Tyranny of Concepts*, *Heresy in the Later Middle Ages*, *History and Social Theory*, other books, and numerous articles.

DONALD MCKENZIE MACKINNON. Professor of Divinity at the University of Cambridge. (Previously Professor of Moral Philosophy at the University of Aberdeen.) Main publications: *Christian Faith and Communist Faith* (editor), *The Notion of a Philosophy of History*, *A Study in Ethical Theory*, *Borderlands of Theology*, *The Stripping of the Altars*, and articles.

NEVILLE MORAY. Professor of Psychology at the University of Toronto. (Previously at the University of Sheffield.) Main publications: *Cybernetics: Machines with Intelligence*, *Listening and Attention*, *Attention: Selection Processes in Vision and Learning*, and articles.

GUNNAR KARL MYRDAL. Director of the Institute of International Economic Studies, Stockholm. (Previously Professor of Economics, Cabinet Minister, Executive Secretary U.N. Economic Commission for Europe.) Main publications: *An American Dilemma*, *Economic Theory and Underdeveloped Regions*, *Asian Drama*, *Objectivity in Social Research*, other books, and numerous articles.

JOHN SYDNEY PYM. Reader in Pure Mathematics at the University of Sheffield. Editor for the London Mathematical Society. Numerous articles on pure mathematics.

SHULAMIT RAMON. Lecturer in Psychopathology at the School of Social Work, University of Tel-Aviv.

TEODOR SHANIN. Senior Lecturer in Sociology at the University of Haifa. (On leave from the University of Sheffield.) Main publications: *Peasants and Peasant Societies*, *The Awkward Class*, and articles.

JAMES PETER THORNE. Reader in English Language at the University of Edinburgh. Articles on theoretical linguistics.

Index